TEXT BOOK
OF
GENERAL PHYSIOLOGY

TEXT BOOK OF GENERAL PHYSIOLOGY

By

Dr. Pradip V. Jabde

M.Sc., Ph.D., D.H.E., F.S.E.S.C.

Reader

Department of Zoology

Mahatma Gandhi Vidya Mandir's

Arts, Commerce and Science College

Manmad (Nasik)

(Maharashtra)

DISCOVERY PUBLISHING HOUSE

NEW DELHI-110002

First Published-2005

ISBN 81-8356-037-7

Published by

DISCOVERY PUBLISHING HOUSE

4831/24, Ansari Road, Prahlad Street,
Darya Ganj, New Delhi-110002 (India)
Phone: 23279245 • Fax: 91-11-23253475
E-mail:dphtemp@indiatimes.com

Printed at
Arora Offset Press
Laxmi Nagar, Delhi–92

Dedicated
To
"Indians"

PREFACE

Physiology as such a vast subject with unlimited scope and which can be studied in different ways. There was a long left need, among students and teachers for a text book with recent information and written according to national syllabus. Efforts have been made to collect recent informations from several standard works and journals. I had tried to add two new topics on "Physiology of Aviation, high altitude, space and deep-sea diving and the "Chronobiology". Attempts have been made to simply the language but in a exhaustive way.

I am grateful to Shri Prashant Hire, General Secretary, M.G. Vidyamandir and Principal R.P. Hire, Arts, Science and Commerce College, Manmad, for their inspiration. Thanks due to my wife Sau. Shubhda for her help in writing and proofing the manuscript.

Thanks to publisher, editor and staff members of Discovery Publishing House, New Delhi for having brought out this book in time in its well designed and attractive form.

Suggestions for improvement are invite with criticism and constructive comments on all errors and defects from expert teachers.

Dr. Jabde P.V.

Contents

(iv) Hibernation

(v) Chill coma

(vi) Heat coma

(B) (i) Role of behaviour

(ii) Pelage

(iii) Sweating

(iv) Panting

(v) Subcutaneous fat, Brown fat

(vi) Counter current heat exchangers

(vii) Shivering and non shivering

(viii) Thermogenesis.

(C) Peripheral and central thermo receptors

6. OSMOREGULATTON **187-215**

(A) Water

(i) Physiological properties

(ii) Biological important ions

(iii) Diffusion

(iv) Osmosis.

(B) Osmoregulation

(i) Organs regulating water and ionic salt balance in the body of aquatic and terrestrial animals

(ii) Hormonal control of osmoregulation.

7. EXCRETION **216-247**

Nitrogenous wastes

(i) Formation and composition of urine

(ii) Counter current multiplier theory

(iii) Blood supply of renal organs

(iv) Hormonal control of kidneys

(v) Modes of excretion.

NUTRITION

(A) BRIEF OUTLINE OF SOURCES OF ENERGY

For the manifestations of life, the intake of food is most essential. The *autotrophic* organisms are able to synthesize all essential organic compounds from inorganic mineral sources; they include the chemosynthetic bacteria (Chemotrophs) and the chlorophyll-bearing green plants (Phototrophs). The *heterotrophic* organisms require organic substances as a food and have limited synthesizing abilities. Almost all animals are heterotrophic and obtain energy for their life processes by swallowing, devouring, or engulfing other animals and plants and by breaking down the complex organic compounds that they contain through hydrolytic processes. Meaning, food provides raw materials for the building up of the body and at the same time constitutes the only source of energy. *A complex of processes which contribute in converting the food into the basic building materials of the body, is known as nutrition or nutrition is supply of food to the tissues and its absorption and metabolism for growth, energy, maintenance and repair of the living body.*

The intake of food within body is called *ingestion*, the ingested food rarely in a form suitable for cellular consumption, and to accomplish this the food must undergo degradation or *digestion*, which convert it into simpler form. This simpler food is then absorbed (absorption) and then transported to the body tissues through blood. The tissue cells utilize (assimilation) these materials for growth and energy release. The undigested and unabsorbed residual part of food is eliminated out side the body (egetion).

For maintenance of a healthy body, food must include carbohydrates, fats and proteins, which can be oxidized to provide heat and energy, in sufficient quantities to suit an individual's metabolic needs, so that some times these organic components are called "proximate principles". They also forms the structural components of the body. In addition to these, vitamins, mineral salts play vital roles in the regulation of several essential metabolic processes in the body. The food may be grouped as *energy food* such as proteins, lipids and carbohydrates, and non-energy food like vitamins, minerals, water and oxygen. Both are interdependent upon one another, in the absence of one type, the utilization of the other becomes practically impossible in organisms.

CARBOHYDRATES

Carbohydrates play a fundamental role in the life of animals and plants. Plants synthesize carbohydrates by a process of photosynthesis and utilize solar energy while animals procure carbohydrates from them. They are an important source of energy (polysaccharides, starch and glycogen) for living organisms as well as a means by which chemical energy can be stored. In addition, some carbohydrates can function as structural units (cellulose and chitin) within the cell.

Carbohydrates are the organic compounds normally made up of carbon, hydrogen and oxygen in the ratio of 1 : 2 : 1. In addition to the above three they are also associated with nitrogen and sulphur.

Main sources of carbohydrates in nature are potatoes, barley, maize, wheat, sugar cane, rice etc.

Carbohydrates may be classified into monosaccharides, disaccharides, oligosaccharides and polysaccharides.

Monosaccharides

Monosaccharides are the carbohydrates having a single ring of carbon, and are sometimes called the simple sugars such as glucose, fructose and galactose. The common sugars are the *pentoses* and *hexoses* and are found in abundance in plants, animals, honey etc. The monosaccharides are grouped according to the number of carbon atoms in their structure, *i.e., trioses* ($C_3H_6O_3$), tetroses ($C_4H_8O_4$), pentose ($C_5H_{10}O_5$), *hexoses* ($C_6H_{12}O_6$) and *heptoses* ($C_7H_{14}O_7$). Except pentoses and hexoses others are less common sugars mentioned in the above lines.

Monosaccharides cannot be hydrolyzed into smaller units under reasonably mild conditions. They are sweet, neutral, crystallizable, readily dialyzable and soluble in water. They can undergo alcoholic fermentation.

Disaccharides

Disaccharides are the compounds formed by the union of the molecules of monosaccharides with the elimination of water. The process is called the *condensation*. During the process an OH group of one monosaccharide joins with one of the carbon atom of the other forming a *glycoside bond.*

$$C_6H_{12}O_6 + C_6H_{12}O_6 \rightarrow C_{12}H_{22}O_{11} + H_2O$$

The glycoside bond is developed either in the two similar or different monosaccharides.

The common disaccharides are *maltose* formed by the combination of two molecules of glucose; *sucrose* formed by the union of glucose and fructose; *lactose* is formed by the combination of glucose and galactose: similarly *phlorhizin* found in the bark of Rosaceae, is a combination of glucose and phloretin; and *amygdalin*, present in the seed of the bitter almond, is a combination of glucose and mandelonitrile. They are sweet crystallizable, soluble and dialyzable compounds.

Polysaccharides

The term polysaccharide refers to a group of compounds that yield a large number of monosaccharides on hydrolysis. The polysaccharides consisting of only one type of monosaccharide units are called *homopolysaccharides* (starch, glycogen, cellulose and dextrins), while those with different types of monosaccharide units are called *hetropolysacchdrides* (mucopolysaccharides). All polysaccharides are insoluble in water. Because of their large size, they form colloidal solution and solids and will not pass across the natural membranes of organisms. They are chemically inert and do not ionize and for this reason very much suited as reserves as starch in plants and glycogen in animals.

Polysaccharides are frequently tasteless, insoluble, amorphous compound with very high molecular weight. The emperical formula is $(C_6H_{10}H_5)_n$ in which the value of n may be even 200 or more. Though most of carbohydrates are true foods and they furnish the energy to our body, but the cellulose is undigestable, so it does not provide the energy. It acts like *roughage*, the substances which are neither digested nor absorbed in gut but their presence is essential to promote the intestinal peristalsis.

CARBOHYDRATE REQUIREMENTS

Carbohydrates supply about 50-80% of the energy requirements, depending upon the economic, status and age of the individual. In balanced diets, about 50-60% of the total energy is derived from carbohydrates. For production of energy, carbohydrates should be converted in to glucose. Although a number of intermediate steps are involved, the net results may be summarised by the equation.

$$C_6H_{12}O_6 + 6O_2 \rightarrow 6\ CO_2 + 6\ H_2O + \text{Energy}$$

On oxidation carbohydrates yields 4.2 cal/g. With the introduction of SI units in 1960, one has to use *kilo Joule (kJ)* as standard measure of heat. The relation between the two units is as follows:

1 Cal (1000 cal) = 4.184 kJ (4184 J)

OR 1J = 0.239 Cal

According to this new system, 386,000 calories correspond to 16.5kJ and 4.2 Cal to 17.6 kJ.

LIPIDS

(a) Composition

The term lipid is applied not only to the fatty substances but also' to those which are soluble in fat solvents such as ether benzene, and chloroform. Like carbohydrates, lipids are composed of the element carbon, hydrogen, and oxygen. Lipids are characterized by the presence of fatty acids, or their derivatives and by their solubility in such solvent as acetone, alcohol, and chloroform. However, a marked difference lies in the relative number of the atoms of the elements in a lipid molecule compared with that found in carbohydrates. From the formula of carbohydrate ($C_6H_{12}O_6$) it is clear that the hydrogen and oxygen atom are in the proportion as found in the water. But it is not true for the lipids. The hydrogen atoms are more in number as compared to oxygen. Chemically they are esters of fatty acids or capable of forming esters. They are found in all animal and plant matter, and at least some of them appear to be an essential constituent of protoplasm. In the animal body they form the main store of reserve food supply, being derived from the fat and carbohydrate diet. The brain and nervous tissues are rich in certain lipids, this fact indicate the importance of these compounds to life.

Lipids occur in many of our food and in nearly all the tissues of our body. Pure fats are odourless and tasteless. The odour of most of the fats with which we are acquainted is generally due to foreign material absorbed by the fat. The percentage of lipids present in different tissue is given below.

Table 1.1 : Chemical composition or lipids.

Tissues	Percentage of lipids
1. Bone marrow	96.0
2. Adipose tissue	83.0
3. Nerve	22.0
4. Egg	12.0
5. Milk	4.0
6. Liver	2.5
7. Blood	0.5

(b) Classification

The lipids can be classified into three groups:

1. ***Simple lipids :*** They are the esters of fatty acid and alcohols.
   (i) *Natural fats and oils* : They are the combinations of glycerol with three molecules of fatty acids. Fats are solid where as oils are liquid at the room temperature.

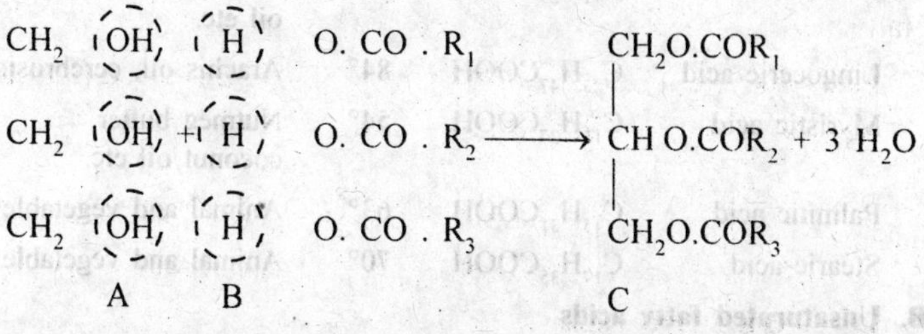

$$\begin{array}{llll} CH_2\ OH & H & O.CO.R_1 & CH_2O.COR_1 \\ CH_2\ OH\ + & H & O.CO.R_2 \longrightarrow & CH\ O.COR_2 + 3\ H_2O \\ CH_2\ OH & H & O.CO.R_3 & CH_2O.COR_3 \\ A & B & & C \end{array}$$

Fig. 1.1: (A) Glycerol, (B) 3-fatty acid molecules (C) triglyceride.

The R in Fig. 1.1 represents the side chain of the fatty acid.

   (ii) *Waxes* : They are similar in structure to triglycerides but instead of glycerol they contain higher aliphatic alcohols; the fatty acids combined with these are longer and possess longer chains than those found in neutral fats. The example is bee wax. They function as protective and impermeable coverings, as in cuticular waxes of several animals.

2. ***Compound lipids :*** These are lipids which on hydrolysis yield compounds other than fatty acid and alcohol, such as phospholipids, glycolipids, terpenes, steroids, etc. For example lecithin, a phospholipid which on hydrolysis gives glycerol, phosphoric acid, choline, and two molecules of fatty acids.

Phospholipids possess both hydrophilic (water attracting) and hydrophobic (water repelling) groups and hence can act as binding agents between the water soluble substances.

They are often found associated with cell membrane, and they are particularly abundant in nerve tissue. There are several kinds of phospholipids. For example lipid containing one of the nitrogenous compounds are choline, *ethanamine*, or serine. The phosphatidyl cholines or lecithin are widely distributed in cells and are important in fat metabolism in the liver. *Cephalins* are simpler than lecithin. *Plasmogens* are similar to lecithins-and cephalins but give a positive reaction to aldehyde with Schiffs test.

Table 1.2 : Showing common fatty acids.

S. No.	Name	Formula	Melting point	Occurrence
A.	**Saturated fatty acid**			
	Arachidic acid	$C_{19}H_{39}COOH$	75°	Peanut oil
	Lauric acid	$C_{11}H_{23}COOH$	44°	Spermaceti, coconut oil etc.
	Lingoceric acid	$C_{23}H_{47}COOH$	84°	Arachis oil, cerebrosides.
	Myristic acid	$C_{13}H_{27}COOH$	54°	Nutmeg butter, coconut oil etc.
	Palmitic acid	$C_{15}H_{31}COOH$	63°	Animal and vegetable fats.
	Stearic acid	$C_{17}H_{35}COOH$	70°	Animal and vegetable fats.
B.	**Unsaturated fatty acids**			
	Oleic acid	$C_{17}H_{33}COQH$	13°	Animal and vegetable fats.
	Linoleic acid	$C_{17}H_{31}COOH$	–5°	Linseed oil, cotton seed oil etc.
	Linolenic acid	$C_{17}H_{29}COOH$	–10°	Linseed oil.
	Arachidonic acid	$C_{19}H_{31}COOH$	–50°	Lecithin, cephalin.

Glycolipids include two major groups *i.e.,* cerebrosides, and the gangliosides. On hydrolysis, glycolipid yields sphingosine, a fatty acid, and a monosaccharide, usually galactose or sometimes glucose. The molecule, however, does not contain phosphoric acid or glycerol. Terpenes, a large and important groups of lipids are related to each other in that the carbon skeleton contain multiples of 5-carbon atoms arranged in simple repeating units of isoprene. Isoprene is not a naturally occurring compound. It is biologically active in the form of isopentenyl phosphate. Condensation of isoprenoid units form the compounds like rubber, carotenes, phytol, various carotenoids and steroids. Steroids are generally found associated with the unsaponifiable residue of fats after saponification. There exist a great diversity of physiological activity among the steroid compounds, as a result they form a sort of group. There is a cyclic nucleus common to all the steroids.

Lipoproteins appear in the blood of mammals as lipids in association with plasma protein.

3. ***Derived lipids :*** These are substances possessing the general physical characteristics of lipids and are obtained by the hydrolysis of simple and compound lipids. Examples are cholesterol and ergasterol. The former is the chief protoplasmic constituent.

   (a) *Fatty acids :* The fatty acids are found in both simple as well as compound lipids. Most of the fatty acids found in the lipids are straight chain acids, although in some cases branched-chain acids have also been found. Many of the important acids are unsaturated and occur in both fats and oils. A few acids, saturated and unsaturated, contain hydroxyl groups and some are cyclic in nature.

   (b) *Soaps :* The metallic salts of the fatty acids are called soaps. This is an important constituent of the lipids.

   (c) *Glycerol :* The common constituent of all fats and oils is glycerol. It is a trihydric alcohol and therefore shows all the chemical reactions of alcohols. Since glycerol is a trihydric alcohol, it will form triple esters with fatty acids. Such esters are the fats and oils.

FAT REQUIREMENT

In the body, lipids serves as the most concentrated and efficient source of energy-both directly, and potentially when stored in the adipose tissue. For example, 1 g of steric acid burned in the bomb calorimeter produces about 40 kJ (9.6 Cal) whereas 1 g of glycogen yield only 16kJ (3.8 Cal). A total of about 40-60 g of fat can be safely consumed daily and in order to obtain the necessary quantities of EFAs the fat intake should include at least 15 g of vegetable oils.

PROTEINS

(a) *Composition :* Proteins are complex nitrogen organic compounds, usually of very high molecular weight. Fundamentally protein molecule consists of carbon, oxygen, hydrogen and nitrogen woven together in an intricate manner in the approximate properties as given in the table below. However, other elements may also be present.

Table 1.3 : Chemical composition of proteins.

S. No.	Elements	Approximate %
1.	Carbon	50% to 55%
2.	Oxygen	21% to 24%
3.	Nitrogen	13% to 17%
4.	Hydrogen	about 7%
5.	Sulphur	0.2% to 7%

The fundamental building block of a protein molecule is the *amino* acid. With one exception, all amino acids obtained from living tissues have their amino group attached to the carbon atom that is nearest to the carboxyl group. Due to this reason they are known as α-amino acids with an emperical formula.

$$R\text{—}CH(NH_2).COOH$$

where R may be one of a variety of organic chain or ring. There are about 20 amino acids which are used by the living organism to form the proteins, but all necessarily do not found in every protein.

On hydrolysis the proteins yield amino acids, water being added to the molecule. The synthesis of protein requires the opposite process, the condensation, because in this water is removed, when two amino acids are joined together.

$$\underset{\displaystyle |\atop R}{H_2N\text{–}CH\text{–}CO}\,(OH) + (H)\text{–}\underset{\displaystyle |\atop H}{N}\text{–}\underset{\displaystyle |\atop R}{CH}\text{–}COOH \rightarrow$$

$$H_2N\text{–}\underset{\displaystyle |\atop R}{CH}\text{–}\underset{\displaystyle \|\atop O}{C}\text{–}\underset{\displaystyle |\atop H}{N}\text{–}\underset{\displaystyle |\atop R}{CH}\text{–}COOH + H_2O$$

The –OC. NH– link so formed is called peptide link. The conjunction of two amino acids in this way is called dipeptide. When third amino acid is joined, tripeptide results. The process continued till a polypeptide chain is formed. The polypeptide chain when contain some 50 amino acids; it begins to show the characteristic properties of proteins. The shape of protein molecule is either spherical or like a long rod. The former is called globular proteins and the latter fibrous proteins. Fibrous proteins are formed in muscles and connective tissue. Biologically active proteins such as enzymes and antigens are usually globular. Proteins tend to polymerize.

(b) Classification

The proteins found as such in the animal body are spoken as native proteins. However, they are classified into three groups, *i.e.,* simple. conjugated and derived proteins.

1. ***Simple proteins :*** The proteins which on hydrolysis yield chiefly α-amino acids or their derivatives are called simple proteins. On the basis of coagulability by heat and solubility, they are further divided as below;

   (a) *Albumin :* Egg albumin, lact-albumin and serum-albumin are of animal origin; legumelin (peas) and leucosin (wheat) are vegetable albumins. They are soluble in pure water. Coagulation occurs by heating. Precipitated by saturation with $(NH)_2SO_4$, but not precipitated by saturation with NaCI or magnesium sulphate.

   (b) *Globulin :* Egg globulin, lact-globulin, serum-globulin, fibrinogen and mycogen and myosin of muscle are of animal origin. Vegetable globulins include legumin (peas), tuberin (potatoes) and edestin (wheat). Globulins are insoluble in pure water but are soluble in dilute salt solutions. They are coagulated by heat and precipitated by saturation with magnesium sulphate or by half saturation of ammonium sulphate.

   (c) *Glutelin :* It is found in the seeds of cereal grains. They are insoluble in water and salt solution. They are soluble in dilute alkalies and acids; coagulated by heat.

   (d) *Protamines :* Gliadin (wheat), zein (corn) and hordein (barley) are the examples of protamines. These are insoluble in water or absolute alcohol but are soluble in 80 per cent alcohol. They are not coagulated by heat.

Protamines are the simplest of all naturally occurring proteins and possess the least complicated structure. They are soluble in water, dilute acids and dilute ammonium hydroxide and are not coagulated by heat. Protamines are strongly basic in reaction and are found in sperm cell.

(e) *Histones* : Histones occur as part of the nucleoprotein and contain predominate of basic amino acids. They are soluble in water and dilute acids but are insoluble in dilute ammonium hydroxide. Not coagulated by heat. Histone is present in the blood corpuscles of bird.

(f) *Albuminoids or scleroproteins* : Albuminoids are among the least soluble proteins and as such the most difficult to digest. In the body they are present in insoluble state. They are tough, yet elastic in nature. Being present in all connective tissue, they confer on the organs and the body as a whole, form strength, rigidity and elasticity. Among the albuminoids are collagen, elastin and keratin. Collagen forms the ground substance of bone and cartilage and is found in white fibrous (inelastic), connective tissue (tendons, aponeuroses,- ligaments, duramater, pericardium and fascia). However, on boiling with dilute acids it is transformed into the gelatin. It digests very slowly. Elastin is found in yellow (elastic) connective tissue in the walls of the blood vessels especially arteries, trachea and lungs. It is very less soluble and hard to digest.

Keratin is found in the outer layer of the skin and in hair, nails, feather, hoops and so on. It is indigestable.

2. ***Compound, complex or conjugated proteins :*** These proteins are composed of a simple united protein with some other non-protein substance (prosthetic group). Conjugated proteins are further divided on the basis of the nature of prosthetic group into chromoproteins, nucleoproteins, glycoproteins, phospho-proteins, lecithoproteins and lipoproteins.

(a) *Chromoproteins* : In chromoproteins the simple protein is united with a pigment for example haemoglobins, cytochromes and flavoproteins.

(b) *Nucleoproteins :* In this the protein is combined with a nucleic acid. The chromatin material of the nuclei of cells and also the substances composing viruses are mostly nucleoproteins.

(c) *Glycoproteins :* It is formed by the union of a carbohydrate with the protein. The most important glycoprotein is the mucin. Mucin is found in saliva, and in the secretions of mucous membranes. It's high viscosity and slimines may be of value as a lubricant and also in furnishing protection of mucous membranes.

(d) *Phosphoproteins :* These are the protein linked with phosphoric acids. Casein in the milk and vitellin in the egg yolk are such phosphoprotein. They are soluble in dilute alkalies, hence the addition of acid causes them to be precipitated.

(e) *Lecithoproteins :* These are the proteins which are linked with the phosphoprotein. It is not a well recognised group but undoubtedly found in the protoplasm.

(f) *Lipoproteins :* These are simple proteins and formed by the combination of fatty substances and protein. Lipoproteins complexes are found in serum and brain tissue.

3. ***Derived proteins :*** Derived proteins are produced by the action of heat, enzyme, or chemical reagents. They are named variously as:

(a) *Primary derived proteins :* They are such proteins in which the size of the protein molecule is not materially altered. They are as follows.

(i) *Proteins :* It is insoluble in water. The first products produced by the action of acids, enzymes, or water, on proteins. Edestan is derived from edestein.

(ii) *Metaprotein :* It is insoluble in water, but soluble in dilute acids and alkali. It is produced by the further action of acid or alkali on proteins into acids or alkali metaprotein.

(iii) *Coagulated proteins :* It is insoluble protein products which are produced by the action of heat or alcohol on protein, for example coagulated egg white.

4. ***Secondary derived proteins :*** These are the derivatives of proteins in which definite hydrolysis has taken place. The molecules are smaller than those of original protein.

   (i) *Proteoses :* It is soluble in water, but not coagulated by heat and precipitated by saturating their solution with $(NH_4)_2SO_4$.

   (ii) *Peptones :* Soluble in water but not coagulated by heat. It is not precipitated by saturating their solution with $(NH_4)_2SO_4$.

Protein Requirement

This depends on age and physiological state of animal. The daily requirements of protein in diet for an adult is about 1 g protein per kg body weight. Young and growing animals obviously need more protein, likewise, the protein needs of females are also greater during pregnancy and lactation than at other times.

The tissues have little capacity for storage of proteins. The proteins will be utilized as a source of energy only if the calorie intake in the form of carbohydrates and fats is insufficient to meet the body's energy needs, (for details see protein metabolism). On complete oxidation protein can yield 23.5 kJ/g, *i.e.,* 5.6 Cal.

Table 1.4 : Protein, fat and carbohydrate content of different foods.

Food	Protein%	Fat%	Carbohy-drate %	Fuel value per 100 gms calories
Apples	0.3	0.4	14.9	64
Asparagus	2.2	0.2	3.9	26
Bacon, fat	6.2	76.0	0.7	712
broiled	25.0	55.0	1.0	599
Beef, medium	17.5	22.0	1.0	268
Beets, fresh	1.6	0.1	9.6	46
Bread, white	9.0	3.6	49.8	268
Butter	0.6	81.0	0.4	733
Cabbage	1.4	0.2	5.3	29
Carrots	1.2	0.3	9.3	45
Cashew nuts	19.6	47.2	26.4	609
Cheese, Cheddar,				
American Chicken	23.9	32.3	1.7	393

Total edible	21.6	2.7	1.0	111
Chocolate	(5.5)	52.9	(18.0)	570
Corn (maize), entire	10.0	4.3	73.4	372
Haddock	17.2	0.3	0.5	72
Lamb, leg, inter-mediate	18.0	17.5	1.0	230
Milk, fresh whole	3.5	3.9	4.9	69
Molasses, medium	0.0	0.0	(60.0)	240
Oatmeal, dry, uncooked	14.2	7.4	68.2	396
Oranges	0.9	0.2	11.2	50
Peanuts	26.9	44.2	23.6	600
Peas, fresh	6.7	0.4	17.7	101
Pork, ham, medium	15.2	31.0	1.0	340
Potatoes	2.0	0.1	19.1	85
Spinach	2.3	0.3	3.2	25
Strawberries	0.8	0.6	8.1	41
Tomatoes	1.0	0.3	4.0	23
Tuna, canned	24.2	10.8	0.5	194
Walnuts, English	15.0	64.4	15.6	702

Energy Requirements for Male

1. Daily food intake must supply total energy requirements for—

1. *Activity* : Special : Individual requirements vary with type of work or play and, from minute to minute, on the intensity of work and frequency and length of Rest pauses.

   Everyday activities : Such as sitting, standing, walking, etc.

2. *Specific dynamic action of food (S.D.A.)* : The mere taking of food stimulates metabolism of cells so that heat production increases (30 % by protein, 4-5 % by carbohydrate and fat). Must allow 10 % above Basal requirements on average mixed diet.

3. *Basal metabolism* : (measured when body is at rest) Energy expenditure of cells doing vegetative processes of living - *e.g.*, tasks involved in respiration, circulation, digestion, excretion, secretion, synthesis of special substances, keeping body temperature at 37°C, growth and repair.

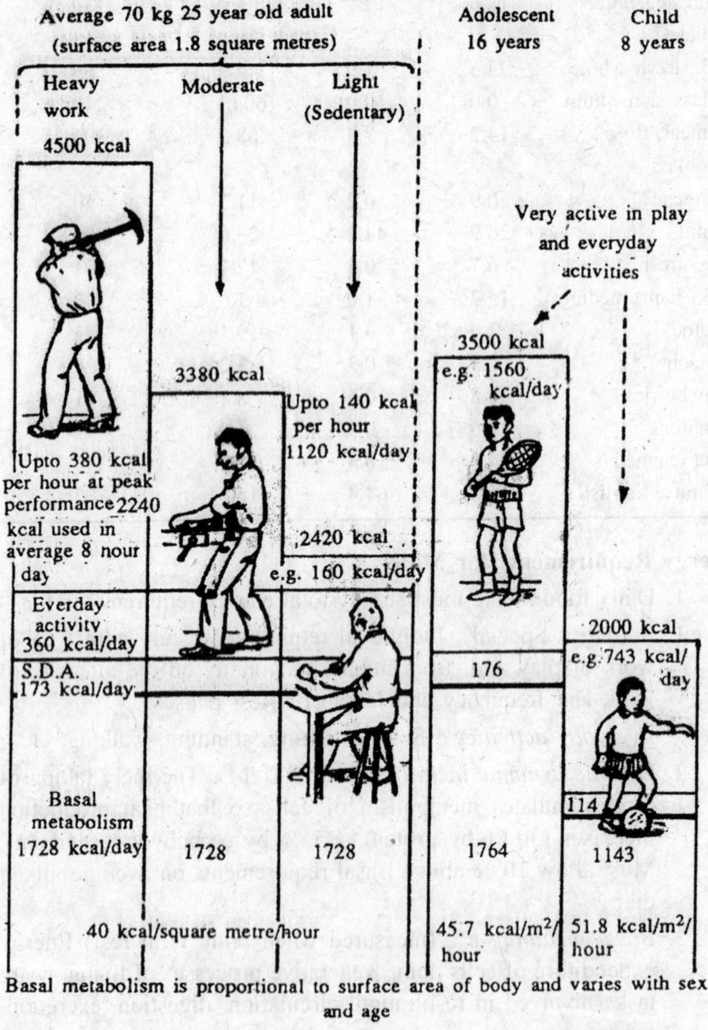

Fig. 1.2 : Showing energy requirements in male at different stages of development.

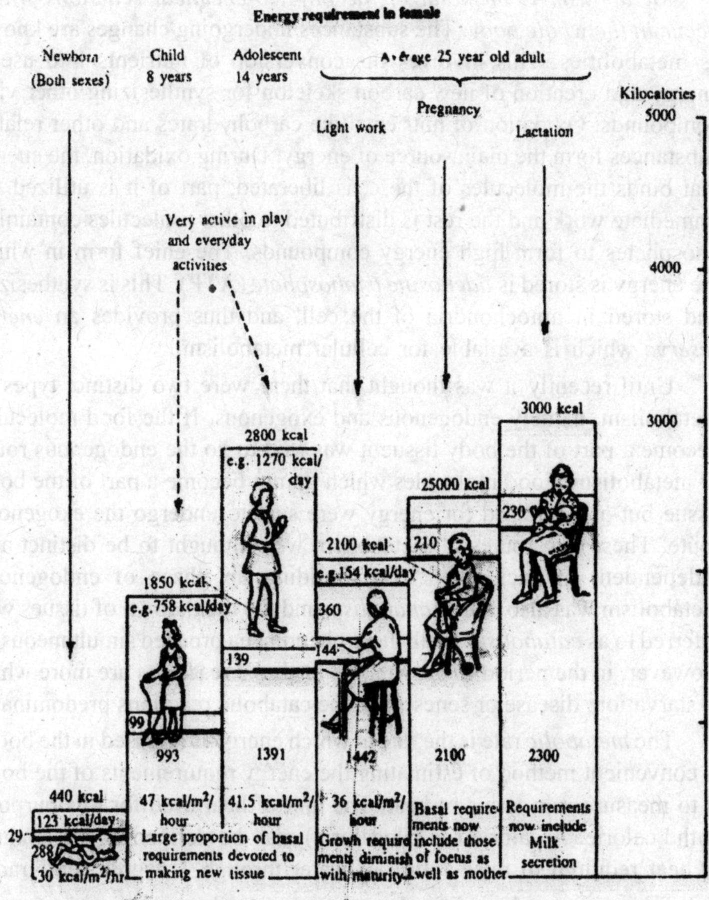

Fig. 1.3 : Showing energy requirements in female at different stages of development.

(B) METABOLISM

Energy is needed for the multitude of activities performed by the body. It is also required for growth, and repair of tissues. This energy is obtained from ingested food, which is first digested and absorbed, and finally metabolized.

Metabolism is the total of the physico-chemical reactions which occur in the whole body. The substances undergoing changes are known as metabolities. This involves the conversion of nutrients into useful energy and creation of new carbon skeleton for synthesizing other vital compounds. Oxidation of nutrients like carbohydrates and other related substances form the main source of energy. During oxidation, the energy that binds the molecules of these, is liberated; part of it is utilized for immediate work and the rest is distributed to other molecules containing phosphates to form high energy compounds. The chief form in which the energy is stored is *adenosine triphosphate* (ATP). This is synthesized and stored in mitochondria of the cell, and thus provides an *energy reserve* which is available for cellular metabolism.

Until recently it was thought that there were two distinct types in metabolism, namely endogenous and exogenous. If the food molecules become a part of the body tissue it was said to go the endogenous route of metabolism. Food molecules which do not become a part of the body tissue but are oxidised for energy were said to undergo the exogenous route. These two routes of metabolism were thought to be distinct and independent of each other. The building up phase of endogenous metabolism was also called *anabolism* and the breakdown of tissues was referred to as *catabolism*. Both these phenomena proceed simultaneously. However, in the period of growth, the anabolic reactions are more while in starvation, disease or senescence the catabolic reactions predominate.

The *metabolic* rate is the rate at which energy is released in the body. A convenient method of estimating the energy requirements of the body is to measure it in terms of heat. The unit of heat used for this purpose is the calorie. A calorie (or kilocalorie) may be defined as the amount of heat required to raise 1 litre of water through 1 degree centigrade.

The energy value of food is also measured in calories:

1 gram of carbohydrate	= 4 calories (16 kJ, or kilo Joules)
1 gram of protein	= 4 calories (17 kJ)
1 gram of fat	= 9 calories (37 kJ).

BASAL METABOLIC RATE—(BMR)

It is the rate of the body's energy expenditure under 'basal conditions'. This means the individual is at rest, mentally and physically, has not eaten for at least 12 hours (*i.e.,* is in the post-absorptive state), and is in a warm comfortable environment. Under these conditions the metabolic needs of the body are at their lowest, energy being used only to sustain vital functions (*e.g.,* breathing, the beating of the heart, maintenance of normal body temperature).

The basal metabolic rate .can be calculated by estimating the amount of oxygen consumed in a given time. Since individuals vary greatly in size, the BMR is expressed in calories per square metre of body surface per hour. The body surface area is calculated from measurements of an individuals weight and height.

Men oxidize food faster than women and therefore have a higher basal metabolic rate. For example, a male in his twenties has a BMR of about 40C per square metre of body surface per hour, whilst a woman of the same age has a BMR of about 37C per square metre of body surface per hour.

Factors influencing metabolism

Age : The metabolic rate of children is relatively greater than that of adults due to high rates of cellular activity and growth. The BMR decreases with increasing age.

Exercise : Exercise requires energy. Strenuous physical exercise can increase metabolic rate as much as a hundred times that of the BMR of an individual for a few seconds at a time.

Body temperature : An increase in body temperature increases the BMR. A decrease in body temperature results in a decrease in the metabolic rate and in oxygen consumption.

Environmental temperature : The average metabolic rate of individuals living in tropical countries is considerably lower than that of people living in cold climates.

Thyroid hormone : This hormone plays an important part in metabolism. When an excess of the hormone is secreted the basal metabolism is increased; when there is a deficiency of thyroid hormone basal metabolism is slow.

Stimulation of the sympathetic nervous system : As in fright or acute anxiety, causes a temporary increase in the metabolic rate in order that the body may cope with an emergency.

Drugs : Certain drugs, such as the amphetamines, or caffeine, can increase the BMR.

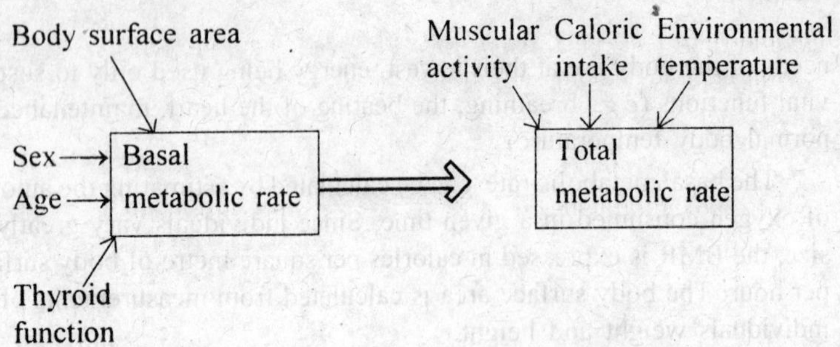

Fig. 1.4 : Relationship between basal metabolic rate and total metabolic rate.

Many of the food entering the blood from digestive tract can be used by the body tissues without alteration, but some tissues requiring special chemicals which are not normally found in the food. To supply these, much of the absorbed food passes to special organs where it is changed into new substances needed by the cells. This process is called intermediate metabolism. Liver can store and split fat and protein into smaller units. It is done by a number of reactions in a definite way called the metabolic pathways.

CARBOHYDRATE METABOLISM

Carbohydrates are the main food stuffs which are synthesized by plants and utilized by animal for their energy requirements. Generally carbohydrates are found in di-and polysaccharides (flour, rice, potatoes, milk, fruits, cane sugar etc.), which are hydrolyzed in the course of digestion into monosaccharides or simple sugars (glucose, fructose and galactose). These are then absorbed in digestive tract and finally transferred into the blood where it is always readily available to all cells for utilization. Excess of glucose is always conveyed to storage depots like liver and muscles, where it stored in the form of glycogen granules.

The normal level of sugar in blood varies from 80 to 100 mg/100 ml. When the blood sugar crosses the level of 180 mg/100 ml, the stage is known as *hyperglycemia*. In several hyperglycemia sugar appears in the urine. This stage is known as glycosuria. In *hypoglycemia*, the blood sugar level falls below the normal value. Such a condition may arise in starvation in normal course or after administration of high dose of insulin. If the blood sugar level falls even below 60 mg/100 ml the individual may fall unconscious, mental confusion and may result death because the brain is the first organ to suffer, as the brain cells are Unable to store any appreciable quantity of glucose and they have only a limited ability to use fats or amino acids as source of energy.

The metabolism of carbohydrate can be studied under the following heads:

Glycogenesis : Glucose is the primary source of energy for all cells and its concentration in the blood must be maintained at a certain minimal value. Excess of glucose is converted into glycogen in liver and muscles. The process of biosynthesis of glycogen from glucose is called glycogenesis. The liver tissue may store glycogen approximately 5-6% of its weight.

Muscle glycogen serves only as a local fuel deposit, available for muscular work and is not available for regulating the blood glucose level as they do not have glucose-6-phosphate to convert glycogen to glucose.

1. During the glycogenesis, the initial step involves the phosphorylation of glucose as a result of which glucose-6-phosphate is formed by the addition of a phosphate group obtained from ATP in the presence of enzyme hexokinase.

   $$\text{Glucose} + \text{ATP} \xrightarrow[\text{mg}^{++}]{\text{hexokinase}} \text{Glucose-6-phosphate} + \text{ADP}$$

2. Glucose-6-phosphate is converted into glucose-1-phosphate by intramolecular rearrangement in the presence of phospho-glycomutase.

   $$\text{Glucose-6-phosphate} \xrightarrow{\text{phosphoglycomutase}} \text{Glucose-1-phosphate}$$

3. Finally, glucose-1-phosphate is converted into glycogen in the presence of an enzyme phosphorylase, with subsequent release of a molecule of phosphoric acid.

   $$\text{Glucose-1-phosphate} \xrightarrow{\text{phosphorylase}} \text{Glycogen+phosphoric acid}$$

Glycogenolysis : Whenever level of blood sugar falls (hypoglycemia) glycogen stored in the liver is reconverted into glucose to maintain its steady state concentration. The sequence of reactions involved in this process is exactly reverse to that described in glycogenesis. The reactions are given below:

1. In initial step glycogen by the addition of inorganic phosphate and an enzyme phosphorylase is converted into glucose-1-phosphate.

   $$\text{Glycogen} \xrightarrow[H_3PO_4]{\text{phosphorylase}} \text{Glucose-1-phosphate}$$

2. The glucose-1-phosphate undergoes intramolecular rearrangement to form glucose-6-phosphate by the action of phosphoglucomutase.

   $$\text{Glucose-1-phosphate} \xrightarrow{\text{phosphoglucomutase}} \text{Glucose-6-phosphate}$$

3. The glucose-6-phosphate is finally hydrolysed to glucose and phosphoric acid by the action of phosphatase present in liver.

   $$\text{Glucose-6-phosphate} \xrightarrow[\text{Liver}]{\text{phosphatase}} \text{Glucose + Phosphoric acid}$$

Gluconeogenesis : When the body's stores of carbohydrates decrease below normal, moderate quantities of glucose can be formed from *amino acids* and from the *glycerol* portion of fat. This process is called gluconeogenesis. Approximately 60 % of the amino acids in the body proteins can be converted easily into carbohydrates, while the remaining 40 % have chemical configuration that make this difficult. Each amino acid is converted into glucose by a slightly different chemical process. For instance, alanine can be converted directly into pyruvic acid by simple deamination; the pyruvic acid then is converted into glucose.

Conversion of glucose into fat: It is another physiological mechanism by which the excess glucose is transformed into fat to maintain the blood sugar at a constant level. The fat so produced is largely stored in the adipose tissue. Fat formation begins when the liver and muscle become incapable of storing more glycogen. This occurs largely in the liver. The glucose is probably metabolized to a 2-carbon compound which is then polymerised into a long fatty acid chain. Glycerol is readily formed from glucose and is combined with fatty acids to form neutral fats.

Catabolism of glucose OR Release of energy from glucose from the glycolytic pathway

Energy is liberated during the cellular breakdown of glucose in major two stages:

(A) The breakdown of glycogen and glucose into pyruvic acid and lactic acids in absence of oxygen. This is called anoerobic state or glycolysis and

(B) The oxidation of pyruvic acid in the citric acid cycle or Kreb's cycle as a result CO_2 and H_2O are produced. This stage requires oxygen for its completion.

(A) Glycolysis : Glycolysis means splitting of the glucose molecule to form two molecules of pyruvic acid. This is also called as *Embden-Meyor hof pathway.*

Successive steps of chemical reactions are illustrated in Fig. 1.5 and can be represented as follows:

1. *Phosphorylation of glucose or ATP consumption phase :* In the liver and muscles, glucose can directly enter into glycolytic series reactions. It starts with the transfer of a phosphate group from ATP to the sixth carbon atom of glucose in the presence of *hexokinase*, Mg^{++} ions, to form glucose-6-phosphate and ADP.

$$\text{Glucose} + \text{ATP} \xrightarrow[\text{Mg}^{++} \;\; \text{ATP} \curvearrowright \text{ADP}]{\text{hexokinase}} \text{Glucose-6-phosphate} + \text{ADP}$$

2. *Glucose-6-phosphate conversion to fructose-6-phosphate :* By intramolecular rearrangement under the influence of an enzyme, phosphoglucose isomerase, glucose-6-phosphate is converted into fructose-6-phosphate.

$$\text{(Glucose-6 phosphate)} \xrightarrow{\text{phosphoglucose isomerase}} \text{Fructose-6-phosphate}$$

3. *Phosphorylation of fructose-6-phosphate to fructose-1, 6-diphosphate.:* A second phosphate group is transferred to the first carbon atom of fructose-6-phosphate from a second ATP molecule ; as a result, fructose-1, 6-phosphate is formed. This is second step that involves ATP consumption. This reaction is catalyzed by the enzyme phosphofructokinase in the presence of ATP and Mg^{++} ions.

$$\text{Fructose-6-phosphate} + \text{ATP} \xrightarrow[\text{Mg}^{++} \;\; \text{ATP} \curvearrowright \text{ADP}]{\text{phosphofructokinase}} \text{Fructose-1, 6-diphosphate} + \text{ADP}$$

4. *Cleavage of fructose-1, 6-diphosphate to triose phosphate:* Fructose-1, 6-diphosphate splits between carbon 3 and 4 into dihydroxy-acetone phosphate and glyceraldehyde-3-phosphate under the influence of an enzyme *aldolase*. The two trioses formed can be reversibly changed into one another by the enzyme *triose-phosphate-isomerase* thereby showing isomerizing reactions.

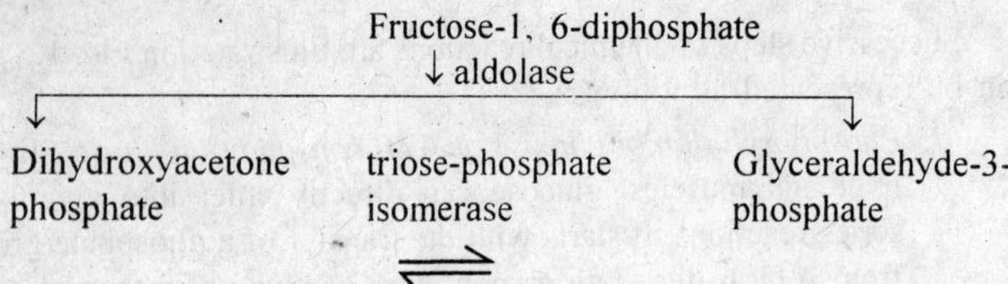

5. *Oxidation of glyceraldehyde-3-phosphate and formation of ATP* : Each molecule of glyceraldehyde-3-phosphate gains a second inorganic phosphate group and becomes 1, 3-diphosphoglyceric acid with concurrent dehydrogenation. The hydrogen atoms thus removed are accepted by NAD (Nicotinamide adenine dinucleotide), a respiratory enzyme which is reduced to NADH + H^+.

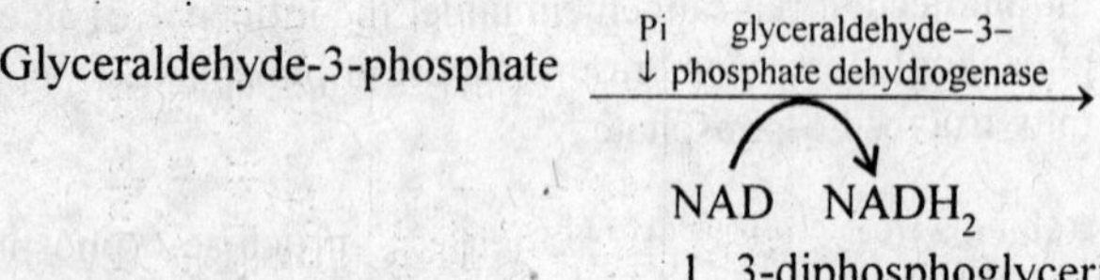

The reaction is catalysed by enzyme glyceraldehyde-3-phosphate dehydrogenase.

6. *Transphosphorylation of l, 3-diphosphoglyceric acid* : 1, 3-diphosphoglyceric acid contains a high energy bond; and in the presence of an acceptor, ADP, magnesium ions, and the enzyme phosphoglycerate kinase, 3-phosphoglyceric acid and ATP are formed.

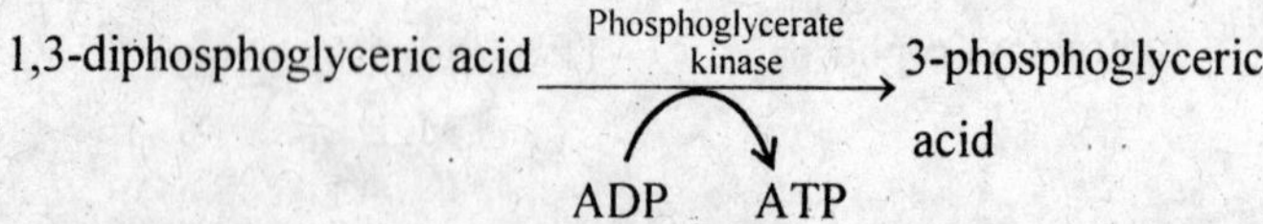

7. *Conversion of 3-phosphoglyceric acid to 2-phospho-glyceric acid* : In the presence of *phosphoglyceromutase*, 3-phosphoglyceric acid is converted into 2-phosphoglyceric acid affecting a shift of the phosphate group from the number 3 carbon to the number of 2 carbon.

3-phosphoglyceric acid $\xrightarrow{\text{phospho glyceromutase}}$ 2-phosphoglyceric acid

8. 2-phosphoglyceric acid is converted to phosphoenol pyruvic acid by dehydration (loss of one molecule of water) in the presence of an *enzyme enolase.*

   2-phosphoglyceric acid $\xrightarrow{\text{enolase}}$ Phosphoenol-pyruvic acid
   $\searrow H_2O$

   Phosphoenol-pyruvic acid contains a higher-energy phosphate bond.

9. High energy phosphate group of phosphoenol-pyruvic acid is transferred to ADP in the presence of enzyme pyruvate kinase, the resulting compound being pyruvic acid and ATP.

10. *Pyruvic acid to lactic acid :* Pyruvic acid forms the main end product of glycolysis in those tissues which are supplied with oxygen in abundance. But in those tissues, where oxygen supply is not sufficient *e.g.,* skeletal muscles, lactic acid forms the usual end product of glycolysis. In such cases, pyruvic acid is reduced to lactic acid under the influence of enzyme lactic dehydrogenase.

    Pyruvic acid $\xrightarrow{\text{lactic dehydrogenase}}$ Lactic acid

ATP Production During Glycolysis

From preceding discussion it is clear that at reactions numbered first and third, ATPs are consumed by the transfer of high energy phosphate groups, as a result fructose 1-6-diphosphate is produced.

The second phase underlines the cleavage of fructose-1, 6-diphosphate into two fragments of three carbon compounds, each one again undergoing further degradation. During sixth and ninth steps two molecules of ATP are regenerated. For each molecule of glucose undergoing glycolysis, 2 ATPs are consumed and (2 + 2) 4 ATPs are generated. Thus there is a net gain of two ATPs.

At reaction five, the compound is oxidized because of the removal of two hydrogen atoms which are subsequently accepted by NAD so that it is converted into NADH + H^+. The hydrogen atoms or electrons are transferred to the electron transfer system in the mitochondria during aerobic phase. Thus for each pair of hydrogen atoms undergoing oxidative phosphorylation three ATPs are produced and during reaction five there is a net gain of 6 ATPs.

In short, as a result of glycolysis (2 + 6) total 8 ATPs are generated.

Reaction		ATP loss/gain per glucose
Glucose → glucose-6-phosphate		–1
Fructose-6-phosphate → Fru. 1, 6-dip.		–1
2 1-3-dip. Glyceric acid → 3p. Gly. acid		+2
2 Phosphoenol py. acid → 2 pyruvic acid		+2
	Net gain	+2
2 $NADH_2$ Electron Transport sys.		+6
	Total	8

Significance of glycolysis : In a number of physiological (inner cells of bulky tissues) and pathological (tumour cells) conditions when the supply of oxygen becomes scarce, energy is mainly generated by glycoletic pathway.

Metabolism of lactic acid : The lactic acid produced in the muscles passes into the liver through blood, where it is converted in glycogen. Some of the lactic acid is excreted in the urine. About 20% is oxidized to carbon dioxide and water. As in the presence of oxygen, lactic acid is normally not detected in the muscle; it is through that pyruvic acid is directly oxidized to CO_2 and water.

The primary pathway of lactic acid is its conversion to CO_2 and H_2O, aerobically by citric acid cycle through acetyl CoA. It may be converted to fatty acids or sterols. Other pathways include transamination to alanine, and carboxylation to malic or oxaloacetic acid. These pathways can be diagrammatically shown as follows:

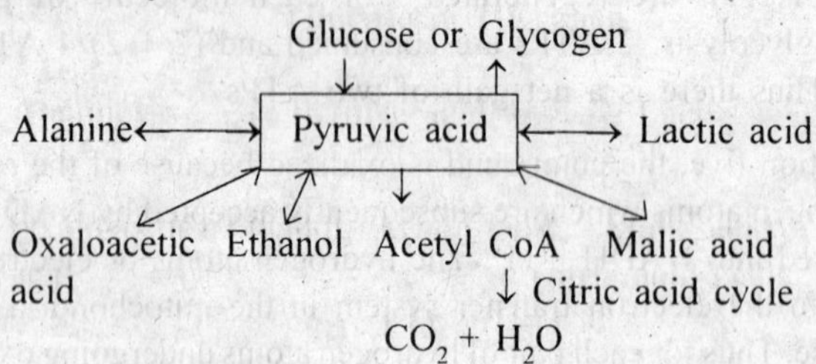

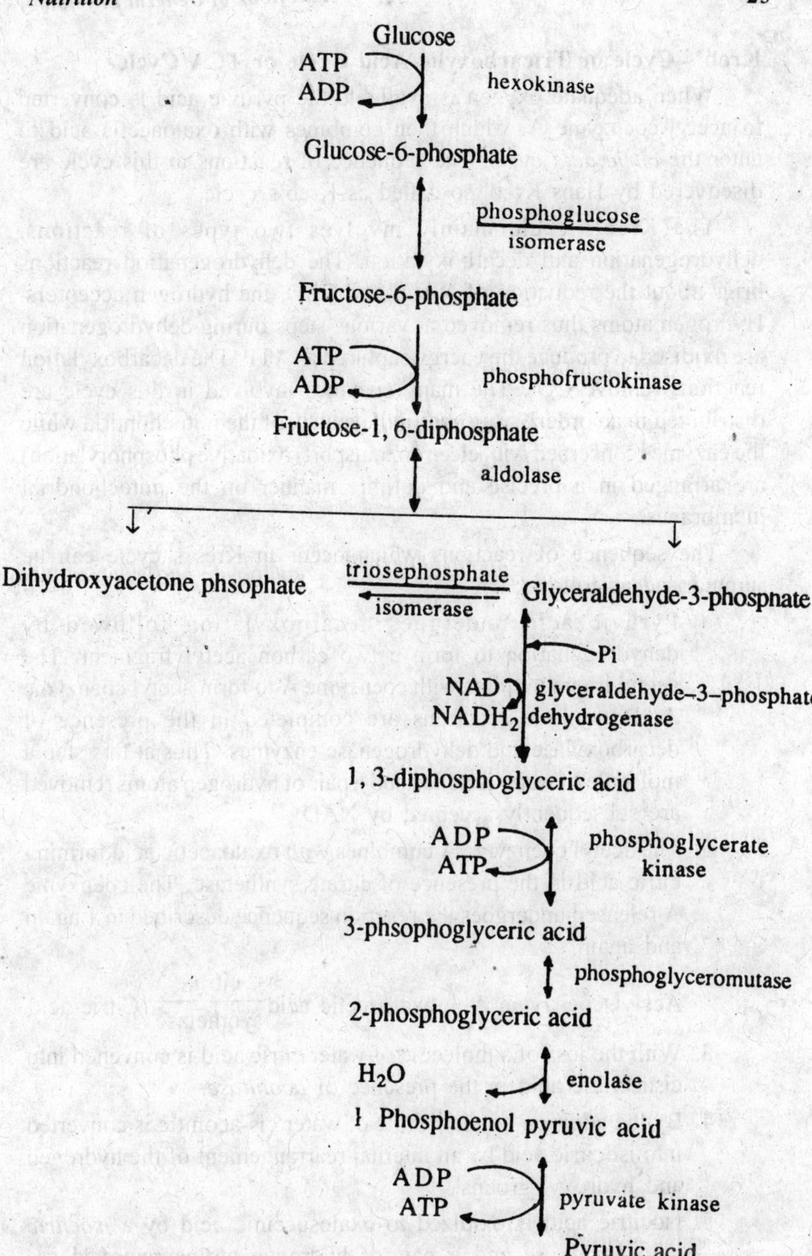

Fig. 1.5 : Sequence of reactions occurring in Glycolysis.

Kreb's Cycle or Tricarboxylic Acid Cycle or TCA Cycle

When adequate oxygen is available the pyruvic acid is converted to acetyl coenzyme A, which then combines with oxaloacetic acid to enter the *citric acid cycle*. The sequence of reactions in this cycle are discovered by Hans Kreb, so called as Kreb's cycle.

The Kreb's cycle mainly involves two types of reactions, dehydrogenation and decarboxylation. The dehydrogenation reactions brigs about the reduction of NAD^+ and FAD, the hydrogen acceptors. Hydrogen atoms thus removed at various steps during dehydrogenation are oxidised to produce the energy captured as ATP. The decarboxylation reactions remove CO_2. The many enzymes involved in this cycle are distributed in an orderly way within the matrix of the mitochondria while the enzymes concerned with electron transport (oxidative phosphorylation) are arranged in a precise and definite manner on the mitochondrial membranes.

The sequence of reactions which occur in Kreb's cycle can be summarised as follows:

1. Pyruvic acid undergoes decarboxylation followed by dehydrogenation to form a two carbon acetyl fragment. The acetyl fragment joins with coenzyme A to form acetyl coenzyme A. Both these reactions are completed in the presence of decarboxylase and dehydrogenase enzymes. Thus at this step a molecule of water is added and a pair of hydrogen atoms removed are subsequently accepted by NAD^+.
2. The acetyl coenzyme A combines with oxaloacetic acid forming citric acid in the presence of citrate synthetase. The coenxyme A released undergoes the reaction sequence described in 1 again and again.

   $$\text{Acetyl coenzyme A} + \text{oxaloacetic acid} \xrightarrow[\text{synthetase}]{\text{citrate}} \text{Citric acid}$$
3. With the loss of a molecule of water citric acid is convened into cisaconitic acid in the presence of *aconitase*.
4. By the addition of a molecule of water cis-aconitic is converted into isocitric acid by an internal rearrangement of the hydrogen and hydroxyl groups.
5. Isocitric acid is oxidized to oxalosuccinic acid by a *isocitric dehydrogenase* and a pair of hydrogen atoms removed are accepted by NAD^+.

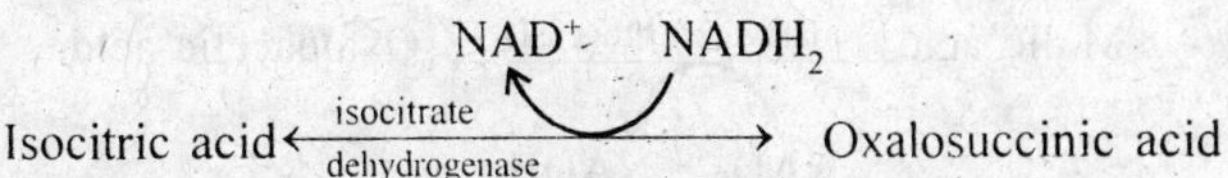

6. Oxalosuccinic acid is decarboxylated in presence of *decarboxylase* to α-ketoglutaric acid and CO_2.

Oxalosuccinic acid $\xrightarrow[CO_2]{\text{decarboxylase}}$ α-ketoglutaric acid + CO_2

7. α-ketoglutaric acid undergoes oxidative decarboxylation forming succinyl coenzyme A. Reaction is catalysed by α-ketoglutarate dehydrogenase. During this reaction a molecule of CO_2 is removed along with a pair of hydrogen atoms which are subsequently accepted by NAD^+.

α-ketoglutaric acid $\xrightarrow[\text{dehydrogenase}]{\alpha-\text{ketoglutarate}}$ Succinyl coenzyme A

CO_2 NAD^+ → $NADH + H^+$

8. Succinyl coenzyme A is convened into succinic acid and the coenzyme A freed undergoes the reaction cycle again and again. During this step a molecule of ATP is generated. This is only step at which ATP is generated similar to glycolysis. Reaction is catalysed by succinyl CoA synthetase.

Succinyl CoA $\xrightarrow{\text{succinyl CoA synthetase}}$ Succinic acid + coenzyme A

Pi   ADP → ATP

9. Succinic acid is oxidised to yield fumaric acid by the enzyme *succinic dehydrogenase* and a pair of hydrogen atoms removed are accepted by FAD.

FAD → $FADH_2$

Succinic acid + FAD $\xrightarrow[\text{dehydrogenase}]{\text{succinic}}$ Fumaric acid + $FADH_2$

10. Fumaric acid is convened into malic acid by the addition of a molecule of water in the presence of *fumerase*.

Fumaric acid $\xrightarrow[H_2O]{\text{fumerase}}$ Malic acid

11. Malic acid finally oxidised to oxaloacetic acid and the hydrogen atoms removed are accepted by NAD^+ in the presence of *malate dehydrogenate*.

$$\text{Malic acid} \xrightleftharpoons[\text{NAD}^+ \quad \text{NADH}_2]{\text{malate dehydrogenate}} \text{Oxaloacetic acid}$$

The oxaloacetic acid is the final product of Kreb's cycle which repeatedly undergoes the cycle again by combining with acetylcoenzyme A.

ATP Production During Kreb's Cycle

1. Oxidation of pyruvic to acetyl CoA via NAD	= 3 ATP
2. Oxidation of isocitric via NAD	= 3 ATP
3. Oxidation of a-ketoglutaric acid via NAD	= 3 ATP
4. Oxidation of succinic acid via FAD	= 2 ATP
5. Oxidation of malic acid via NAD	= 3 ATP
Total	14 ATP
6. Conversion of succinyl CoA to succinic acid	= 1 ATP
Grand total	= 15 ATP

One mole of pyruvic acid when oxidized to CO_2 and H_2O by Kreb's cycle thus leads to formation of 15 moles of ATP. Since two moles of pyruvic acid may be obtained per mole of glucose entering into glycolytic reaction, 30 moles of ATP may be synthesized in all.

In the anaerobic oxidation of glucose via glycolysis into pyruvic acid liberates 8 moles of ATP of which two are consumed in the formation of glucose-6-phosphate and fructose-1, 6-diphosphate. Therefore, the net gain of ATP in the both cycles is 8 + 30 = 38 –2 = 36 moles.

Other Pathways of Carbohydrate Metabolism

Glycolysis and TCA cycle together form the principal (90% of the glucose is metabolised) but not the only pathway by which animal tissue oxidize glucose to CO_2 and H_2O with the production of useful energy in the form of ATP, yet alternate pathways exist. Even when glycolysis and citric acid cycle are blocked by inhibitors-iodoacetate and fluoride, mammalian tissues can metabolize glucose at a reduced rate. One of the most important alternative routes is the *pentose phosphate pathway or warburg Dickens pathway* or *phosphogluconate shunt* or *hexose monophosphate shunt*. This pathway is the major pathway for the biosynthesis of pentoses, sedoheptulose, the hexosamine, uronic acids, neuraminic acid and some other carbohydrate derivatives. It also serves for the oxidation of glucose to CO_2 and formation of $NADH_2$ and ATP.

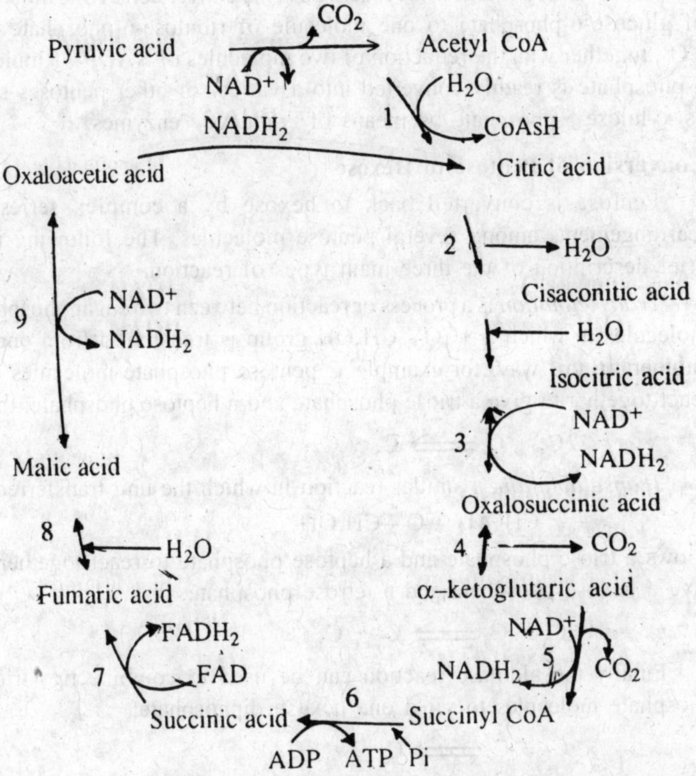

Fig. 1.6 : Citric acid cycle. Citrate Enzymes: (1) citrate synthetase (2) aconitase (3) isocitric dehydrogenase (4) decarboxylase (5) a-ketoglutarate dehydrogenase (6) succinyl CoA synthetase (7) succinic dehydrogenase (8) fumarase (9) malate dehydrogenate.

The cycle can be divided into two phases : The conversion of hexose to pentose and the conversion of pentose to hexose.

Conversion of Hexose to Pentose

Glucose-6-phosphate is oxidised to 6-phosphogluconic acid by *glucose-6-phosphate dehydrogenase* and NADP. In a second dehydrogenation by NADP, 6-phosphogluconic acid is further oxidised to an unstable intermediate which loses CO_2 to give the pentose, ribulose-5-phosphate.

The overall effect of these reactions is the conversion of one molecule of glucose-6-phosphate to one molecule of ribulose-6-phosphate and CO_2, together with the reduction of two molecules of $NADP^+$. Ribulose-5-phosphate is readily converted into a variety of other pentoses such as xylulose-5-phosphate by means of *epimerase* enzymes.

Conversion of Pentose to Hexose

Pentose is converted back to hexose by a complex series of rearrangements among several pentose molecules. The following is a brief description of the three main types of reaction:

Transketolation is a process or reaction between two sugar phosphate molecules in which a—CO—CH_2OH group is transferred from one to another. In this way, for example, 2 pentose phosphate molecules can react together to give a triose phosphate and a heptose phosphate, thus:

$$C_5 + C_5 \rightleftharpoons C_3 + C_7$$

Transaldolation, a similar reaction in which the unit transferred is

—CHOH—CO—CH_2OH

allows a triose phosphate and a heptose phosphate to react together to give a hexose phosphate and a tetrose phosphate:

$$C_3 + C_7 \rightleftharpoons C_6 + C_4$$

Finally the aldolase reaction can be used to combine two triose phosphate molecules to yield one hexose diphosphate:

$$C_3 + C_3 \rightleftharpoons C_6$$

These three reactions can be employed to convert pentose quantitatively to hexose in the following manner.

In the starting, six pentose phosphate molecules arranged in pairs, then two of these pairs undergo transketolation followed by transaldolation to yield two hexose phosphates and two tetrose phosphates. The latter .then undergoes transketolation with the remaining pair of pentose phosphates to give two more hexose phosphates and two tetrose phosphates. Under the influence of *aldolase* the two triose phosphates combine to give fructose 1, 6-diphosphate, which is hydrolysed by fructose 1, 6-diphosphatase to give another hexose monophosphate. Thus the overall reaction is the conversion of 6 molecules of pentose phosphate to 5 of hexose phosphate:

$$6\ C_5 \rightarrow 5\ C_6$$

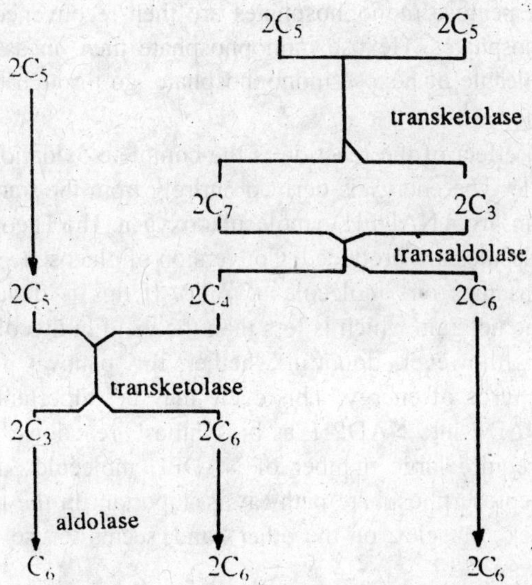

Fig. 1.7 : Summary of transketolase and transaldolase reactions.

Overall Reaction

In this pathway the two reaction sequences are combined. Six hexose monophosphates are oxidized to give six pentose monophosphates and

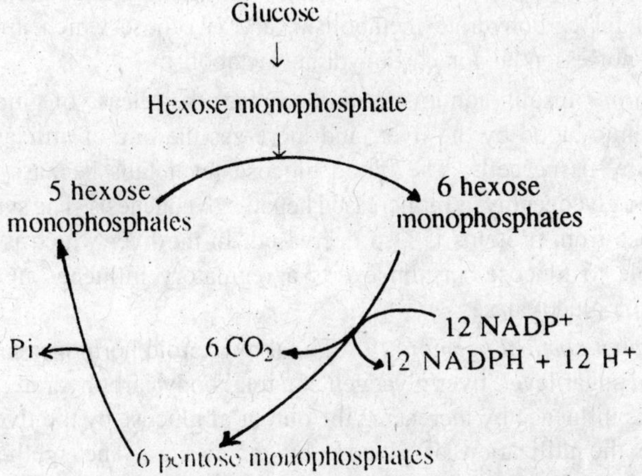

Fig. 1.8 : Summary of reactions of the pentose phosphate pathway.

6 CO_2. The six pentose monophosphates are then reconvened to five hexose monophosphates. Hexose monophosphate then, in association with a fresh molecule of hexose monophosphate, go through the cycle again (Fig. 1.8).

The overall effect of the reaction is the complete oxidation of one glucose molecule. The energy is derived entirely from the transport of 24 hydrogen atoms from NADPH to molecular oxygen. The Theoretically, $12 \times 3 = 36$ molecules are produced. Conversion of glucose to glucose-6-phosphate consumes one molecule of ATP. If this is deducted 35 molecules are the net gain which is less than the yield in glycolysis and TCA cycle. It is, however, doubtful whether, this pathway functions primarily as a source of energy. This cycle may be important for the conversion of NADP into NADPH, as biosynthesis reactions like fatty acid synthesis require large number of NADPH molecules. It seems likely that the pentose phosphate pathway is important in the liver and the adrenal cortex. Muscles, on the other hand, seems to use only the glycolytic pathway.

Hormonal Control of Carbohydrate Metabolism

The supply of glucose to the blood by the liver and its utilization in the tissues must be regulated for the 'smooth' functioning of the metabolic processes in the body. Hormones secreted by the endo-organs play an important role in the metabolism. They can be classified into two varieties, (i) those which regulate the normal function and are essential for carbohydrate metabolism, and (ii) those which influence and are not essential for carbohydrate metabolism.

Insulin : Insulin administration decreases the release of glucose to the systemic blood by the liver, and increases the rate of utilization of glucose by tissue cells. The blood glucose level falls because of the decreased glycogenolysis or increased hepatic glycogenesis. The synthesis of glucose from proteins is also decreased. In the liver which is freely permeable to glucose, insulin exerts a regulatory influence upon the activity of glucokinase.

Adrenal cortical hormones : Adrenal oxysteroid hormones increase the blood sugar level, liver glycogen and total body carbohydrate. These hormones influence by increasing the output of glucose by the liver, and decrease the utilization of glucose by the tissues. The synthesis of carbohydrates from protein is also increased by the stimulation of activity of certain transaminases.

Adrenohypophyseal factors : The adrenocorticotrophic hormones (ACTH) and thyroid stimulating hormones increase the secretions of adrenal cortex and thyroid glands by stimulating them, which on their turn effect the carbohydrate metabolism. Anterior pituitary extracts increase the blood sugar and decrease the respiratory quotient. These 'diabetic' symptoms are due to somatotropin which depresses the utilization of glucose.

Epinephrine : The action of epinephrine is to increase the blood sugar and lactic acid, which is due to an increase in the rate of glycogenolysis in the liver and muscles. Epinephrine stimulates phosphorylase activity and diminishes the uptake of glucose by tissue cells.

Thyroxine : The thyroid hormone increases the breakdown of glycogen and thereby the blood sugar. Thyroxine also increases the absorption of hexoses from the intestine.

Glucagon : The physiolog cal importance of this substances is not known. It is produced by the α-cells of islets of Langerhans and causes an increase in blood sugar by accelerating hepatic glycogen breakdown.

LIPID METABOLISM

A number of different chemical compounds in the food and in the body are classified as *lipids*. These include (1) neutral fat, known also as *triglycerides*, (2) the *phospholipids*, (3) *cholesterol*, and (4) a few others of less importance. Chemically, the basic lipid moity of both the triglycerides and the phospholipids is fatty acids, which are simply long chain hydrocarbon organic acids. A typical fatty acid, palmitic acid, is the following:

$$CH_3(CH2)_{14}\ COOH$$

Though cholesterol does not contain fatty acid, its sterol nucleus, is synthesized from degradation products of fatty acid molecules, thus giving it many of the physical and chemical properties of other lipid substances.

The triglycerides are used in the body mainly to provide energy for the different metabolic processes. In human body, the three fatty acids most commonly present in neutral fat are (1) *stearic acid*, which has an 18-carbon chain and is fully saturated with hydrogen atoms, (2) *oleic acid* which also has an 18-carbon chain but has one double bond in the middle of the chain, and (3) palmitic acid, which has 16 carbon atoms and is fully saturated.

Fats are hydrolyzed into glycerol and fatty acids during the process of digestion. These and some of the unhydrolyzed fats are absorbed in a finely emulsified form by the lymphatic system into the blood, where it appears in the form of minute droplets of neutral fat. Most of the fatty acids and glycerol are also absorbed into the blood stream in combination with the bile salts. The fate of the ingested food fat after absorption is its deposition in the fat depots of the body of which the mesenteries, intramuscular and subcutaneous connective tissue are the most important sites. The total amount of fat in human body varies from 10-20% of the body weight but in a very obese person it may be as high as 50% of the body weight. Of the total fat stored in the adipose tissues, about 50% exists in the subcutaneous tissues, 10 to 15% in the abdominal cavity, 10 to 15% in the renal space and remaining 5 % in the inter muscular space. All the fat in the body does not come from dietary food but it is readily synthesized from the excess of carbohydrates not stored as glycogen.

Fat has certain definite advantages over proteins and carbohydrates as a reserve food or fuel. It is richer in carbon and hydrogen, so that there is more combustible material in fat than either in protein or carbohydrates. If one gram of protein and carbohydrate are combusted in a bomb calorimeter, 5,600 calories and 4,200 calories of-energy respectively are evolved. On the other hand, one gram of fat on combustion yields 9,300 calories of energy. Fats on hydrolysis give out glycerol and fatty acids.

Hydrolysis of Triglycerides

The first stage in the utilization of triglycerides for energy purposes is its hydrolysis into fatty acids and glycerol. The glycerol is immediately converted into glyceraldehyde which can subsequently enter into the phosphogluconate pathway of glucose metabolism. On the other hand fatty acids are utilized for energy purposes as follows.

Use of Triglycerides for Energy and Formation of ATP or Oxidation of Fatty Acids

Most of the dietary fatty acids as well as those derived from the hydrolysis of triglycerides undergo a process called Beta *oxidation*; termed owing to the carbon atom next to that to which the carboxyl group is attached is attacked first. By a series of reactions involving several enzymes and coenzymes, the fatty acid with two less carbon atoms than the original one is produced. Thus, during this process a fatty acid molecule is degraded by progressive release of two carbon segments into the form of acyl-CoA. The successive stages in the beta oxidation can be summarised as follows (Fig. 1.9):

1. $RCH_2CH_2CH_2COOH$ + Co-A + ATP $\xrightleftharpoons{\text{thiokinase}}$
(fatty acid)

$RCH_2CH_2CH_2COCo\text{-}A$ + AMP + pyrophosphate
(fatty acyl Co-A)

2. $RCH_2CH_2CH_2COCo\text{-}A$ + FAD $\xrightarrow[\text{dehydrogenase}]{\text{acyl}}$

$RCH_2CH_2CH = CHCOCo\text{-}A + FADH_2$
(Enoyl-Co-A compound)

3. $RCH_2CH = CHCOCo\text{-}A + H_2O$ $\xrightleftharpoons{\text{enoyl hydrase}}$

$RCH_2CHOHCH_2COCo\text{-}A$
(3-hydroxy acyl-CoA compound)

4. $RCH_2CHOHCH_2COCo\text{-}A$ + NAD $\xrightleftharpoons[\text{acyl dehydrogenase}]{\beta-\text{hydroxy}}$

$RCH_2COCH_2COCo\text{-}A + NADH + H^+$
(3-oxyacyl-CoA comp.)

5. $RCH_2COCH_2COCo\text{-}A$ + Co-A $\xrightleftharpoons{\text{thiolase}}$

(3-oxyacyl-Co-A comp.) $RCH_2COCo\text{-}A + CH_3COCo\text{-}A$
(fatty acyl Co-A) (Acetyl Co-A)

R-represents the saturated aliphatic chain of the fatty acids: $CH_4(CH_2CH_2)_{n-1}$. (n-number of two carbon fragments).

Fig. 1.9 : Beta oxidation of fatty acids to yield acetylcoenzyme A.

1. The fatty acid molecule first combines with coenzyme A to form a fatty acyl-CoA molecule.
2. Fatty acyl-CoA loses two hydrogen atoms from the alpha and beta carbons leaving double bonds there. The hydrogen atoms which are removed are accepted by the flavoproteins which subsequently undergo oxidative phosphorylation.
3. The unsaturated double bond formed in the above reaction is hydrated so that a hydrogen atom attaches to the alpha carbon and a hydroxyl radical to the beta carbon.
4. Two additional hydrogen atoms removed, one from the beta carbon and one from the hydroxyl radical, are accepted by DPN which, in turn, undergoes oxidative phosphorylation.

5. In general, during a cycle of beta oxidation, compound splits between the alpha and beta carbons, the long portion of the chain combines with a new molecule of coenzyme A, while the shorter acetyl portion remains combined with original coenzyme A in the form of acetyl-CoA.

The new fatty acyl CoA, which now has two carbon atoms less than the original fatty acyl-CoA, re-enters in the second cycle of reaction as described above, until another acetyl-CoA molecule is released and still a new fatty acyl CoA is formed with two carbon atoms less. This process is repeated again and again until the entire fatty acid molecule is split into acetyl-CoA. For example for each molecule of stearic acid, nine molecules of acetyl-CoA are formed.

Oxidation of Acetyl Coenzyme A : The acetyl CoA molecules produced as a result of beta oxidation enter into the Kreb's cycle by combining with the oxaloacetic acid to form succinic acid that in turn, is degraded into carbon dioxide and water on the common metabolic pathway. Thus, the net reaction that each molecule of acetyl-CoA undergoes can be presented as:

$CH_3CO.CoA$ + oxaloacetic acid + $3H_2$ + ADP $\xrightarrow{TCA}$ $2CO_2$ + 8H + H-CO-A + ATP + oxaloacetic acid

In summary, after the initial oxidation of fatty acids to acetyl-CoA, their subsequent degradation is precisely the same as that of the acetyl-CoA formed from pyruvic acid during the glucose metabolism.

ATP Formed by Oxidation of Fatty Acids

In Fig. 1.9 note that 4 hydrogen atoms are released each time a molecule of acetyl-CoA is formed from the fatty acid chain. Therefore, for every stearic acid molecule that is split, a total of 32 hydrogen atoms is removed. In addition, for each acetyl-CoA degraded by the citric acid cycle, 8 hydrogen atoms are removed, making an additional 72 hydrogens for each molecule of stearic acid metabolised. This added to the above 32 hydrogen atoms, makes a total of 104 hydrogen atoms. Of this group 34 are removed from the degrading fatty acid by flavoproteins and 70 are removed by NAD^+ as NADH and H^+. These two groups of hydrogen atoms are oxidised in the mitochondria, but they enter the oxidative system at different point, so that upto 1 molecule of ATP is synthesized for each of the 34 flavoprotein hydrogens and upto 1-5 molecules of ATP are synthesized for each of the 70 NADH and H^+ hydrogens. This makes 34 plus 105, or a total of 139 molecules of ATP formed by the oxidation of hydrogen derived from each molecule of stearic acid. And another 9 molecules of ATP are formed in the citric acid cycle, one for each of the 9 acetyl-CoA molecules metabolized. Thus, a total of 148 molecules of ATP is formed during the complete oxidation of 1 molecule of stearic acid. However, 2 high energy bonds are consumed in the initial combination of coenzyme A with the fatty acid molecule, making a net gain of 146 molecule of ATP.

Ketosis

In circumstances when the metabolism of carbohydrates is impaired or operated at a slow level, the fate of the acetyl CoA is altered for two reasons:

1. the oxalacetate available to condense with acetyl CoA is in limited supply, and
2. a much greater proportion of the body's energy needs is being supplied by the oxidation of fatty acids, leading to the production of acetyl CoA is greater than normal amounts. Because of these reasons, two molecules of acetyl CoA condense to form acetoacetyl CoA. The enzymes *deacylases* in the liver hydrolyze acetoacetyl CoA to coenzyme A and acetoacetic acid. Acetoacetic acid is reduced to β-hydroxybutyric acid or decarboxylated to form acetone. These three compounds are *ketone bodies* and the process is known as *ketogenesis*.

2 acetyl coenzyme A → acetoacetyl-COA →

Acetoacetic acid

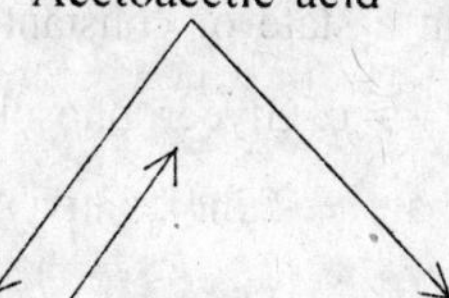

β-Hydroxybutyric acid Acetone

The accumulation of these substances in the blood results in ketosis. Ketosis is a dangerous condition as acetoacetic acid and p-hydroxybutyric acid reduce the alkalinity of the blood and produce a condition known as acidosis.

Further stages in the breakdown of acetoacetic acid to carbon dioxide and water occur largely in tissues other than the liver and involve the participation of coenzyme A and the reactions of the Kreb's tricarboxylic acid cycle.

Fatty Acid biosynthesis

The biosynthesis of fatty acids can be well expected to follow the reversal of the beta oxidation pathway, however, this does not occur to an appreciable extent. No doubt the carbon atoms of a fatty acid are derived, two at a time, from the acetyl groups of acetyl-CoA molecules and that many of the reactions leading to the fatty acid synthesis resemble closely to those of the degradation reactions.

The synthesis of fatty acids then involves two important processes; one is the formation of new carbon to carbon bonds between acyl radicals and the second is the reduction of ketone groups to the hydrocarbon stage. Both of these processes are endergonic and the energy is directly supplied by TPNH. Under biological conditions, the methyl group of one acetyl-CoA is apparently not sufficiently reactive for combination with another acetyl group so that acetyl-CoA units cannot directly condense to produce longer carbon chains. This difficulty is overcome with the formation of malonyl-CoA as a more reactive intermediate, with ATP furnishing the required energy. It is synthesized by the addition of CO_2 (actually HCO_3) to a molecule of acetyl-CoA.

The reaction sequence goes as follows (Fig. 1.10).

Fats are also synthesized from excess of carbohydrates. This is possible under two conditions; when large quantities of acetyl-CoA formed from the carbohydrates are available and there is low concentration of free fatty acids in the adipose tissue. The process involves conversion of acetyl-CoA into fatty acids. Thus excess of carbohydrates in the diet increase the stores of the fat. It represents a best example of the fact that living matter is always in a state of constant flux.

1. Glycerol + ATP → α-Glycerophosphate
2. α-Glycerophosphate + 2 mol. fatty Acid CoA → L-α-phosphatidic acid

```
H2COH                              H2C–O–C–R
  |                                  |   ||
H–COH + 2R–C–SCoA → R2–C–O–C–H O
  |        ||                        |
H2CO–PO3H2  O                      H2C–O–PO3H2
```

3. L–α–phosphatidic acid $\xrightarrow[+H_2O]{\text{phosphatase}}$ D–1, 2-Diglyceride + Pi

4. D-l, 2–Diglyceride + $R_3–\underset{\underset{O}{\|}}{C}–S\text{-}CoA$ → Triglyceride

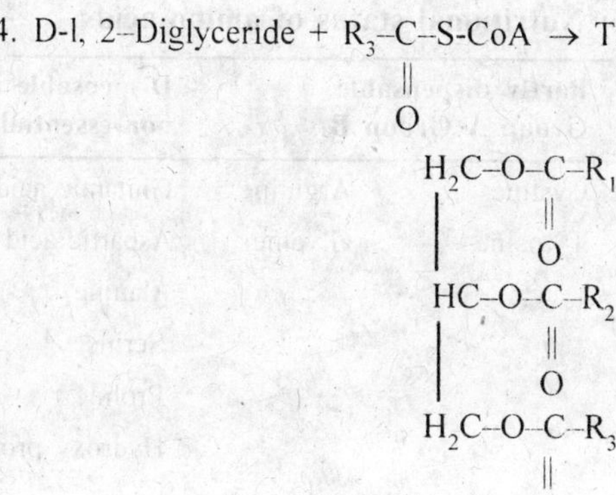

Fig. 1.10: Synthesis of fat.

Hormonal Control of Fat Metabolism

Fat metabolism is coordinated and controlled by the endocrine system through the hormones.

The release of free fatty acids from the adipose tissue is controlled by insulin. Insulin stimulates the utilization of glucose-6-phosphate by the pentose phosphate pathways, thus increasing the supply of NADPH and this in turn promotes fatty acid synthesis.

Adrenaline increases the movement of fat from the fat deposits and this causes an increase in the concentration of blood non-esterified fatty acids. Fat mobilization is also stimulated by ACTH, TSH and glucagon. Prostaglandin has an opposite effect.

PROTEIN METABOLISM

Proteins are essential dietary components forming the building blocks for the formation of new cells and growth. About three quarters of the body solids are proteins. These include *structural proteins*, enzymes, nucleoproteins, proteins that transport oxygen, proteins of the muscle that cause contraction, and many other types that perform specific functions both intracellularly and extracellulariy throughout the body.

Amino acids are the end products "of protein digestion. There are about 20 naturally occurring amino acids, which are categorised as *essential amino acids*, which cannot be synthesized in the body and their intake from outside is essential and *non-essential* amino acids which ordinarily be synthesized in the body and hence their presence in the diet is not essential. Both are given in Table 1.5.

Table 1.5: Nutritional status of amino acids

Indispensable or essential	Partly dispensable Group A	Group B	Dispensable or non-essential
Histidine	Cystine	Arginine	Glutamic acid
Lysine	Tyrosine	Glycine	Aspartic acid
Tryptophan			Alanine
Phenylalanine			Serine
Methionine			Proline
Threonine			Hydroxy proline
Leucine			
Isoleucine			
Valine			

Use of Proteins for Energy

Proteins are rarely oxidized for the energy purposes. It is known that there is an upper limit to the amount of protein that can accumulate in each particular type of cell. Once the cells are filled to their limits, any additional amino acids in the body fluids are degraded and used for energy or stored as fat. This degradation occurs almost entirely in the liver and kidney.

The removal of amino group from an amino acid constitutes the first step in the utilization of proteins for energy purposes and it is a prominent feature of protein metabolism. The process is carried out by several different means; however, two of which are the most important;

1. **Deamination**
2. **Transamination**

1. *Deamination :* Deamination means removal of the amino group from the amino acids and usually is transferred to the other carboxylic acid. To help in this process, the excess amino acids in the cells, especially in the liver, induce the production of large quantities of *aminotransferases*, the enzymes responsible for initiating most deamination. Deamination enables inter-conversions of amino and carboxylic acids. The deamination may be *oxidative* or *non-oxidative*. Removal of the amino group by oxidation which converts the amino acid into a keto acid is

called as oxidative deamination. The conversion is catalysed by the enzymes *amino acid oxidases*. In non-oxidative deamination alanine is converted into the pyruvic acid and glutamic acid into the alpha keto-glutaric acid in the presence of catalytic enzyme like flavoproteins.

Proteins ← Amino acids → α-ketoglutaric acid
↓ glutamic dehydrogenase
α keto acid → Glutamic acid
] Ammonia (NH_3)

The liberated ammonia is highly poisonous; therefore, it is either immediately expelled out of the body or it is converted into urea and uric acid to be subsequently given out of the body through the excretory organs. Or, as it happens in many cases, this ammonia combines with an amino acid called glutamic acid to form another amino acid, glutamin.

2. *Transamination* : Transamination is even important than deamination, in which an amino group of one amino acid is transferred to a α-keto acid, forming a new amino acid and a keto acid without the formation of ammonia in the free state. Thus, an amino group after removal from the amino acid alanine is transferred to keto-glutaric acid which now becomes glutamic acid, and what is left behind is pyruvic acid. Pyruvic acid then joins citric acid (Kerb's) cycle.

$$\text{Alanine} + \text{ketoglutaric acid} \xrightarrow{\text{transa min ase}} \text{pyruvic acid} + \text{Glutamic acid}$$

The synthesis of a large number of amino acids is made possible by this method, provided a suitable source of nitrogen is available.

Removal of Ammonia

The ammonia released during deamination is removed from the blood almost entirely by conversion into urea, two molecules of ammonia and one molecule of CO_2 combining in accordance with the following net reaction:

$$2\,NH_3 + CO_2 \rightarrow H_2N\text{–}\underset{\underset{\displaystyle O}{\|}}{C}\text{–}NH_2 + H_2O$$

Urea

Essentially all urea formed in the human body is synthesized in the liver. In the absence of the liver or in serious liver disease, ammonia accumulates in the blood. This in turn is extremely toxic, especially to the brain, often leading to a state called *hepatic coma.*

The stages in the formation of urea are essentially the following:

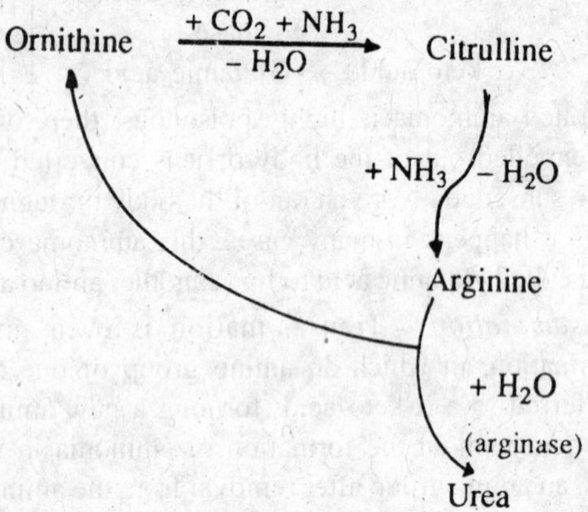

The reaction begins with the amino acid derivative *ornithine* which combines with one molecule of CO_2 and one molecule of ammonia to form a second substance, *citrulline.* This in turn combines with still another molecule of *ammonia* to form *arginine* which then splits into *ornithine* and *urea.* The *urea* diffuses from the liver cells into the body fluids and is excreted by the kidneys, while the ornithine is reused in the cycle again and again.

3. *Transmethylation :* It is the transfer of methyl group of methionine to other suitable acceptors. The phenomenon of transmethylation was discovered by *Vignaud* and his colleagues, the reactions are enzymatically catalyzed by *transmethylases.* Methionine is first activated and then converted into S-*adenosylamethionine* (active methionine) by an ATP dependent enzyme system. Methyl group can also be transferred to sulphur atom showing the sulphur metabolisms.

   Methionine which a methyl group donor supplies its methyl group while synthesizing choline from glycine as shown in the following lines.

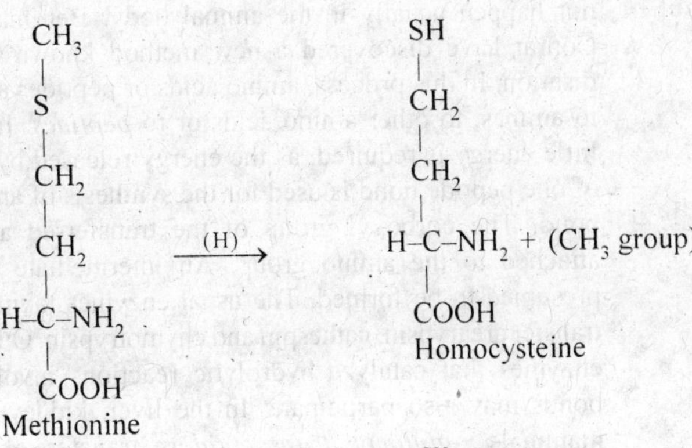

$$H_2N.CH_2COOH \rightarrow H_2N.CH_2CH_2OH \xrightarrow[(CH_3)_2NH_2CH_2OH.OH]{CH_2\ \text{groups}}$$

Glycine Ethanolamine Choline

4. *Decarboxylation* : Decarboxylation is a process in which certain amines are formed by the removal of CO_2 from the COOH group of amino acid. The process is catalyzed by *amino acid decarboxylases and pyridoxal phosphate is required* as a co-factor. Some of the amines formed as a result of decarboxylation have important physiological affects, probably not in man. Decarboxylation reactions are involved in the synthesis of histamines, dopamines, amino butyric acid etc. These substances are important neurohumors (chemical transmitters). Decarboxylation reactions are irreversible. Some reactions are given below:

$$\text{Tyrosine} \xrightarrow[\text{kidney}]{\text{tyrosine decarboxylase}} \text{Tyramine}$$

(increases blood pressure)

$$\text{Histidine} \xrightarrow[\text{(kidney, liver, lungs, intestine)}]{\text{histidine decarboxylase}} \text{Histamine}$$

(stimulates gastric secretion)

$$\text{Glutamic acid} \xrightarrow[\text{(liver, muscles \& brain)}]{\text{glutamic acid decarboxylase}} \gamma\text{-aminobutyric acid}$$

(inhibits synaptic transmission)

5. *Transpeptidisation* : The conversion of peptides into amino acids is a reversible reaction. Amino acids, therefore, can combine to form peptides. But the equilibrium favours only the formation of amino acids and, not peptides. Peptides can be synthesized by removing them as soon as they are formed and by using amino acids which yield insoluble peptides. However, this does

not happen usually in the animal body. Bergman and Frack-Conrat have discovered a new method known as transpeptidisation. In this process, amino acids or peptides are transferred to amines, to other amino acids or to *peptides*. In this process little energy is required, as the energy released by the breaking of one peptide bond is used for the synthesis of another peptide bond. The corboxyl group of the transferred amino acid is attached to the amino group. An intermediate compound is presumed to be formed. The usual enzymes taking part in this transfer are trypsin, cathespin and chymotrypsin. Other hydrolytic enzymes that catalyze hydrolytic reactions involving peptide bonds may also participate. In the liver, kidney and brain of mammals *γ-glutamyl transpeptidase* transfers the γ-glutamyl radical from glutathione to amino acids.

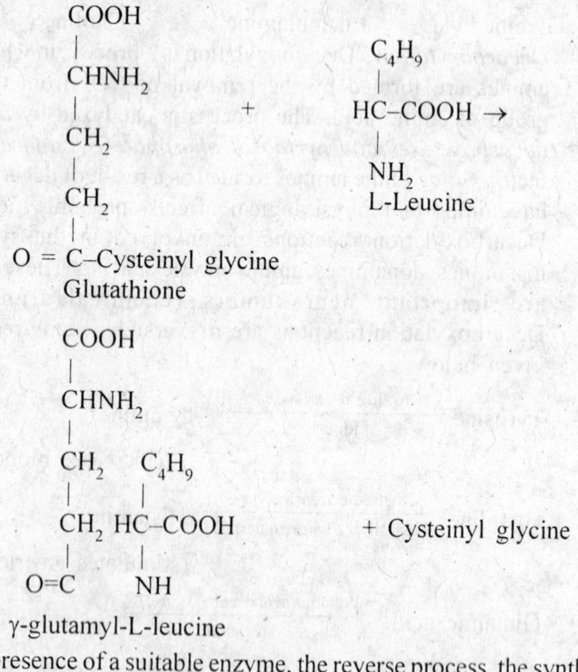

```
      COOH
       |                          C4H9
      CHNH2                        |
       |              +         HC–COOH →
      CH2                          |
       |                          NH2
      CH2                         L-Leucine
       |
  O = C–Cysteinyl glycine
      Glutathione

      COOH
       |
      CHNH2
       |
      CH2    C4H9
       |      |
      CH2  HC–COOH              + Cysteinyl glycine
       |      |
    O=C      NH

  γ-glutamyl-L-leucine
```

In the presence of a suitable enzyme, the reverse process, the synthesis of glutathione can also be accomplished. ATP is required.

γ-glutamylglycine + Cysteinylglycine → Glutathione + Glycine

Regulation of Protein Metabolism

Protein metabolism is influenced and regulated by the following factors.

Food : The nature of food exerts considerable influence on the protein metabolism. Meat food gives rise to greater amounts of uric acid, creatinine and ammonia.

Water : The amount of water available to the organism has its own effect on metabolism. Aquatic animals excrete ammonia which is converted into urea in *terresterial* animals getting sufficient amount of water. Animals living in xeric conditions excrete uric acid.

Hormones : Hormonal regulation is most significant. Different hormones have different effects as given in the following lines:

(i) *Insulin* : Whenever the amount of glucose falls in the blood and under secretion of insulin occurs, the breakdown of protein is promoted, especially in muscles. It rises the amino acid concentration in blood and they are deaminated in liver to form glucose or acetoacetate. The amino group of amino acid is converted to urea resulting a negative nitrogen balance. Increased protein metabolism is associated with tissue hypoxia resulting the excretion of K^+ in the urine.

(ii) *Thyroxine* : Thyroxine greatly influences the intensity of protein metabolism. In hyperthyroidism or if the excess of (hyroxine is taken orally, the catabolism of protein is increased resulting the increased nitrogen loss in the urine and loss-in the body weight.

(iii) *Growth hormone* : It is the pituitary hormone and increases transcription or the formation of mRNA that on the other hand promotes the synthesis of protein from the'amino acids. It lowers the amino acid concentration in blood.

(iv) *Cortisol* : Adernal hormone cortisol promotes the catabolism of proteins. and thus causes a negative nitrogen balance. It also increases the excretion of creatine. Other effects are retardation of growth, thining of skin and body and wasting of muscles.

Integration of Metabolism

Supply of various food materials is not always constant, moreover at the same time a definite proportion of mainly three, proteins, fats and carbohydrates, is maintained in the body. This proportionate constancy of various body "constituents is maintained with the help of labile enzyme system and there exists a common metabolic pathway on which various food stuffs are interconverted or degraded as shown in Fig. 1.11.

Carbohydrates constitute primary source of energy. Among others, fats have a high energy potential and are stored as energy reservoirs. Proteins are rarely utilized for the production of energy.

In general there are mainly three phases during the energy production.

Phase I : It involves hydrolysis of triglycerides into fatty acids and glycerol, polysaccharides into hexoses and proteins into constituent amino acids. Thus, ultimately fatty acids, glycerol, monosaccharides and amino acids are produced at the end of this phase.

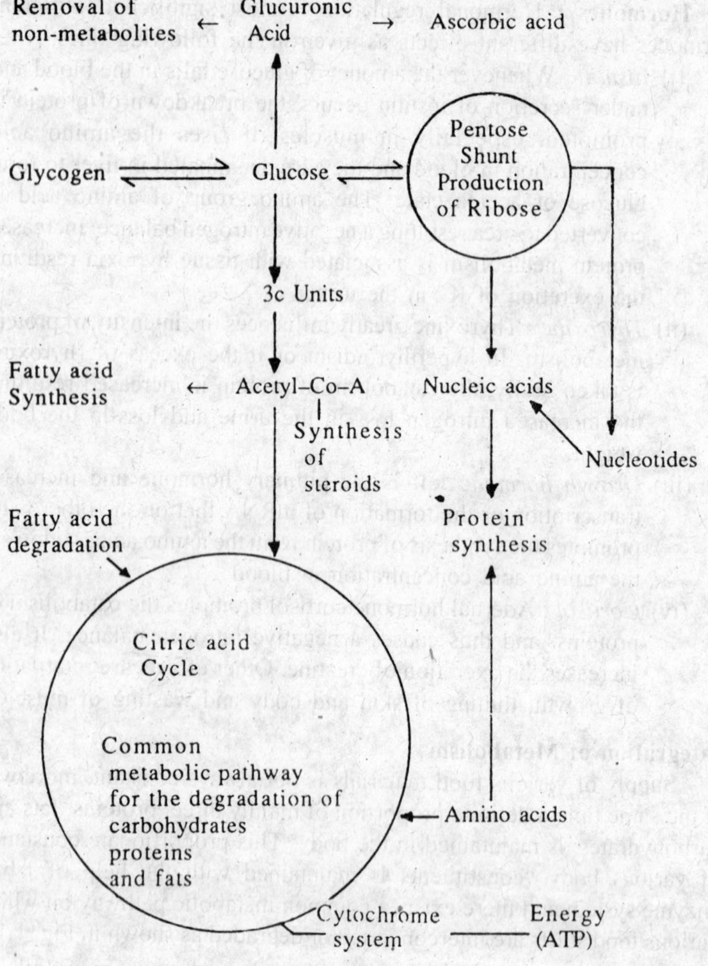

Fig. 1.11 : An outline of the interrelations of the major metabolic pathways.

Phase II : The second phase involves the conversion of various hydrolytic products to different compounds which are key intermediates of the common metabolic pathway.

The monosaccharides, particularly hexoses are convened into acetyl coenzyme A via pyruvic acid formation. During this process (glycolysis) some high energy phosphate bonds are also generated.

Similarly long chain fatty acids are oxidized to acetyl coenzyme A while glycerol is converted to pyruvate and acetyl coenzyme A by means of the glycolytic pathway.

Among different amino acids alanine, serine and cystenine are converted into pyruvate acid. Other amino acids like proline, histidine arginine are converted into glutamic acid which in turn, undergoes transamination to produce keto glutaric acid, a member of the TCA cycle. Aspartic acid is also transaminated to yield oxaloacetic acid, another intermediate of TCA cycle. Some amino acids like leucine yield acetyl coenzyme A on degradation. Similarly, phenylalanine and tyrosine on oxidative degradation produce acetyl coenzyme A and oxaloacetic acid through fumeric acid. To summarize, carbon skeletons of essentially all the amino acids yield either an intermediate of the TCA cycle (oxaloacetic acid or ketoglutaric acid) or acetyl coenzyme A which in turn, are oxidized on TCA cycle.

Phase III : During this phase various intermediate degradation products formed in phase II are oxidized on Kreb's tricarboxylic acid cycle. The hydrogen atoms and electrons removed undergo oxidative phosphorylation liberating energy that is captured and stored as ATP.

PHYSIOLOGY OF DIGESTION

The food on which the body lives, with the exception of small quantities of substances such as vitamins and minerals, can be classified as carbohydrates, fats, and proteins. However, these generally cannot be absorbed in their natural forms through the gastrointestinal mucosa and, for this reason, are useless as nutrients without the preliminary process of digestion. Digestion is a series of physical and chemical changes by which the complex and non-diffusible food is transformed into simple and diffusible forms with the help of enzymes. It is also known as the progressive enzymatic hydrolysis as the complex substances are broken down by the addition of water molecules in presence of specific enzyme during the process.

$$R - R + H_2O \xrightarrow[\text{enzyme}]{\text{digestive}} R - OH + H - R$$

All the digestive enzymes are proteins and show specificity in their action according to type of food.

Ingestion of Food

The amount of food that a person ingests is determined principally by the intrinsic desire for food called hunger. The type of food that a person preferentially seeks is determined by appetite. This mechanical aspects of food ingestion includes mastication and swallowing.

Mastication (Chewing)

The teeth are admirably designed for chewing, the anterior teeth (incisors) providing a strong action and the posterior teeth (molars) a grinding action. All the jaw muscles working together can close the teeth with a force as great as 55 pounds on the incisors and 200 pounds on the molars or it may increase in small object.

Most of muscles (abductor and adductor) of jaw are voluntary in their action and under the control of 5th cranial (trigeminal) nerve. During mastication the food is broken up by the teeth into small bits or pieces which is suitable for swallowing and increases surface for enzyme to act.

When food is chewed, it is mixed with saliva which convert the food into a semisolid mass.

Saliva : This is colourless viscous fluid having specific gravity 1.002 to 1.008 and pH of 6.8. It contains 99.5% water and a little *mucin* which helps to lubricate the food and makes the particles adhere to one another, saliva also contains a few salts including bicarbonates, and an enzyme *ptylin* (α-amylase). An adult may secrete from 1 to 1.5 litres of saliva per day.

Functions of Saliva

1. It keeps the mouth and teeth clean and acts as a lubricant for the mouth cavity.
2. It subserves the sense of taste by acting as a solvent.
3. Lubrication of food which facilitates swallowing of masticated food.
4. It acts as a buffering system due to presence of bicarbonate, phosphate and mucin.

5. It also contains an antibacterial substance Lysozyme, which control the bacterial population in mouth within limit.
6. The enzyme *ptylin* secreted mainly by parotid glands, hydrolyzes starch into the diasaccharide *maltose* and other small polymers of glucose containing 3 to 9 glucose molecules (such as maltotriose and α limit dextrins) that are the branch points of the starch molecule, but the food remains in the mouth only a short time and probably not more than 3 to 5% of all the starches that are eaten will have become hydrolyzed by the time the food is swallowed.

Nervous regulation of salivary secretion (Fig. 1.12) : Activity of the salivary glands to secrete saliva is controlled by the facial and *glassopharyngeal* nerves by the centres known as *salivary nuclei* located in brain at about the juncture of the medulla and pons. These nuclei are under the overall control, of the *appetite area* of cerebral cortex and are excited by when the person smells or eats favourite foods (especially sour taste). It is the nervous centres which evoke salivation of the mouth. Each salivary gland receives both sympathetic and parasympathetic fibres. Parasympathetic fibres generally stimulate secretion and digestion.

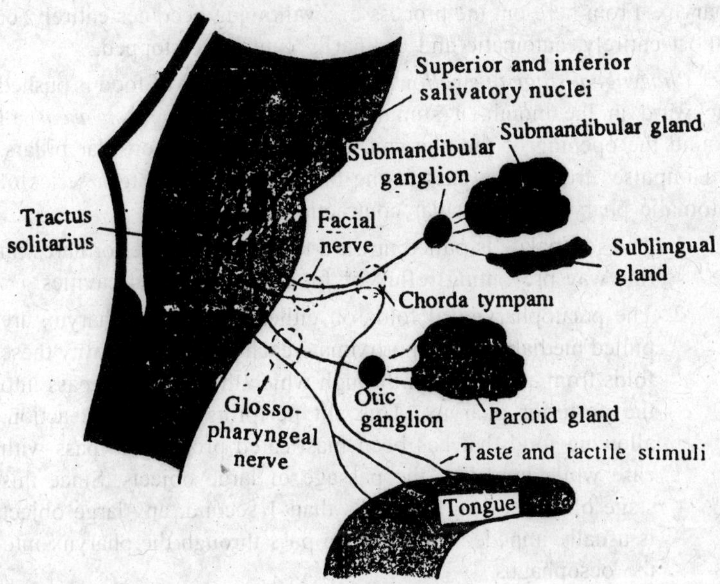

Fig. 1.12 : Nervous regulation of salivary secretion.

Swallowing (Deglutition)

The semifluid masticated food then passes down the oesophagus through the pharynx. Action of the tongue musculature rolls the food mass into bolus of convenient size which is then swallowed.

Swallowing is a complicated mechanism, principally because the pharynx most of the time subserves several other functions besides swallowing and is converted for only a few seconds at a time into a tract for propulsion of food. Especially it is important that respiration not be seriously compromised during swallowing.

In general, swallowing can be divided into–

1. the *voluntary stage*, which initiates the swallowing process,
2. the pharyngeal stage, which is involuntary and constitutes the passage of food through the pharynx into the oesophagus and
3. the *oesophageal stage*, another involuntary phase which-promotes passage of food from the pharynx to the stomach.

Voluntary stage of swallowing : When the food is ready for swallowing, it is voluntarily squeezed or rolled posteriorly in the mouth by pressure of the tongue upward and backward against the palate, as shown in Fig. 1.13. Thus, the tongue forces the bolus of food into the pharynx. From here on, the process of swallowing becomes entirely, or almost entirely, automatic and ordinarily cannot be stopped.

Pharyngeal stage of swallowing : When the bolus of food is pushed backward in the mouth, it stimulates *swallowing receptor areas* all around the opening of the pharynx, especially on the tonsillar pillars, and impulses from these pass to the brain stem to initiate a series of automatic pharyngeal muscular contractions as follows:

1. The soft palate is pulled upward to close the posterior nares, in this way preventing reflux of food into the nasal cavities.
2. The palatopharyngeal folds on either side of the pharynx are pulled medialward to approximate each other. In this way these folds from a sagittal slit through which the food must pass into the posterior pharynx. This slit performs a selective action, allowing food that has been masticated properly to pass with ease while impeding the passage of large objects. Since this stage of swallowing lasts less than 1 second, any large object is usually impeded too much to pass through the pharynx into the oesophagus.

3. The vocal cords of the larynx are strongly approximated, and the hyoid bone and larynx are pulled upward and anteriorly by the neck muscles, causing the epiglottis to swing backward over the superior opening of the larynx. Both these effects prevent passage of food into the trachea. Especially important is the approximation of the vocal cords, but the epiglottis helps to prevent food from ever getting as far as the vocal cords. Destruction of the vocal cords or of the muscles that approximate them can cause strangulation. On the other hand, removal of the epiglottis usually does not cause serious debility in swallowing.

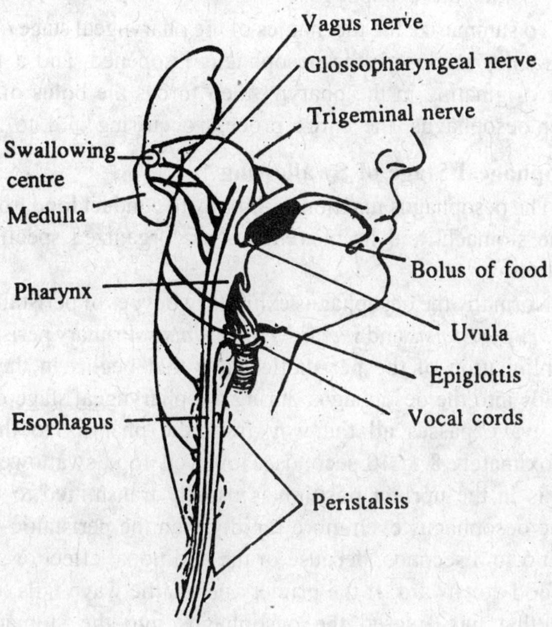

Fig. 1.13 : The swallowing mechanism.

4. The upward movement of the larynx also stretches the opening of the oesophagus. At the same time, the upper 3 to 4 centimetres of the oesophagus, an area called the *upper esophageal sphincter, the pharyngeoesophageal sphincter*, or the cricopharyngeal muscle, relaxes, thus allowing food to move easily and freely from the posterior pharynx into the upper oesophagus. This sphincter, between swallows, remains tonically and strongly contracted, thereby preventing air from going into the oesophagus

during respiration. The upward movement of the larynx also lifts the glottis out of the main stream of food flow so that the food usually passes on either side of the epiglottis rather than over its surface; this adds still another protection against passage of food into the trachea.

5. At the same time that the larynx is raised and the pharyngoesophageal sphincter is relaxed, the superior constrictor muscle of the pharynx contracts, giving rise to a rapid peristaltic wave passing downward over the middle and inferior pharyngeal muscles and into the oesophagus, which also propels the food into the oesophagus.

To summarize the mechanics of the pharyngeal stage of swallowing– the trachea is closed, the oesophagus is opened, and a fast peristaltic wave originating in the pharynx then forces the bolus of food into the upper oesophagus, the entire process occurring in 1 to 2 seconds.

Oesophageal Stage of Swallowing

The oesophagus functions primarily to conduct food from the pharynx to the stomach, and its movements are organized specifically for this function.

Normally the oesophagus exhibits two types of peristaltic movements *primary peristalsis* and *secondary peristalsis*. Primary peristalsis is simply a continuation of the peristaltic wave that begins in the pharynx and spreads into the oesophagus during the pharyngeal stage of swallowing. This wave passes all the way from the pharynx to the stomach in approximately 8 to 10 seconds. However, food swallowed by a person who is in the upright position is usually transmitted to the lower end of the oesophagus even more rapidly than the peristaltic wave itself, in about 5 to 8 seconds, because of the additional effect of gravity pulling the food downward. If the primary peristaltic wave fails to move all the food that has entered the oesophagus into the stomach, secondary peristaltic waves, generated by the enteric nervous system of the oesophagus, result from distension of the oesophagus by the retained food. These waves are essentially the same as the primary peristaltic waves, except that they originate in the oesophagus itself rather than in the pharynx. Secondary peristaltic waves continue to be initiated until all the food has emptied into the stomach.

Nervous Control of Deglutition

The successive stages of the swallowing process are reflexly controlled by neuronal areas in the medulla and the pons. These areas are collectively called the deglutition or swallowing centre. Impulses generated by the presence of food at the pharyngeal opening are transmitted to the swallowing centre by the trigeminal and glosso-pharyngeal nerves. Motor impulses originating from the swallowing centre reach the pharynx and upper oesophagus through the 5th, 9th, 11th and 12th cranial and a few of the cervical nerves, and cause swallowing.

The peristaltic waves of the oesophagus are controlled almost totally by vagal reflexes that are part of the overall swallowing mechanism. These vagal afferent fibres from the oesophagus to the medulla and then back again to the oesophagus through vagal *efferent fibres*.

Digestion in the Stomach

As swallowing occurs, the stomach relaxes reflexly to make room for the food. Here food undergoes further mechanical disintegration and chemical changes primarily in the protein constituents.

Stomach is a muscular bag and physiologically divided into two major parts:

1. the *corpus,* or *body* and
2. the *antrum*

Stomach has three motor functions:

1. Storage of large quantities of food until it can be accommodated in the lower portion of the gastrointestinal tract,
2. Mixing of this food with gastric secretions until it forms a semifluid mixture called chyme and
3. Slow emptying of the food from the stomach into the small intestine at a rate suitable for proper digestion and absorption by the small intestine.

1. *Storage function* : Stomach wall is highly distensible due to presence of smooth muscles. As food enters the stomach, it forms concentric circles of the body and fundus of the stomach, the newest food lying closest to the oesophageal opening and the oldest food lying nearest the wall of the stomach. Normally, when food enters the stomach, a vagal reflex greatly reduces the tone in the muscular wall of the body of the stomach so that the wall can bulge progressively outward, accommodating greater and greater quantities of food up to a limit of about 1 litre. The pressure in the stomach remains low until this limit is approached.

2. *Mixing function* : The digestive juices of the stomach are secreted by the *gastric glands*, which cover almost the entire outer wall of the body of the stomach. These secretions come immediately into contact with that portion of the stored food lying against the muscosal surface of the stomach; when the stomach is filled, weak peristaltic *constrictor waves*, also called mixing waves, move toward the antrum along the stomach wall approximately once every 20 seconds. As the waves move down the stomach, they not only cause the secretions to mix with stored food but also provide weak propulsion to move these mixed contents into the antrum.

As the constrictor waves progress from the body of the stomach to antrum, they become more intense, some becoming extremely intense and providing powerful *peristaltic constrictor rings* that force the antral contents under high pressure towards the pylorus.

Chyme : After the food has become mixed with the stomach secretions, the resulting mixture that passes on down the gut is called chyme. The degree of fluidity of chyme depends on the relative amounts of food and stomach secretions and on the degree of digestion that has occurred. The appearance of chyme is that of a murky, milky semifluid or paste.

Emptying of the stomach : Basically, stomach emptying is opposed by resistance of the pylorus to the passage of food, and it is promoted by peristaltic waves in the antrum of the stomach. The pyloric antrum and pylorus can be together regarded as a pyloric or gastroduodenal pump" which moves fluid from the stomach to the duodenum. During emptying pyloric sphincter is more or less relaxed. It allows several millilitres of the suitably liquified chyme to spurt into the duodenum when the antrum contracts and then closes only on the peristaltic wave passes over it. The hormone *gastrin* from antral mucosa also enhances the activity of the pyloric pump, relaxes the pylorus and thus has a strong promoting effect on stomach emptying.

Process of Digestion in Stomach

The gastric mucosa consists of a simple branched tubular glands packed tightly together and arranged perpendicularly to the surface. Groups of glands, open into *gastric pits*, which in turn open on to those mucosal surface. Functionally glands can be distinguished into those producing mucus (cardiac and pyloric glands and those secreting digestive fluids (gastric glands).

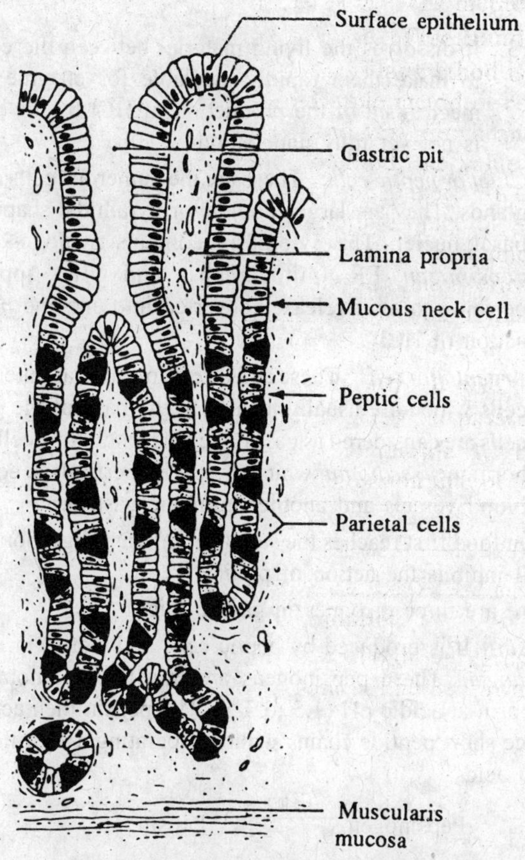

Fig. 1.14 : Showing gastric gland in stomach mucosa.

Mucus secreted by cardiac and pyloric gland provides lubrication for the back and forth movement of the chyme during digestion.

The gastric gland proper contains four types of cells:

1. *Mucus cells* : as above.
2. *Parietal cells or oxyntic cells* : are the main source of hydrochloric acid, having a pH of approximately 2.0. The ions exists as H^+ and Cl^- in the gastric juice. HCl has following functions:
   1. It kills the detrimental bacteria which have been taken in along with food.
   2. It provides favourable medium in which the enzymes of gastric juice can do their work rapidly.

3. It dissolves the living material between the cells in order to make them rapidly available for enzyme action. The mechanism of the production of HCl by the parietal cells is not yet fully understood.

3. *Chief or peptic cells :* These are the numerous cells of the gastric glands. They are large cuboidal or pyramidal shaped cells with basal nuclei. The cytoplasm contains zymogen granules of *pepsinogen*, ER., mitochondria and golgi apparatus. The pepsinogen after release converted into enzyme *pepsin* by the action of HCl

4. *Argentaffin cells :* These cells are also called as enterochromaffin cells which are usually located at the base of the gland. These cells are considered as gastrointestinal endocrine cells and secrete hormone *serotonin* which helps in peristalsis contraction of blood vessels and another hormone gastrin.

When food first reaches the stomach, salivary digestion is continued until HCl inhibits the action of ptylin.

There are three enzymes in gastric juice.

Pepsin : It is produced by peptic cells and stored in inactive state as *pepsinogen.* These pepsinogens are transferred automatically into active pepsin at acidic pH (1.5 to 3.5). The pepsin then acts on protein to produce short peptide chains without liberating a significant quantity of amino acids.

$$\text{Pepsinogen} \xrightarrow[\text{pH } 1.5\,-\,3.5]{\text{HCl}} \text{Pepsin}$$

Proteins + pepsin → proteoses, peptons and polypeptides

Renin : It is also known as *rennet* or *chymosin*, possessed by infants that curdles milk. It is found in the inactive form prorenin which on coming in contact with HCl is converted into active renin. Its optimum pH of action ranging from 5 to 6. It acts upon the milk proteins casein (soluble) and converts into its insoluble form *calcium paracaseinate* (curd) in the presence of calcium. This is called that the milk has curdles. This curdles are then accessible to pepsin for digestion.

$$\underset{\text{(Inactive)}}{\text{Pro-renin}} \xrightarrow[\text{pH } 5-6]{\text{HCl}} \underset{\text{(Active.)}}{\text{Renin}}$$

$$\text{Renin + Casein} \xrightarrow{\text{Calcium}} \text{calcium-paracaseinate (curd)}$$

$$\text{Curdles} \xrightarrow{\text{Pepsin}} \text{Proteoses, peptones, polypeptides}$$

The curdling of milk in the stomach is important in digestion, because in curdle form the milk remains in stomach for a longer period of time than uncurdled milk would. This gives the gastric enzymes a longer time to act on milk.

Gastric lipase : The gastric secretion also contains a fat hydrolyzing enzyme known as gastric lipase. The amount of fat hydrolysed in the stomach is small, and only fats which are in an emulsified form are attacked. A good example of such a fat is that form in milk. Fats do not emulsify well in an acidic medium; hence emulsification does not take place to any great extent in the stomach. Gastric lipase is most active at pH 5 – 0.

Evacuation of stomach : As gastric digestion proceeds, the food become more or less liquified and in the form-of acidic paste called *chyme*. It is the end product of gastric digestion. Now the stomach wall begins to contract, producing a peristaltic wave which moves towards the pyloric opening into the intestine. As digestion proceeds; these peristaltic waves become more powerful, and more liquid chyme is forced into the intestine. Finally, all the food is liquified, and all the chyme is forced into the intestine jet by jet slowly.

Control of gastric secretion : The digestive events occurring in the stomach are controlled by an interplay of both nervous and hormonal mechanisms. These events may be distinguished into three phases:

1. *Cephalic phase :* This is entirely nervous and starts before the food enters the stomach and results due to the appetite generating signals perceived through smell, sight, taste or even thought of food. The appropriate motor signals originate in the brain and are transmitted through the vagus nerve to the wall of the stomach. Under vagal influences there is secretion of acid, mucus, and enzymes in the stomach. Vagal stimulation also elicits the release of gastrin.
2. *Gastric phase :* Presence of food in the stomach triggers this phase during which over two-thirds of the total gastric secretions are produced. The initial response is activation of the gastrin mechanism which cause a sustained release of gastric juice that continues throughout the period during which the food remains in the stomach. Furthermore, the presence of food in the stomach also stimulates the vagal reflex arc and the myenteric plexus, resulting in parasympathetic stimulation of the gastric glands. Gastric phase has thus both, nervous and hormonal components.

3. *Intestinal phase :* Distention of particularly the duodenum due to presence of food also causes the stomach to produce small quantities of gastric juice. This probably occur due to the release of gastrin from the duodenal mucosa. Finally, as the stomach is being drained of the acidified food into the duodenum, the latter secretes yet another hormone enterogastrone which inhibits the gastric secretions, thus, "switching off" the stomach. Intestinal phase is thus predominantly hormonal in nature.

DIGESTION IN INTESTINE

The small intestine is divided into three parts. The first part is the *duodenum* into which open the ducts from liver and pancreas, this is followed by *jejunum* which is particularly rich in intestinal glands ; and this is followed by the *ileum* characterised by the vast number of villi which increase the absorptive surface area of the intestine.

The small intestine, into which the *chyme* passes by the force of the peristaltic waves in the stomach, is the part where greater part of enzymatic digestion and almost all absorption occur here. Once the food enters the intestine from the stomach, it remains there for a considerable time. In man, depending upon the type of food, it may stay there from 12 to 24 hours. The food in small intestine is more or less constantly in motion. The purpose of this movement is to mix and churn the intestinal contents or *chyle* and propel it towards the large intestine.

Movements of the small intestine : The movements of the small intestine, is elsewhere in the gastrointestinal tract, can be divided into the *mixing contractions* and the *propulsive contractions*. However, to a great extent this separation is artificial because essentially all movements of the small intestine cause at least some degree of both mixing and propulsion. Yet, the usual classification of these processes is the following :

Mixing Contractions (Segmentation Contractions)

When a portion of the small intestine becomes distended with chyme, the stretch of the intestinal wall elicits localized concentric contractions spaced at intervals along the intestine. The longitudinal length of each one of the contractions is only about 1 cm so that each set of contraction causes "segmentation " of the small intestine, as illustrated in Fig. 1.15 dividing the intestine into spaced segments that have the appearance of a chain of sausages. As one set of segmentation contractions relaxes a new set begins, but the contractions this lime occur at new points between the previous contractions.

These segmentation contractions "chop" the chyme as often as 8 to 12 times a minute, in this way promoting progressive mixing of the solid food particles with the secretions of the small intestine.

The maximum frequency of the segmentation contractions in the small intestine is determined by the frequency of the *slow waves* in the intestinal wall, which is the basic electrical rhythm (BER). Since this frequency is about 12 per minute in the duodenum, the maximum frequency of the segmentation contractions in the duodenum is also about 12 per minute. However, in the ileum, the maximum frequency is usually 8 to 9 contractions per minute.

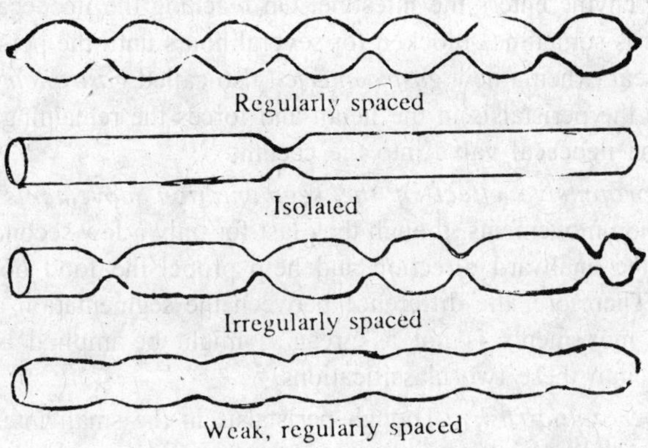

Fig. 1.15 : Segmentation movements of the small intestine.

PROPULSIVE MOVEMENTS

Peristalsis in the small intestine : Chyme is propelled through the small intestine by peristaltic waves. These can occur in any part of the small intestine, and they move analward at the velocity of 0.5 to 2 cm per second, much faster in the proximal intestine and much slower in the terminal intestine. However, they are normally very weak and usually die out after travelling less than 10 cm, so that movement of the chyme is also very poor, so poor in fact that the net movement of the chyme along the small intestine averages only 1 cm per minute. This means that normally 3 to 5 hours are required for passage of chyme from the pylorus to the ileocecal valve.

Peristaltic activity of the small intestine is greatly increased after a meal. This is caused partly by the beginning entry of chyme into the duodenum but also, by the so-called *gastroenteric reflex* that is initiated by distension of the stomach and conducted principally through the myenteric plexus from the stomach down along the wall of the small intestine. This reflex increases the overall degree of excitability of the small intestine, including both increased motility and secretion.

The function of the peristaltic waves in the small intestine is not only to cause progression of the chyme toward the ileocecal valve but also to spread out the chyme along the intestinal mucosa. As the chyme enters the intestine from the stomach and causes initial distension of the proximal intestine, the elicited peristaltic waves begin immediately to spread the chyme along the intestine, and this process intensifies as additional chyme enters the intestine. On reaching the ileocecal valve the chyme is sometimes blocked for several hours until the person eats another meal, when a new *gastroenteric* (also called *gastroileal*) reflex intensifies the peristalsis in the ileum and forces the remaining chyme through the ileocecal valve into the cecum.

The propulsive effect of the segmentation movements : The segmentation movements, though they last for only a few seconds, also travel in the analward direction and help propel the food down the intestine. Therefore, the difference between the segmentation and the peristaltic movements is not as great as might be implied by their separation into these two classifications.

The peristaltic rush : Though peristalsis in the small intestine is normally very weak, intense irritation of the intestinal mucosa, as occurs in some severe causes of infectious diarrhoea, can cause both very powerful and rapid peristalsis called the *peristaltic rush.* This is initiated mainly by extrinsic nervous reflexes to the brain stem and back again to the gut. The powerful peristaltic contractions then travel long distances in the small intestine within minutes, sweeping the contents of the intestine into the-colon and thereby relieving the small intestine of either irritative chyme or excessive distention.

For digestion, the most important part of the small intestine is the *duodenum.* Three juices enter the intestine in the duodenum. They are the *intestinal juice*, secreted by the duodenal wall itself ; the pancreatic juice, the external secretion of the pancreas ; and the bile, which comes from liver. All are alkaline in reaction and play an important role in complete digestion.

Digestive role of the liver : One of the important function of liver is secretion of bile (choleresis) which is stored in contractile gall bladder. Bile is viscous, greenish yellow, bitter and alkaline fluid. In man bile is secreted at a rate of about 1000 ml/day. Table 1.6 shows composition of liverbile and gallbladder bile. During digestion the gall bladder rapidly pumps (*Cholecystokinesis*) bile into the duodenum where it mixes with the pancreatin secretion. Bile does not contain any enzymes.

The liver cells produce bile salts, their precursor cholesterol is converted mainly into *cholic* and some *deoxycholic*, *chenodeoxycholic* and *lithocholic acids*. These bile acids are conjugated to glycine or taurine. In this form the bile acids are water soluble. They enter bile as ionised salts of sodium *e.g., sodium glycocholate* and *taurocholate*.

The bile pigments are *bilirubin* and *bitiverdin*. These are formed by the decomposition of haemoglobin. These are excretory products and are expelled out along with undigested food.

Bile which is alkaline in nature, helps to neutralise the chyme. Bile salts have two major actions. The first is related to their considerable ability to affect the surface tension of water and lipids. The polar part of bile salt is highly soluble in water and its sterol half part in fat. Consequently the bile salts aggregate at the surface of the fat droplets. This decreases the surface tension of the fat so that with the mixing action of the gut wall, small fat globules are produced (emulsification). The lipases which are also water-soluble can now brings about their lipolytic action.

Bile salts also facilitate the absorption of fatty acids, glycerols, cholesterol, and other lipids including the fat soluble vitamins, over the intestinal mucosa.

Table 1.6 : Concentration of the constituents of hepatic and gallbladder bile (mmol/1).

Compound	Liver bile	Gall-bladder bile
Bile salts	26	145
Bilirubin	0.7	5.1
Cholesterol	2.6	16
Fatty acids	3.6	29
Lecithin	0.5	3.9
Na^+	145	130
K^+	5	12
Ca^{2+}	5	23
Cl	100	25
HCO_3	28	10

Regulation of bile Secretion

Liver and gall bladder functions are controlled by certain gastrointestinal hormones.

Cholecystokinin : is a powerful agent that induces rhythmic contractions and emptying of the gall bladder. Now this hormone is known to be biochemically identical with pancreozymin and the polypeptide is now known as *cholecystokinin-pancreozymin (CCk-PZ)*. This also stimulates release of the pancreatic hormones insulin and glucagon.

Recently it has been suggested that *Hepatocrinin*, secreted by the duodenal mucosa stimulates the liver, leading to the production of dilute bile. A minor vagal effect also exists.

Digestion by pancreatic juice : Digestive secretions of the pancrease are formed in its exocrine (acinar) tissue and brought to the duodenum via pancreatic duct. Pancreatic juice is nonviscous fluid with pH 7.5-8.0 or higher. This alkalinity is due to presence of bicarbonates and this property serves to neutralize the acidity of chyme.

About 70 per cent of the pancreatic secretions are proteolytic (protein splitting) enzymes. These include both *endopeptidases* (trypsin, chymotrypsin and clastases) and *exopeptidases* (carboxypeptidases A and B). All are secreted in an inactive form (trypsinogen, chymotrypsinogen, proelastase and procarboxypeptidases).

In the intestine the enzyme *enterokinase* of intestinal juice converts some trypsinogen to trypsin, the active enzyme. This trypsin then activates autocatalytically remainder of trypsinogen and all of the other proteolytic zymogens.

$$\text{Trypsinogen} \xrightarrow{\text{enterokinase}} \text{Trypsin}$$

$$\text{Proteins, peptones and proteoses + trypsin} \xrightarrow{\text{7.8 pH}} \text{amino acids}$$

Chymotrypsin : About a series of four pancreatic *chymotrypsins* are known which are secreted in their inactive form *chymotrypsinogen*. The chymotrypsinogen becomes active in alkaline medium (pH 7 to 8) in the presence of trypsin.

$$\text{Chymotrypsinogen + Trypsin} \xrightarrow{\text{pH 7 to 8}} \text{Chymotrypsin}$$

Proteins, peptones and proteoses + Chymotrypsin → Polypeptids, amino acids

Carboxypeptidases : They are found in pancreatic juice in inactive form procarboxypeptidase. There are two viz., Carboxypeptidases A and B, both contain zinc atom per molecule.

$$\text{Procarboxypeptidases} \xrightarrow{\text{tryp sin}} \text{carboxypeptidase}$$

$$\text{Polypeptides} \xrightarrow[\text{pH 5.0}]{\text{carboxypeptidase}} \text{Lower polypeptides, free amino acids}$$

Pancreopeptidase E or Elastase : This enzyme hydrolyses fibrous protein elastin.

Amylase or amylopsin : This is the carbohydrate digesting enzyme. It is maximally active in the pH range 6.2 to 7.2. It converts starch, dextrin and glycogen into maltose. For amylase, chloride and phosphate act as co-enzymes.

$$\text{Starch, Dextrin, Glycogen} \xrightarrow[\text{pH 6.2 - 7.2}]{\text{amylase}} \text{Maltose}$$

Lactase, sucrase and maltase have also been reported in pancreatic juice in small quantities hydrolysing lactose, sucrose and maltose respectively.

$$\text{Lactose} \xrightarrow{\text{lactase}} \text{Glucose + Galactose}$$

$$\text{Sucrose} \xrightarrow{\text{sucrase}} \text{Glucose + Fructose}$$

$$\text{Maltose} \xrightarrow{\text{maltase}} \text{Glucose}$$

Lipase or steapsin : It is the fat splitting enzyme of pancreatic juice. It is secreted in the active form. It splits dietary fats and oils into glycerol, fatty acids, monoglycerides, and diglycerides. Its action is highly promoted by bile salts, soaps, calcium salts and certain peptides. It shows maximum activity at a pH 7 to 8.

$$\text{Fats and oils} \xrightarrow[\text{Ca}^{++}\text{, bilesalts}]{\text{steap sin}} \text{Fatty acids, glycerol, glycerides}$$

pH 7-8

Pancreatic juice has also been shown to contain two more lipolytic enzymes in addition to lipase. They are:

(a) *Phospholipase :* Also known as *lecithinase*. It removes two fatty acids from phospholipids.

(b) *Cholesterol-esterase :* It catalyses the conversion of free cholesterol into cholesterol-esters in the presence of fatty acids.

Nucleolytic enzyme : Pancreatic juice also contains two enzymes hydrolyzing nucleic acids (RNA and DNA):

(a) *Ribonuclease or RNase :* It degrade RNA into simple nucleotides.

(b) *Deoxyribonuclease or dornase or DNAase :* It dissociates DNA into simple nucleotides.

Regulation of pancreatic secretion : Pancreatic secretion, is regulated by both nerves and hormonal mechanisms but hormonal regulation is by far the more important.

Nervous Regulation

When the cephalic and gastric phases of stomach secretion occur, parasympathetic impulses are simultaneously transmitted along the vagus nerves to the pancrease, resulting in acetylcholine release followed by secretion of moderate to large amounts of enzymes into the pancreatic acini.

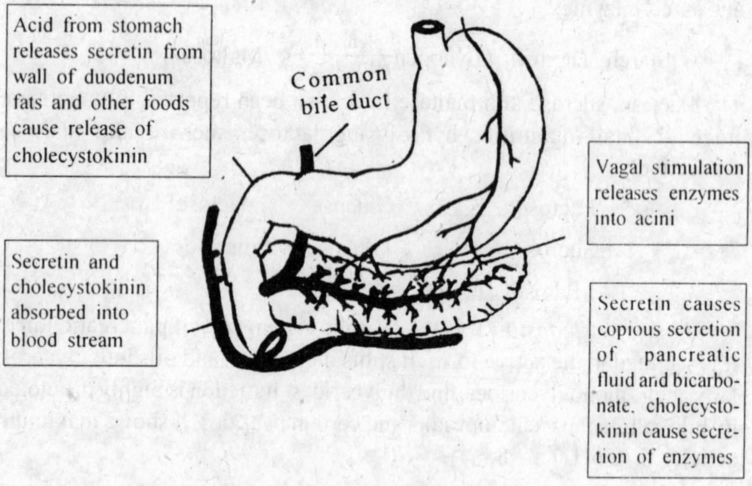

Fig. 1.16 : Regulation of pancreatic secretion.

Hormonal Regulation

After chyme enters the small intestine, "pancreatic secretion becomes copious, mainly in response to hormone *secretin*. In addition, a second hormone, *cholecystokinin*, causes still far more increase in the secretion of enzymes.

Secretin is released by the duodenal mucosa under the stimulus of acidic pH, fat or bile. It acts directly upon the acinar cells of the pancrease causing a copious flow of watery and alkaline with high concentration of bicarbonate ions but enzyme-deficient pancreatic juice.

Cholecystokinin is a powerful hormone secreted by upper small intestinal mucosa. In presence of partially digested products of protein-proteoses and peptones, mucosa secrete cholecystokinin, which passes by way of the blood to pancrease, and induce acinar cells to secrete large quantities of digestive enzymes.

Recently, it has been suggested that hormone *chymodenin*, secreted by duodenal wall which can selectively elicit rapid secretion of *chymotrypsinogen.*

Digestion by Intestinal Juice (Succus entericus)

Two distinct types of glands are found in the small intestine:

1. the *Brunner's* gland found only in the submucosae of the duodenum, produce an alkaline secretion containing mucous but no enzymes.
2. the *intestinal glands* or *crypts of Lieberkuhn*, present throughout the small intestine, these are simple tubular glands which open into the spaces between neighbouring villi. Intestinal glands secrete large number of enzymes which act upon all sort of food material. These enzymes are called *succus entericus*. It is clear yellow fluid secreted about 2 to 3 litres/day. It has a pH of 7.6, *i.e.,* slightly alkaline and contains 98.5% water, and 1.5% solid matters, mucus, and enzymes that complete the digestion of carbohydrates, proteins and fats.

Enzymatic Activities

Intestinal juice consists of group of enzyme peptidases collectively called *erepsin* which hydrolyze various peptides to amino acids. They do not act on native proteins but only complete the digestion started-by other proteolytic enzyme. Additionally, intestinal juice also contains traces of maltase and lipase.

Two peptidases are found associated with succus entericus:

(a) *Amino polypeptidase :* It hydrolyses polypeptides to amino acids at pH about 8.0. The repeated action of aminopolypeptidase results the formation of dipeptide, tripeptide and free amino acids. Some of the peptidases are activated by Mg^{++}, Co^{++}, Mn^{++} and Zn^{++} ions.

(b) *Dipeptidase and tripeptidases :* They hydrolyze dipeptides and tripeptidases, upto the stage of amino acids. Co^{++} ions activate the dipeptidase. Dipeptidase has a pH optimum of 7.6.

$$\text{Polypeptides} \xrightarrow[\text{pH 7.5 to 8.5}]{\text{amino polypeptidase}} \text{Tripeptides}$$

$$\text{Tripeptides} \xrightarrow[\text{pH 7.5 to 8.5}]{\text{tripeptidase}} \text{Dipeptides}$$

$$\text{Dipeptides} \xrightarrow[\text{pH 7.5 to 8.5}]{\text{dipeptidase}} \text{Amino acids}$$

Enterokinase : It is an enzyme secreted by crypts of Leiberkuhn is also present in intestinal juice. It activates pancreatic trypsinogen into active trypsin at optimum pH of 7.5.

Carbohydrases : They include disaccharide - splitting enzymes (sucrase, maltase, and lactase). They can completely hydrolyse the carbohydrates.

Sucrase or invertase : This enzyme breaks sucrose (cane sugar) into a molecule of glucose and a molecule of fructose. It shows maximum, activity at a pH of 5.0 to 7.0.

$$\text{Sucrose} \xrightarrow[\text{pH 5 to 7}]{\text{sucrase}} \text{Glucose + Fructose}$$

Maltase : Maltose is derived from the partial hydrolysis of starch by amylase of saliva and of pancreatic juice. Maltase splits maltose into two molecules of glucose. Its optimum pH varies from 6.7 to 7.2.

$$\text{Maltose} \xrightarrow[\text{pH 6.7 to 7.2}]{\text{maltase}} \text{Glucose (2)}$$

Lactase : Lactose is found in milk. Lactase digests lactose into a molecule of glucose and a molecule of galactose. It acts best at pH 5.4 to 6.0.

$$\text{Lactose} \xrightarrow[\text{pH 5.4 to 6.0}]{\text{lactase}} \text{Glucose + Galactose}$$

Nucleolytic enzymes : Three enzymes responsible for the hydrolysis of nucleic acid are present in the intestinal juice. They are:

1. *Polynucleotidase* : These enzymes hydrolyze nucleic acids into nucleotides or mononucleotides.

   $$\text{Nucleic acid} \xrightarrow{\text{polynucleotidase}} \text{Nucleotides}$$

2. *Phosphatases* : These break the nucleotide into nucleoside and phosphoric acid or in other words they remove phosphoric acid from nucleotide,

   $$\text{Nucleotide} \xrightarrow{\text{phosphatase}} \text{Nuclcoside + Phosphoric acid}$$

3. *Nucleosidases* : These enzymes hydrolyses nucleosides into free nitrogenous bases and pentose sugar.

Nucleoside $\xrightarrow{\text{nucleosidase}}$ Nitrogenous bases + pentose sugar

In short, result of digestion is formation of diffusible products like *monosaccharides* (glucose), the amino acids, and the fatty acids, glycerides and glycerols from dietary foodstuffs.

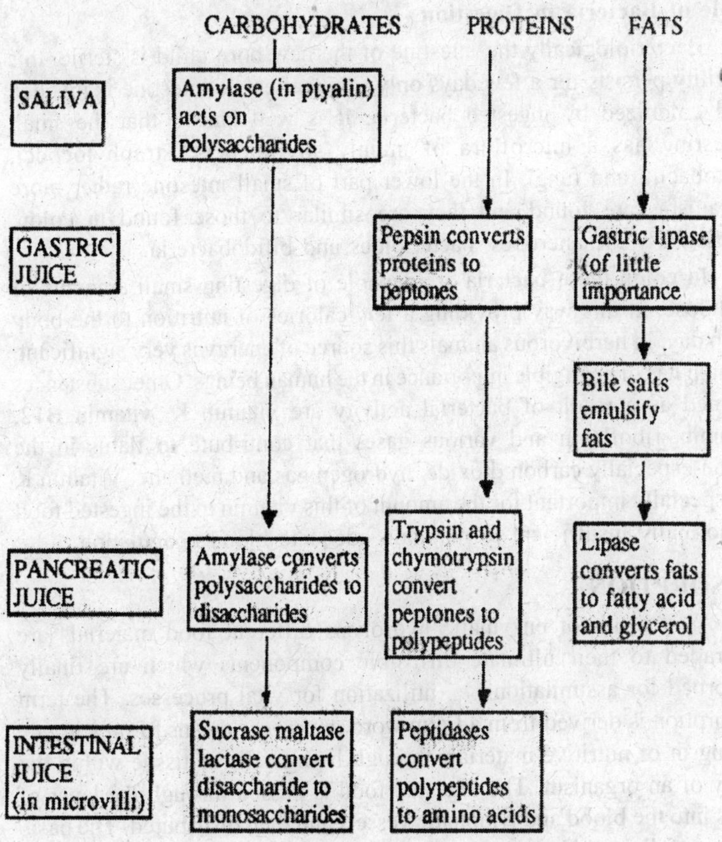

Fig. 1.17 : Summary of digestive enzymes.

Regulation of Small Intrestinal Secretion

Local stimuli : By far the most important means for regulating small intestinal secretion are various local nervous reflexes, especially reflexes initiated by tactile or irritative stimuli. Therefore for the most part, secretion in the small intestine occur simply in response to the presence of chyme in the intestine-the greater the amount of chyme, the greater the secretion.

Hormonal regulation : Some of the same hormones that promote secretion elsewhere in the gastrointestinal tract also increases small intestinal secretion, especially secretin and chotecystokinin.

Role of Bacteria in Digestion

Bacteriologically the intestine of the new born child is sterile, this sterility persists for a few days only ; thereafter the intestine is invaded and colonized by ingested bacteria. It is well known that the small intestine has a microflora of mainly streptococci, straphylococci, lactobacilli and fungi. In the lower part of small intestine rather more organisms are found and they are similar to those found in colon, particularly the anerobes, bacterioides and bifidobacteria.

In colon these bacteria are capable of digesting small amounts of cellulose, in this way providing a few calories of nutrition to the body each day. In herbivorous animals this source of energy is very significant, though it is of negligible importance in the human beings. Other substances formed as a result of bacterial activity are vitamin K, vitamin B12, thiamin, riboflavin and various gases that contribute to flatus in the colon-especially carbon dioxide, hydrogen gas and methane. Vitamin K is especially important for the amount of this vitamin in the ingested food is normally insufficient to maintain adequate blood coagulation.

ABSORPTION

As a result of enzymatic hydrolysis different food materials are degraded to their ultimate diffusible components which are finally absorbed for assimilation *i.e.,* utilization for vital processes. The term absorption is derived from a Latin word *absorbere* means to *suck* in *i.e.,* taking in of nutritive materials through living cells or tissue within the body of an organism. The digested food is passed through the layer of cells into the blood and lymphatic vessels and then distributed. The basic process followed in absorption is diffusion but it has been observed that diffusion and osmotic laws are not followed very strictly as the hexose sugar diffuses more rapidly than the pentose sugar in the body. Therefore, the differential absorption is taking place.

The process of absorption is mainly confined to the small intestine. No absorption takes place in mouth and oesophagus. To a limited extent absorption of water, alcohol, simple salts, glucose and chlorides, takes place in stomach. Small intestine is well adopted for absorption. The mucosal layer of intestine has undergone a marked surface enlargement. In mammals there is a three-fold increase in the surface area due to the formation of mucosal folds. Again, on each fold densely spaced 1 mm long villi cause a further ten fold increase (Total 30 fold increases). Finally, the lumenal sides of the epithelial cells are covered with microvilli about one micron long (In man each epithelial cell has 1000 microvilli). This situation still increases the total area of absorbing surface at least 20-30 times. Thus the surface area of small intestine increase about 600 times. In the human small intestine the total mucosal surface has been estimated at about 75,000 sq. cm. In human being the length of small intestine is about 25 feet long. About 5 million villi has been estimated. Each villus contains an arteriole and a venule with their communicating capillary plexus and also a blind ending lymphatic vessel or lacteal. The veins ultimately open into the portal vein going to the liver, about 1.4 litres of blood flows through this vein per minute, during the digestion of a meal this amount increases by one third.

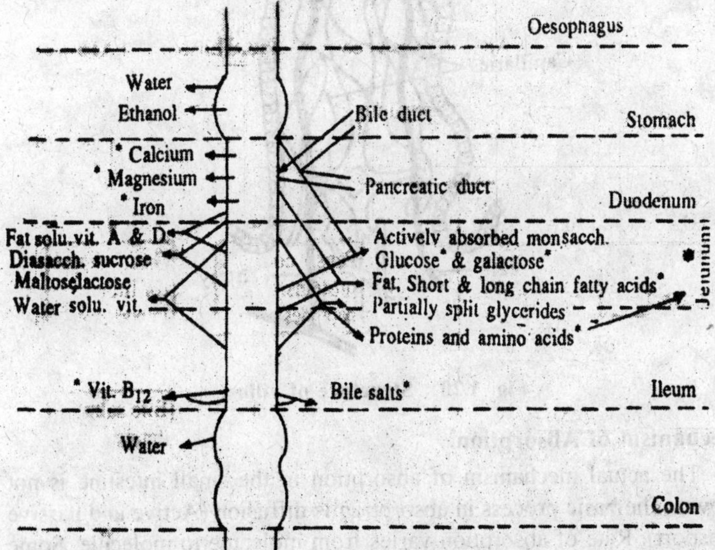

Fig. 1.18 : Known sites of absorption in the alimentary canal.
*** Indicates substances known to be actively transported.**

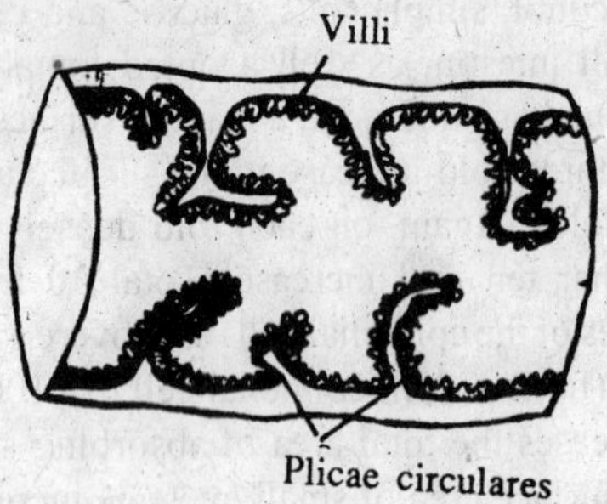

Fig. 1.19 : Section of small intestine illustrating mucosal folds and villi.

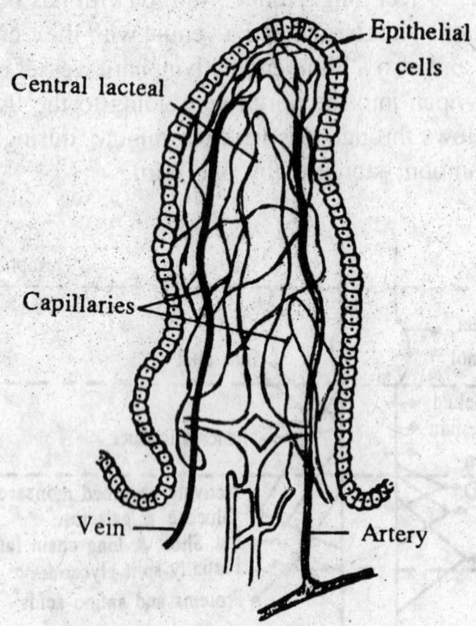

Fig. 1.20 : Structure of villus.

Mechanism of Absorption

The actual mechanism of absorption in the small intestine is not known. The basic process in absorption is diffusion (Active and passive transport). Rate of absorption varies from molecule to molecule. Some molecules like fructose, glucose and galactose are the same in their size and chemical composition but are absorbed at different rates. This is the differential absorption. There are some evidence that white blood cells pass through the intestinal wall, become loaded with food and .carry it back into the blood and lymph and thus help in absorption. It has also been reported that during digestion and absorption, the villi contract fairly quickly at irregular intervals and relax slowly. The contraction probably helps to pump lymph into the lacteal of the submucosa.

Carbohydrate Absorption

Carbohydrates are broken down and absorbed in the form of monosaccharides. Various kinds of monosaccharides are absorbed at different rates. The rate of absorption of the different sugars has been found in the following decreasing order: galactose, glucose, fructose, mannose, xylose and arabinose. The pentoses (ribose, deoxyribose) have smaller molecules and therefore diffused more rapidly than hexoses. The mucosal cells are also capable of absorbing diasaccharides as such when these are present in excess, however, the extent of such an absorption is very small. Most of the dietary disaccharides which are absorbed in the intact form are hydrolysed within the mucosal cells into their constituent monosaccharides, and subsequently carried further. Undigested disaccharides may serve as food for intestinal organisms in large intestine.

Some of the monosaccharides are absorbed by the passive transport. In this process the concentration of mono-saccharides is more in the intestine than that of blood capillaries, hence, the molecule diffuses passively from lumen of the intestine to the blood. In this process energy is not required.

Monosaccharides are also absorbed by the active transport. The absorption depends on the presence of Na^+. During transport the sugar combines with a mobile carrier to form the sugar-carrier complex that brings the sugar across the lipid barrier of the cell membrane and release the sugar inside the cell. Carrier needs energy. Na^+ affects the supply of energy from ATP probably by activating ATPase in the cell membrane.

It is believed that during absorption the sugars combine with phosphoric acid to form hexose phosphate. Before entering the blood stream the hexose phosphates are apparently hydrolysed, since hexose are found in the blood rather than hexose phosphates.

The rate of absorption of sugar is influenced by the amount of anterior thyroxine, ant pituitary hormone, vitamin B complex and the state of mucous membrane and the time for which the carbohydrate remains in contact with it.

Protein Absorption

Proteins are broken down into amino acids by the action of *proteases*. Amino acids are absorbed into the intestinal capillaries and these enter the portal vein, to be carried into the general circulation by way of the liver. The amino acids are absorbed at different rate of speed depending upon the molecular weight. The glycine is absorbed more rapidly followed by alanine, cystine, glutamic acid, valine and so on. The d-amino acids are absorbed passively but the L-forms are absorbed actively. The transport system of amino acids contains a complex of carrier, its specific amino acid, and Na^+. Vitamin B_6 is involved in the active transport of the L-amino acids. Its deficiency shows a lowered rate of uptake of the L-amino acids.

Sometimes minute quantities of dipeptides are absorbed and rarely whole protein particles can be absorbed by the process of *pinocytosis*. Proteoses and peptones though soluble, are not absorbed by the intestinal mucosal cells. Many conditions such as asthma, eczema and hay fever are known to be aggravated by certain food proteins. It is believed that in these cases certain protein particles are absorbed in a partly digested form. If undigested or partly digested proteins are repeatedly injected into the blood or tissue of an animal, the animal may receive a severe shock or even the after an injection of some protein later on.

Absorption of Fats

The fats on hydrolysis yield a mixture of glycerol, diglycerides, monoglycerides and free fatty acids. Since glycerol is water soluble, there is no difficulty in explaining its absorption. The absorption of fatty acids depends upon their molecular weight. Low molecular weight fatty acids are relatively hydrophilic whereas the high molecular weight fatty acids are hydrophobic. Low molecular weight fatty acids are absorbed without much difficulty. The high molecular weight fatty acids cannot be absorbed till they are brought about into soluble form (*fatty acid-bile salt complexes*). About 25-60% of the fat appears to be fully hydrolyzed before it is absorbed. The action of bile salt in forming water soluble complexes with fatty acids is known as *hydrotrophic action*. The fatty acids can also be absorbed in combination with the steroids by forming more soluble esters. As soon a absorption takes place, this complex breaks down, the fatty acids liberated from complex, and the bile salt is eventually carried to the liver, where it is re-secreted in the bile. Experimentally it has been proved that if fats are fed to an animal whose bile duct has tied off, about 80 per cent of fatty acids are found in the faeces.

The absorbed or resynthesized long chain fatty acids enter the lymphatic system as triglycerides specially in the form of *chylomicrons*. The chylomicrons are about one micron in diameter and consist of 2% protein, 7% phospholipid, 9% cholesterol, and 82% triglycerides. The particles of emulsified fat having dimensions 0.1 to 0.5% are called the *micelles* that can be easily absorbed as such without undergoing hydrolysis.

The villi through a process of contraction force pour chyle into the large lymphatics, and the chyle finally enters the blood stream at the junction of the subclavian and jugular veins under the left shoulder by way of the thoracic duct.

The blood carries the fats to the tissues.

Absorption of Vitamins

Water soluble vitamins are absorbed by a simple process of diffusion. Only vitamin B_{12} requires certain intrinsic factors secreted by the stomach. Fat soluble vitamins are absorbed along with emulsified fat in the presence of bile.

Absorption of Nucleic Acids

Nucleic acids are first hydrolyzed in the gut into nucleosides of RNA and DNA in the presence of ribonuclease and deoxyribonuclease respectively. Thus, nucleoside is the diffusible form of nucleic acid.

Absorption of Water and Electrolytes

In human being about 15-20 litres of water can be absorbed in ileum in 24 hours. The process of movement of water in the intestine is called the *gastro intestinal circulation.*

The mucosa of large intestine is the main organ for the sodium absorption. Chloride is absorbed along with the sodium ions. Iron is absorbed in the duodenum while calcium along the entire length of the intestine. The absorption of calcium is 50 times slower than that of the sodium. Bicarbonate is absorbed by different areas of the intestine.

ASSIMILATION

The absorbed food materials enter into two draining systems:

1. circulation of blood via the portal route and
2. circulation through the lymphatic route. The portal circulatory route transports blood from the intestine along with absorbed

nutrients into the liver. The non essential as well as excess of substances are removed from blood and are conveyed to kidney for their subsequent excretion. Fat soluble substances are taken into the lymphatic route or may be deposited in lymph nodes before getting to the general circulation.

Glucose and other carbohydrates when in excess are stored as glycogen in the liver and muscle. However, the major amount of glucose is primarily utilised as an instant energy source.

Most of the fatty acids and glycerol are deposited in the form of neutral fats (triglycerides) after their synthesis in the adipose tissues. Neutral fats are also used as supplementary energy source because of their high energy potential.

Most of the amino acids are primarily utilized to build up proteins characteristic of an organism. Very rarely, for instance, during starvation, proteins are degraded and utilized as supplementary energy source.

Fate of various food materials after intestinal absorption is summarized below. Glucose and other carbohydrates:

1. Stored as glycogen when in excess in liver and muscles.
2. Glucose in the circulation is used as an instant energy source.

Fatty Acids and Glycerol

1. Synthesis of neutral fat and its deposition in the adipose tissue.
2. Used as supplementary energy source because of high energy potential.

Amino Acids

1. Synthesis of proteins, building blocks of the body.
2. Under emergency degraded as supplementary energy source.

The generalizations, outlined above regarding fate of various food constituents after their absorption does not form a rigid rule. As a matter of fact, in the body, continuous interconversions of various food substances go on or in other words, various body constituents are present in a state of flux.

Faeces

As the contents of the small intestine enter the large intestine, they are semi-liquid and consist largely of undigested food, residues and the remains of digestive juices. Much of the water of the intestinal contents is absorbed here. The contents of the large intestine are called the faeces. The composition of the faeces depends very little on the constitution of the diet. The faeces normally are about 3/4 water and 1/4 solid matter containing 30 per cent dead bacteria, 10 to 20 per cent fat, 10-20 per cent inorganic matter, 2 to 3 per cent protein and 30 per cent undigested food. The colour of the faeces is due to stercobilin, an oxidation product of bile pigment; their odour is due mainly to the *indole* and *skatole*, derived from the action of bacteria on certain amino acids; and to gases produced by fermentation of carbohydrates. The volume of intestinal gases may vary from about 10 ml to 2500 ml. High milk diet increases hydrogen, high vegetable diet methane, non-vegetarian diet-nitrogen and hydrogen sulfide. At high altitude, gas formation is increased. The amount of faeces produced in twenty four hours varies widely, according to the diet, from about 80 to 200 gm, but is usually about 100 gm. The reaction is usually slightly alkaline on the surfaces (pH-7.0 to 7.5).

Defecation

Mass peristaltic movement pushes faecal matter into the rectum. The resulting distension of the rectal wall stimulates pressure-sensitive receptors initiating a reflex which is *gastrocolic reflex for defecation*, which is emptying of the rectum. Contraction of the longitudinal rectal muscles shortens the rectum, thereby increasing the pressure inside it. The pressure forces the sphincters open, and the faeces are expelled through the anus. Voluntary contractions of the diaphragm and abdominal muscles and defecation by increasing pressure inside the abdomen, which pushes the walls of the signoid colon and rectum inward. If defecation does not occur, the faeces remain in the rectum until the next wave of mass peristalsis again stimulates the pressure-sensitive receptor, creating the desire to defecate.

2

CIRCULATION

All the multicellular and higher animals which are large in size and active in movement acquired some sort of transport system so that necessary fluids, gases and nutrients could reach to all the cells. Such a circulatory system comprises of heart which pumps an efficient transporting agent *i.e.*, blood through arteries, veins and capillaries.

I. BLOOD

Blood is a liquid connective tissue and acts as the main transporting system of the body. It consists of a fluid intercellular substance called *plasma*, in which are freely suspended various *blood cells* or *corpuscles*. Blood is somewhat sticky, viscous and colour ranges from the bright red in oxygenated to the dark red in deoxygenated blood. It is slightly alkaline (7.4 pH), has a distinctive odour and a salty taste. It makes up from 8 to 10 per cent of the total body weight. The specific gravity of blood is 1.057 in males and 1.053 in females.

PLASMA

It is fluid portion of the blood from which corpuscles have been removed and constitutes about 55% of total blood volume. It is a straw coloured, slightly alkaline, 2.2 times more viscous than water and 9 % solids. The solids either get dissolved or suspended and are in the form of organic and inorganic substances.

ORGANIC CONSTITUENTS

1. *Proteins* (7.5%) are serum albumin and globulin, fibrinogen, prothrombin etc.

Albumin (4.5%) is the major component of plasma proteins. It is soluble in distilled water and with molecular weight about 69,000. It is made up of polypeptide chain containing 575 amino acids. It is synthesized in liver. Its isoelectric pH is 4.7. It is heat coagulable. It performs many functions which are as follows:

1. The albumin released from the liver is circulated to all tissues which can utilize the amino acids of albumin for the synthesis of their own proteins. Thus it serves as a source of amino acids.
2. Nearly half of the calcium present in blood is loosely bound to albumin at different sites.
3. It helps in the transport of thyroxine and steroid hormones.
4. It binds to the toxic products of metabolism and carries to the sites of excretion.
5. It plays a major role in osmotic regulation of the fluid distribution.

Globulins (2.5%) due to their high content of carbohydrates, it is highly soluble and not coagulated by heat. It is a mixture of several globulins

(i) α_1 and α_2 *globulin* : Molecular weight ranges from 41,000 to 200,000 with isoelectric pH 5.1. α_1 globulin is present in small amount, and has an inhibitory effect on trypsin. It consists of two functions :

(a) one fraction combines with bilirubin,

(b) another fraction helps in the carriage of lipids, steroids and glycoproteins. α_2, globulin consists of α_2 macroglobulins, mucoproteins, ceruloplasmin and hepatoglobulins.

(ii) *β-globulin* : It has molecular weight varying from 90,000 to 1,300,000. Its isoelectric pH is 5.6. It is concerned with carriage of the insoluble lipid along with fat soluble vitamins. It is also concerned with iron transport. Prothrombin is a β-globulin.

(iii) *γ-globulin* : It has molecular weight ranging from 150,000 to 190,000. Its isoelectric pH is 6.0. Antibodies belong to this class.

Fibrinogens (0.3%) : It is another glycoprotein, it has molecular weight of 340,000 daltons and has an isoelectric pH of 5-8. It is synthesized by the liver at a rate of 4-5 gm per day. It is primarily concerned with blood clotting.

2. *Carbohydrates (1%)* - Glucose, fructose, galactose, etc.
3. *Lipids* - Neutral fats, phospholipids. cholesterol and cholesterides etc.
4. Non protein nitrogenous substances (NPN) urea, uric acid, xanthine, hypoxanthine, creatine, creatinine, ammonia, amino acid etc.
5. *Other substances* - Hormones, antibodies and various enzymes.

INORGANIC CONSTITUENTS (0.9%)

This constituent includes various anions and cations such as chloride, bicarbonate, phosphate, sulphate, sodium, potassium, calcium and magnesium. Small amounts of iron and iodine are also found.

Apart from this the plasma contains a small amount of bilirubin, carotine and xanthophyllin which impart the characteristic yellow colour to the plasma.

Blood Corpuscles

There are three types of blood corpuscles are present in plasma viz,, (i) Red blood corpuscles (Erythrocytes); (ii) white blood corpuscles (Leucocytes) and (iii) platelets or thrombocytes.

(I) Red Blood Corpuscle (RBCs)

Erythrocytes are present in most of vertebrates. These are circular biconcave and non-nucleated in human beings and contain a respiratory pigment called *haemoglobin* in cytoplasm. The biconcave shape increases the surface area, while the absence of nucleus increases the haemoglobin content. Human RBCs average 7.5 μ in diameter; 2.4 μ in thickness at the edge but only 1 μ in centre, and a volume of 90 cu μ. One erythrocyte contains 30 μ gm of haemoglobin which constitutes 90% of the dry weight. The erythrocytes smaller than 6 μ are called microcytes and those larger than 9-12 μ are called *macrocytes*. The erythrocytes with variable shape and size are called *poikilocytes*. The total area of an individual's erythrocytes amounts to about 3000 sq. m. which is 1500 times the whole surface area of the body.

The erythrocytes are acidophilic and stained with eosin. These are very flexible; and able to squeeze through capillaries of only half their diameter and then regain their original shape. Mammalian mature RBCs lack mitochondria, golgi body, endoplasmic reticulum and other cell organelles, the human erythrocytes has a highly oriented structure of lipids, proteins and haemoglobin consisting of approximately 64% water, 28% haemoglobin, 7% lipids or fatty materials and the remaining 3% sugars, salts, enzymes and other proteins.

Number : The number of erythrocytes differs in different animals as well as the physiological state of an individual. There are about 5 million red blood cells per cubic millimetre of blood in the adult human male and 4.5 million per cubic millimetre of blood in the adult female. In infants the count is 6 to 7 million, whereas in foetus 7–8 millions. In the first ten days of postnatal life large number of red cells are destroyed. This is one Of the cause of *jaundice* in the new born.

The R.B.C. count decreases in human females during pregnancy and during and just after menstruation. The erythrocyte count of a normal individual may vary at least 5% during the course of a day. It is low during sleep and after meals and high during activity and high environmental temperature., The erythrocyte count is high in animals living at high altitudes. Whenever the number of erythrocytes increases much above the normal value, the stage is called *polycythemia*. This is the reason that the persons living at high altitudes (Kashmir, Tibet etc.) have rosy cheeks.

Life span : The life span of RBCs is about 100-120 days. Worn out red cells are removed from circulation and destroyed by spleen and liver. In one second there is a destruction of about 2.5 million of erythrocytes. The destruction of RBCs in healthy person produces about 250 mg of bile salt per day.

Erythropoises : Formation of erythrocytes is called erythropoises. These are produced in haemopoietic organs like yolk sac, kidney, spleen, liver and bone marrow. The production needs a hormone called erythropoietin synthesized in kidney. In higher animals the red cells are produced in bone marrow in adults.

Function : It helps in respiration due to presence of a respiratory pigment-haemoglobin which have a affinity towards oxygen.

II. WHITE BLOOD CORPUSCLES

White blood corpuscles are nucleated, non pigmented Or colourless cells also known as *leucocytes*. They are described as wandering cells and are not always confined to the blood channels. Due to their amoeboid properties they can easily pass through the unruptured blood vessels wall by a process of *diapedesis*. These cells are attracted to areas of infection or inflammation by chemical substances released during tissue destruction. An important function of W.B.C. is *phagocytosis*. Phagocytic white blood cells protect the body by engulfing disease producing micro-organisms and digesting them with lysosomal hydrolytic enzymes.

Number : The average number of white blood cells in a healthy person ranges from 5,000 to 10,000 per cubic millimetre of whole blood. In an acute infection, such as appendicites or pneumonia, the total leucocytes increase considerably upto 20,000 or 30,000 per cubic millimetre of blood. During pregnancy and in the new born also, the number increases above 10,000 per cubic mm. This increase, is the *leucocytosis*. In contrast to this, if the number falls below 4000 the term leucopenia is applied. Leucopenia occurs in persons with certain diseases, such as tuberculosis. *Leukemia* is a pathological increase in number and the term is used today to denote one type of neoplastic disease (blood cancer).

One of the most important function of leucocytes is the body defence against infection. This is achieved by three processes :

(1) phagocytosis,

(2) production of antibodies and

(3) destruction and removal of toxins of protein origin.

Leucocytes are manufactured in spleen, lymph nodules, tonsils, peyer's patches etc. According to *Osgood* and *Sabin* the life span of the different varieties of leucocytes differs as shown in the following lines :

(i) Granulocytes	1-2 days (Sabin)	
(ii) Neutrophils	2-4 days	Osgood
(iii) Eosinophils	8-12 days	
(iv) Basophils	12-15 days	
(v) Lymphocytes	1-2 or 3 days	

White blood cells are sub-divided into two categories, granular and non-granular leucocytes, based on the presence or absence of cytoplasmic granules:

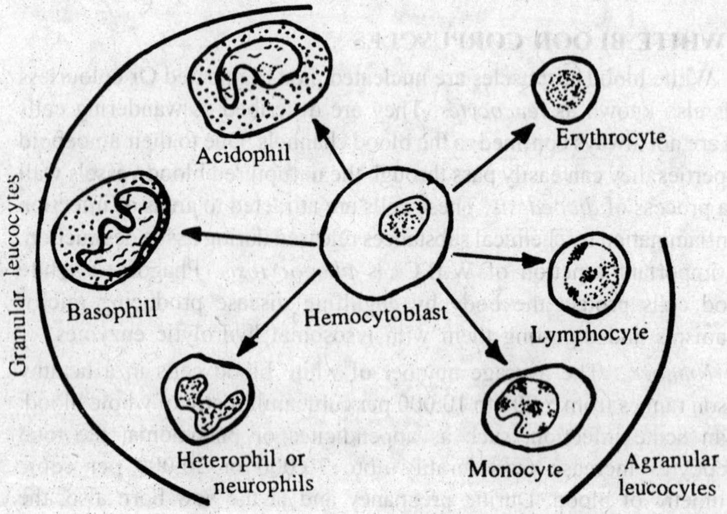

Fig. 2.1 : Various types of blood cells differentiated from haemocytoblasts.

(a) **Granular leucocytes :** The leucocytes containing cytoplasmic granules and lobulated nuclei are the *granulocytes*. The granulocytes arise in red bone marrow from precursor cells called *myeloblasts*. The nuclei of granulocytes appear in many shapes that-is-why also called *polymorphonuclear leucocytes*. The *granules* can be stained with Wright's stain, eosin or methylene blue. They are classified as neutrophils, eosinophils, or basophils on the basis of the shapes or their nuclei or the staining reactions of their granules.

Neutrophils

Neutrophils comprise about 60 to 70% (or 3000-6000 per cubic mm.) of all white blood cells in peripheral circulation. They are about 10 to 12 microns in diameter and contain nuclei that have form three to five lobes. The cytoplasm of the mature neutrophil is filled with fine lysosomal granules containing phosphatase, nucleotidase, protease, amylase, lipase etc. They show amoeboid movement, and can move upto 40 microns per minute. Neutrophils are the chief phagocytic cells of the body. They are not confined to blood vessels, but throughout the entire body where they function as *scavengers*. Neutrophils survive more than a few days after leaving the blood stream. If the infection is massive or the bacteria are very virulent, many neutrophils die; an accumulation of dead neutrophils and bacteria is known as *pus*. A localised accumulation of pus is called as *abscess*.

Some physiologists have described certain sex differences in the nuclei of neutrophils. About 3-5 % of neutrophils from a female show the sex chromatin attached to one of the nuclear lobes by a thin stalk forming the so called "*drumstic bodies*".

Eosinophils

Also known as acidophils and comprise only 2 to 4 % of all white blood cell. 100-400 per cubic mm. They are about 10 to 15 microns in diameter. They have bilobed nuclei, and contain large lysosomal granules that stain red with Wright's stain. Eosinophils phagocytize antigen-antibody complexes: the number of eosinophils is in the peripheral blood increases in allergic diseases, such as asthma or hay fever, and in parasitic infections, such as trichinosis. Some people believe that the eosinophils contain much of the histamine that is present in the blood. Histamine causes the symptoms of allergic reactions.

Basophils

Basophils are also known as *cyanophils* are even rarer and make up only about 0.5 to 1% of all white blood cells or 25 to 200 per cubic mm. They are about 8 to 10 microns in diameter (smallest among W.B.C.) have bilobed or kidney shaped nuclei and contain large granules that stain dark blue with Wright's blood stain. These granules contain *histamine* and *heparin*, which are released into the blood stream under conditions of stress or allergy. Basophils are non-phagocytic; they are similar to the most cells in loose connective tissue. They possibly has some role in local anticoagulation and formation of ground substance. They are believed to belong to cells of the reticulo-endothelial system. The .number of basophils increases in chicken pox.

The increase of granulocytes in the blood is called as *granulocytosis*. Diminution of granulocytes in the blood is known as *granulocytopenia*. Complete disappearance of granulocytes is known as *agranulocytosis*.

(b) **Agranular leucocytes :** These are non-granular white blood cells contain simple spherical non-lobulated nuclei. These cells comprise about 25-30 % of all leucocytes, these cells include *monocytes*, which are formed in lymph nodes and the spleen and *lymphocytes* which are formed in all types of lymphoid tissue, including lymph nodes, spleen, tonsils and possibly the thymus.

Monocytes : These are the largest among all white cells ranging from 16-22 microns in diameter. Monocytes make up about 5 per cent of all white cells. The number of monocytes varies from 100-400 per-cubic mm of blood. The number increases in tuberculosis. Their nuclei are indented to horse shoe shaped and stain purple. The nucleus is eccentric with a large amount of clear non-granular cytoplasm, may be, with vacuoles in it. They arise in the red bone marrow from precursor cells called *monoblasts*. The monocytes are motile and have the power of engulfing bacteria. These are most active in acid environment (pH ranges below 7). In general, they are found around walled off abscesses and infections which have been brought under control. They are also found in tissues, and in these locations the cells are differentiated into *macrophages* or scavanger cells. Monocytes live as macrophages for several months in the tissues and are commonly found at sites of chronic infection or inflammation. They play a vital role in removing damaged tissue and thus preparing the way for regeneration processes of the body.

Lymphocytes : They make up about 25% of all white blood cells. The number varies from 1500-2700 per cubic mm of blood. The number increases in tuberculosis. Two types of lymphocytes have been reported. *Small lymphocytes* are most common in blood. They have a diameter of 8 microns. They have relatively large somewhat spherical nuclei. Large lymphocytes have a diameter of 12 microns. They are primitive, proliferative cells, residing in the lymph nodules that give rise to the active small, lymphocytes. Both small and large lymphocytes have a spherical nucleus surrounded by a thin rim of cytoplasm. Lymphocytes arise from *lymphoblasts*. Mature lymphocytes are released into the lymphatic system and ultimately enter the cardiovascular system, which they leave very rapidly to enter the tissues. In the tissues, lymphocytes live only a few days but they may survive for years in the lymphatic system.

Lymphocytes are non phagocytic and neutralize the toxicity produced in the body. The important function of these cells is to produce antibodies. They also contribute to scar formation after injury and thus facilitate wound healing.

(c) **Blood platelets :** Blood platelets are also known as *thrombocytes*. These are the smallest of the formed elements in the circulating blood. In mammals the platelets are fragments of protoplasm and are also called as *cytoplasmic bodies*. These are derived from giant cells called *megakaryocytes* in bone marrow. Although platelets lack a nucleus, they do possess a variety of metabolic enzymes and cellular oganelles. There are approximately 200,000 to 300,000 platelets per cubic millimetre of blood. A marked decrease in the number of circulating platelets is called thrombocytopenia. Persons with *thrombocytopenia* have a tendency to bleed from capillaries all over their bodies; then skin is covered with many small purple blotches, called *petechiae*, which represent haemorrhages of skin capillaries. When the platelets count drops below 70,000 per cubic millimetre of blood, spontaneous bleeding becomes a serious problem. In peripheral circulation, the platelets survive for about a week.

Platelets initiate the blood clotting process at the site of vascular injury. If the rupture of the blood vessel is small, the formation of a platelet plug is sufficient to close off the vessel. If the rupture is larger, the *release reaction* initiated by the platelets stimulates the series of reactions leading to the formation of fibrin from fibrinogen and the formation of a fibrin clot. Platelets also release vasocontriction substance such as serotonin, which causes the blood vessels to constrict.

II. FUNCTION OF THYMUS AND BONE MARROW IN IMMUNE MECHANISM

The human body has the ability to resist almost all types of organisms or toxins that tend to damage the tissues and organs. This capacity is called immunity. Much of the immunity is caused by a special immune system that forms antibodies and activated lyrmphocytes that attáck and destroys die specific organisms or .toxins. This type of immunity is called acquired *immunity*. However, an additional portion of the immunity results fròm general processes rather than from processes directed at specific disȩase organisms. This is called *innate immunity*.

Role of lymphoid tissue in acquired immunity : Acquired immunity is the product of the body's lymphoid tissue. The lymphoid tissue is located most extensively in the *lymph nodes*, but it is also found in special lymphoid tissues such as that of the spleen, *submucosal areas* of *gastrointestinal tract* and the bone marrow. The lymphoid tissue is distributed very advantageously in the body to intercept the invading organisms or toxins before they can spread too widely. For instance, the lymphoid tissue of the GIT is exposed immediately to antigens invaling through the gut. The lymphoid tissue of the throat and pharynx (the tonsils and adenoids) is extremely well located to intercept antigens that enter by way of upper respiratc:y tract. The lymphoid tissue of the spleen ànd bone marrow plays the specific role of intercepting antigenic agents that have succeeded in reaching the circulating blood.

Though most of the lymphocytes in normal lymphoid tissue look alike when studied under the microscope, these cells are distinctly divided into two major populations. One of the population is responsible for forming the activated lymphocyte that provide cell-mediated immunity and the other for forming the antibodies that provide humoral immunity.

Both of these types of lymphocytes are derived originally in the embryo from *pluripotent haemopoietic stem cells* that differentiate and become committed to form lymphocytes. The lymphocytes that are formed eventually end up in the lymphoid tissue, but before doing sc they are further differentiated or "preprocessed" in the following ways

Those lymphocytes that are eventually destined to form activatec lymphocytes first migrate to and are preprocessed in *thymus gland*, for which reason they are called T *lymphocytes*. These are responsible for cell mediated immunity *i.e.,* they attack foreign materials (tissue transplants, fungi, parasites) by direct cell to cell contact.

The other population of lymphocytes those that are destined to form antibodies are preprocessed in some unknown area of the body, probably in the liver during midfetal life and in the bone marrow in late fetal life and after birth. This type of cells were firstly discovered in birds in which the preprocessing occurs in the *bursa of fabricius*, for this reason lymphocytes are called B lymphocytes, and they are responsible for humoral immunity *i.e.,* these B lymphocytes stimulate plasma cells to secrete antibodies that circulate in blood and inactivate antigen molecules produced by bacteria.

Thymus gland, in addition to formation of T lymphocytes, also secretes a hormone, called *thymopoetin*, that circulates through the body fluids and increases the activity of the T lymphocytes. This hormone is believed to cause further proliferation and increased activity of these lymphocytes. T cells are classified into 3 major groups:

1. *Cytotoxic T cells or killer cells :* attack directly on microorganisms and release a cytotoxic substance directly into the attacked cell. The cytotoxic substances are probably mainly lysosomal enzymes manufactured in T cells. These cells play an important role in destroying cancer cells, heart transplant cells or other types of cells that are 'foreign' to the person's own body.
2. *The helper T cells :* As their name implies they' help' in functions of the immune system in multiple ways:
   (a) Increasing the action of B cells, cytotoxic T cells and suppressor T cells by antigens.
   (b) These cells secrete a substance called interleukin –2, one of the lymphokines, that increases the activity of other T cells.
   (c) They activate macrophage system for efficient phagocytosis.
3. *Suppressor T cells :* Much less is known about the suppressor T cells, but they are capable of suppressing the functions of both cytotoxic and helper T cells, because excessive immune reactions that might be severely damaging to the body, so that these cells are also called as *regulatory T cells*.

Coagulation or Clotting of Blood

Since humans are liable to injury and the shedding of blood, a mechanism is provided within the body whereby there is a spontaneous tendency for the loss of blood to be limited. The process by which there

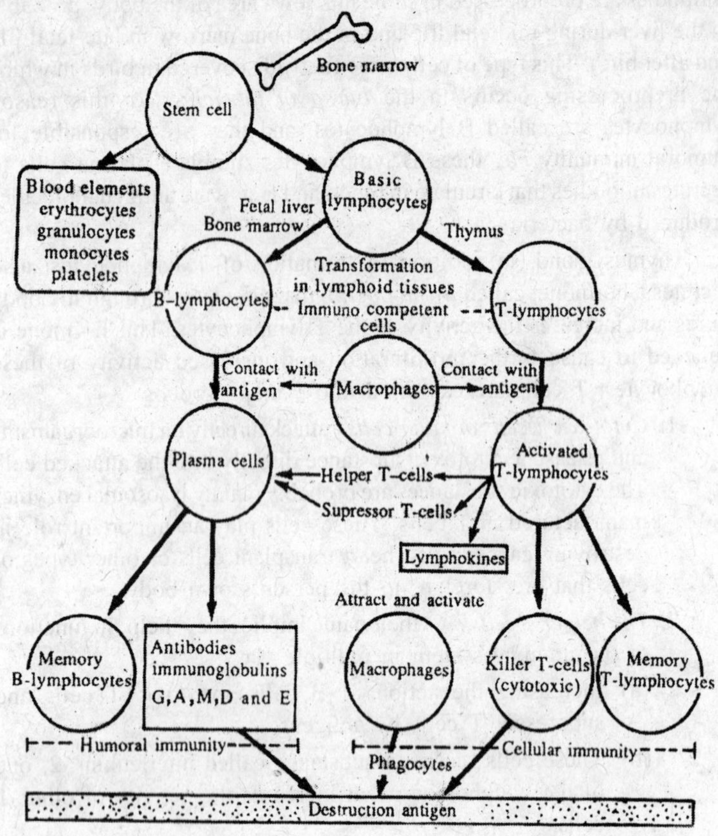

Fig. 2.2 : The immune system, a simplified schematic diagram.

is prevention of excessive loss of blood from the body is called *coagulation of blood*.

The actual mechanism is a complicated one, but the general principles are simple and important. Shortly after being shed, the blood becomes sticky and sets into a jelly-like mass. After a few hours this mass contracts and from it is squeezed a yellowish fluid, the *serum*. When this process is studied at ultramicroscopic level, the sequence of observed events is: first, small granules appear at the site of injury. On joining in chain they form needles which again unite to form long threads passing along the cut surface. The threads cross one another and form a sort of network into the meshes of which the blood cells get entangled. The clot so formed slowly gets retracted squeezing out *serum*.

Inside the blood vessels the blood does not clot due to presence of an anticoagulin substance-the *heparin* secreted by liver. In normal circulating blood it prevents the conversion of prothrombin into an active form thrombin.

Process of clotting can be described in a sequence of three stages. Stage I is concerned with the formation of a substance called *thromboplastin.* Stage II involve the conversion of prothrombin, a plasma protein, into *thrombin*, an enzyme. This stage requires the presence of thromboplastin and several other plasma coagulation factors. In stage III, thrombin catalyzes the conversion of *fibrinogen* into *fibrin.* Fibrin forms the threads of the clot.

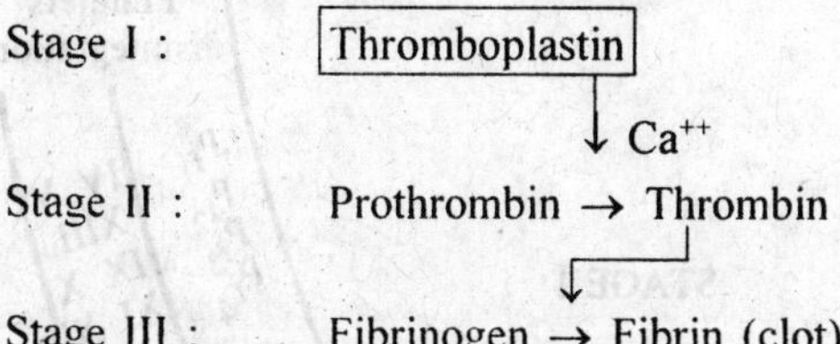

(i) *Thromboplastin (Thrombokinase)* : wounded tissue on disintegration of blood cells and platelets release this substance. The release of thromboplastin is the initiating step of the coagulatory process. In normal circulating blood this substance is totally absent.

(ii) *Prothrombin* : This is another factor synthesized in the liver with the help of vitamin K and present in the normal circulating blood. It is a precursor form of another active substance, thrombin, which is an enzyme. In the presence of calcium ions prothrombin is activated and transformed into active enzyme thrombin.

(iii) *Fibrinogen* : It is a plasma protein supplying main raw material for the clot formation. During the process, fibrinogen is converted into fibrin which forms a meshwork to seal the exposed .injured surface.

In this process, Stages II and III are relatively well understood. By contrast. the formation of thromboplastin (Stage I) is complex and is still not completely understood.

Thromboplastin may arise through a series of reactions that follow the rupture of blood platelets (Intrinsic pathway), or it may develop following the injury of blood tissues (Extrinsic pathway). These processes, by which intrinsic or extrinsic thromboplastin is formed, involve four to eight different steps or reactions. MacFarlane (1964) suggested that in this series, a succession of factor acts sequentially, each molecule of one factor activates progressively more molecules of the succeeding factors ; this exponentially increasing involvement forms a *coagulation Cascade*.

Means, for thromboplastin formation there are two sources in the body. The *extrinsic* and *intrinsic* sources or pathways.

Extrinsic pathway : It is released by tissues like brain, lung, placenta, blood vessels when injured. However, to convert prothrombin to thrombin, extrinsic thromboplastin requires two or more factors like V, VII and

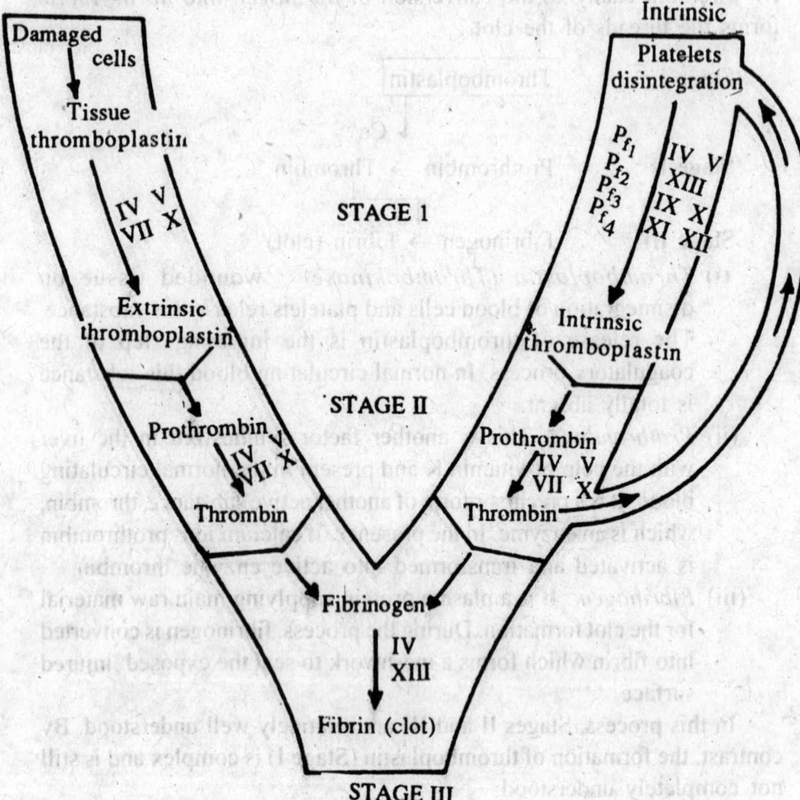

Fig. 2.3 : Diagrammatic representation of the stages in the process of coagulation with extrinsic and intrinsic factors.

X, in addition to calcium. Factor V is a plasma glycoprotein, synthesized in liver; factor VII is a plasma protein, synthesized in liver and requires vit. K for its synthesis. Factor X is a glycoprotein and synthesized in liver in presence of vit. K. All these factors accelerate the conversion of prothrombin to thrombin. This is stage I of the extrinsic pathway. In stage II prothrombin becomes active and called thrombin. This activation requires extrinsic thromboplastin and several plasma factors such as IV, V, VII and X. In stage III fibrinogen is converted to fibrin in the presence of factors IV and XIII (Fig. 2.3).

Intrinsic pathway : The intrinsic thromboplastin is formed when four platelet coagulation factors (Pf_1, Pf_2, Pf_3, Pf_4) react with seven plasma coagulation factors (IV, V, VIII, IX, X, XI, XII). It happens in stage I. In stage II, prothrombin is converted to thrombin in the presence of intrinsic thromboplastin and plasma factors IV, V, VII and X. The stage III involve the conversion of fibrinogen into fibrin in the presence of thrombin and plasma coagulation factors IV and XII.

Table 2.1 : Clotting factors in blood and their synonyms.

Clotting Factor	Synonyms
Fibrinogen	Factor I
Prothrombin	Factor II
Tissue thromboplastin	Factor III : tissue factor
Calcium	Factor IV
Factor V	Proaccelerin; labile factor; Ac-globulin; Ac-G
Factor VII	Serum prothrombin conversion accelerator, proconvertin; SPCA; stable factor
Factor VIII	Antihemophillic factor; AHF; antihemophillic globulin; AHG; antihemophillic factor A
Factor IX	Plasma thromboplastin component; PTC; antihemophillic Christmas factor; antihemophilic factor B
Factor X	Stuart factor; Stuart-Prower factor,
Factor XI	Plasma thromboplastin antecedent; PTA; antihemophilic factor C
Factor XII	Hageman factor.
Factor XIII	Fibrin-stabilizing factor
Platelets	

Platelet coagulation factors : There are four platelet coagulation factors as given below :

(i) Platelet factor I : (Pf_1) or *platelet accelerator*. Essentially same as plasma coagulation factor V.

(ii) *Platelet factor II* : (Pf_2) or *thrombin accelerator*. Accelerates formation of thrombin in stage I of intrinsic pathway and conversion of fibrinogen to fibrin.

(iii) *Platelet factor III* : (Pf_3) or platelet thromboplastic factor.

(iv) *Platelet factor IV* : (Pf_4) Birds heparin, an anticoagulin during clotting.

HAEMODYNAMICS

Haemodynamics is the study of blood flow and blood pressure. Many of the principles involved are the purely physical principles of the movement of fluids through tubular channels. Haemodynamics considers the factors like force, viscosity, the velocity of blood flow through vessels, total blood flow, lateral pressure, elasticity of the blood vessels etc. We will consider here some important factors only.

Blood Volume

Blood contains both extracellular fluid (the fluid of the plasma) and intracellular fluid (the fluid in the red blood cells). However, since blood is contained in a closed chamber all its own-the circulatory system-its volume and its special dynamics are exceedingly important.

The average blood volume of a normal adult is almost exactly 5,000 ml, on the average approximately 3,000 ml of this is plasma, and the remainder, 2,000 ml is red blood cells. However, these values vary greatly in different individuals; also, sex, weight, and many other factors affect the blood volume.

Effect of Weight and Sex on Wood Volume

In persons who have a minimum of adipose tissue the blood volume varies almost directly in proportion to the body weight, normally averaging about 79 ml/kg ± 10 per cent for both lean males and lean females. However, the greater the ratio of fat to body weight, the less the blood volume per unit weight, because fat tissue has little vascular volume.

Blood Volume Regulation

Even after severe haemorrhage, it is generally found that the blood volume is restored to the normal range. Thus, the volume of blood remains constant. A dynamic balance is maintained between the plasma volume and the fluid in the tissue spaces. The plasma volume is dependent on the fluid taken in and loss of fluid. The output of urine can also be varied within a broad range and thus a balance is maintained in the fluid despite wide fluctuations in fluid intake. During haemorrhage there is a rapid movement of fluid from the tissues into the blood and the urine output is reduced.

The concentration of red .blood corpuscles is also regulated during haemorrhages by extra supplies of red cells by spleen and if this is not sufficient, the bone marrow increases its rate of production, so that the original volume is maintained.

Blood Pressure

The very fact of the circulation of the blood shows that it is always under pressure which is constantly highest in the arteries and lowest in the veins. The blood pressure can be defined as '*the pressure that the blood exerts against the walls of its containing vessels*'. The force of the heart contraction is the cause of blood pressure. But this force alone would not furnish a sustained pressure if unaided by other factors. One of them is the pressure that arterial wall exerts upon their contents. The second important factor in the sustaining of arterial pressure is the resistance to the passage of blood through the small blood vessels, specially the arterioles and capillaries. This factor is commonly called as *peripheral resistance*. The cause of this resistance is the friction produced by the passage of the viscous blood through minute tubes. This resistance brings up liquid pressure in existance. The third factor, which is of course minor and which modify the blood pressure is the *breathing*. During inspiration, the thorax enlarges and some suction is exerted upon all the blood within thorax specially upon the large veins near the heart. The veins are affected largely, because veins possesses comparatively less sturdy and elastic walls. Another modifying factor is gravity. This force tends to increase pressure in arteries at levels below that of the heart and to decrease pressure in arteries at level above that of heart.

Arterial Blood Pressure

Arteries distribute blood through the body under certain pressure. As it exists in the arteries, it is called *arterial blood pressure*. At the height of *ventricular contraction* (ventricle systole) pressure in the arteries reaches a maximum. This is the *systolic blood pressure*. During the relaxation of ventricle (ventricular diastole) blood pressure tends to fall to minimum. This is the *diastolic blood pressure*. The difference between these two pressures gives an index of the capacity of the circulatory system to sustain pressure.

In the adult human, the actual pressure Observed for the large arteries of arm normally vary between 115 to 150 mm Hg. The pressure is less in smaller arteries and larger in aorta. The pressure varies with sex, higher in male than female. It also varies during mental and physical work. It shows a tendency to fall in fatigue, also it shows more or less fluctuations during physical and psychological conditions.

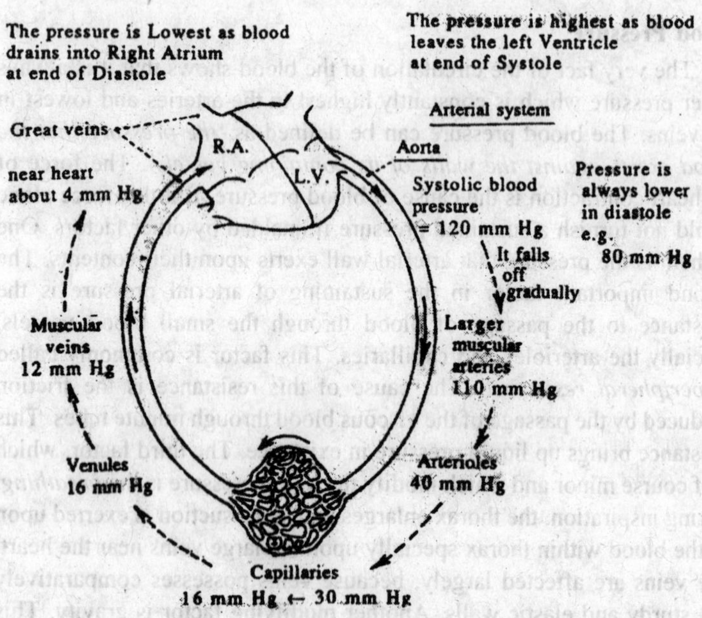

Fig. 2.4 : Showing systolic and diastolic blood pressures.

Venous Blood Pressure

The pressure observed in veins of the limb^ of mammals is usually less than 10 mm Hg and shows a fairly regular tendency to decrease along the venous system toward the heart. In jugular vein pressure less than 1 mm Hg.

Capillary Pressure

The capillary pressure in different animals is roughly measured and the figure has been obtained between 18 to 40 mm Hg in mammals; means it is much lowerer than the arteries.

Measurement of Arterial Blood Pressure

The arterial blood pressure is measured in man by means of a sphygmomanometer. This consists of a rubber bag (covered with a cloth envelope) which is wrapped round the upper arm over the brachial artery.

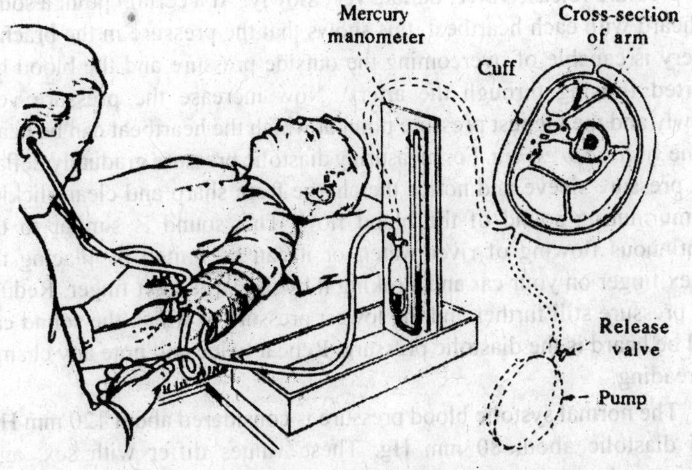

Fig. 2.5 : Showing method for measurement of blood pressure.

One tube connects the inside of the bag with a manometer containing mercury. Another tube connects the inside of the bag to a hand operated pump with a release valve.

Method (Fig. 2.5) : Ask your partner to sit at ease on a table with the arm resting upon the table and at about the level of the heart. After removing the shirt sleeve from his left arm, place the pressure sleeve snugly on the upper left arm without much pressure and wrap the remaining strip of cloth around the arm and tuck it under the pressure sleeve. There are two methods by which blood pressure can be measured; the *palpatory* or by *auscultatory* method.

The palpatory method : Only systolic blood pressure can be measured by this method. Place the armlet in proper position and by using the rubber bulb and screw valve closed, inflate the pressure sleeve ; at the same time by using the finger tips of your left hand, feel the radial pulse. Inflate the pressure sleeve (up to 155 mm Hg) until the pulse disappears. Now slowly deflate the pressure sleeve by using the pressure release valve and when the pulse appears, note the reading on the mercury column. This is the systolic pressure.

The Ausculatory method: Both the systolic and the diastolic pressures can be measured by this method. Follow the method described above and place a stethoscope bulb over the brachial artery close to the pressure sleeve. Now inflate the pressure sleeve upto 150 mm Hg and by using the pressure release valve, deflate very slowly. At a certain point a sound is heard with each heartbeat, this shows that the pressure in the brachial artery is capable of overcoming the outside pressure and the blood has started flowing through the artery. Now increase the pressure very slowly and the highest pressure point at which the heartbeat can be heard is the *systolic pressure*. For measuring diastolic pressure gradually deflate the pressure sleeve and notice the charge from sharp and clear clicking to murmuring sound of the blood flow. This sound is similar to the continuous flowing of river water, or it can be imited by placing the index finger on your ear and stroking it by the large next finger. Reduce the pressure still further and the lowest pressure at which the sound can still be heard is the diastolic pressure. Repeat twice and note any change in reading.

The normal systolic blood pressure is considered about 120 mm Hg, and diastolic about 80 mm Hg. These values differ with sex, age, exercise, sleep etc.

(II) HEART

The blood vascular system begins and ends in the heart. This structure is developmentally and structurally an extremely modified blood vessel. It is a hollow muscular structure that pumps blood to various parts of body through the blood vessels. The basic purpose of circulation is to supply oxygen, heat, metabolic fuels, hormones and vitamins to every cell and to remove their metabolic end products. The heart is located in the *mediastinum* the space in the thoracic cavity between the two pleural sacs.

Anatomy of the Heart

The human heart is a pyramidal structure, it has a base, an apex, two surfaces, two borders, several grooves. Its pointed end, the *apex,* projects downward, forward, and to the left and lies superior to the central depression of the diaphragm. Its broad end, or *base* , projects upwards, backward and to the right and lies just inferior to the second rib. The atrio-ventricular (coronary) sulcus marks the division between the atria and ventricles. The anterior and posterior interventricular sulci mark the division between the right and left ventricles.

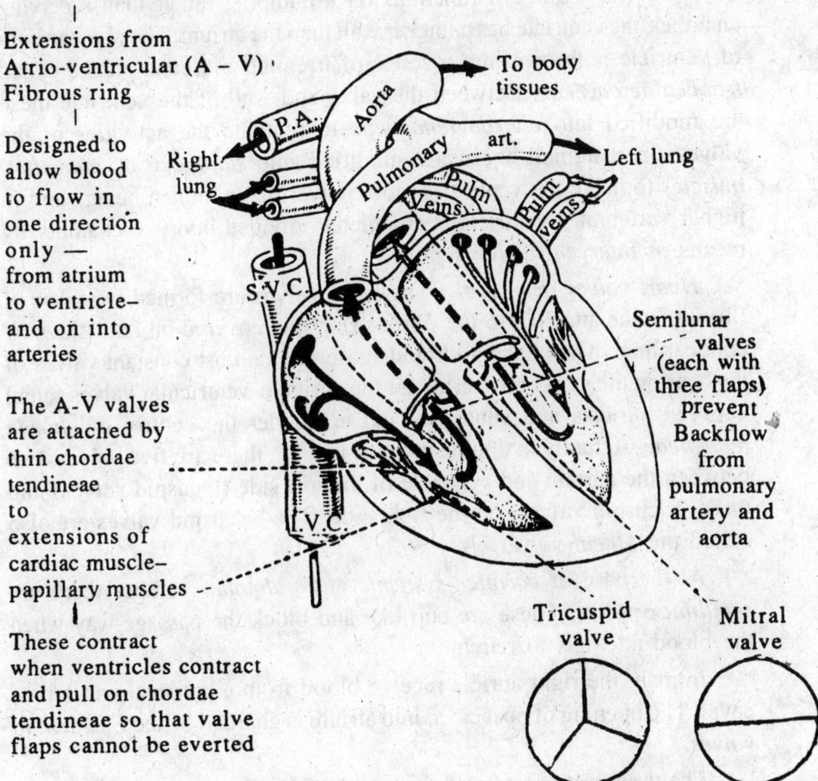

The Great Veins do not have valves guarding their entrance to the heart. Thickening and contraction of the muscle around their mouths prevent Backflow of blood from heart.

Fig. 2.6 : Showing internal structure of heart and its valves.

The heart is composed of two chambers; upper small thin walled chamber-*auricle* or *atrium* and receives blood from various parts of body that is why also known as receiving chamber; and lower large thick walled well muscularized ventricle that supplies blood to various body organs thus also called the *distributing chamber*.

Auricle : It is divided into right and left atria by means-of *inter-auricular septum* which is made up of two walls : the *septum primium* and *septum secundum*. Right auricle receives deoxygenated blood while left one receives oxygenated blood.

Ventricle : Since it functions on a pumping rather than receiving chamber, the ventricle has a thicker wall than the atrium. The myocardium of ventricle is thrown into a series of irregular muscular ridges called *trabeculae carneae*. Between the valve and wall of the ventricle these are modified into *chorda tendeneae* to regulate the activities of the valves. In mammals these are modified into *papillary* or *mammary muscles* to make the ventricles more powerful. In human beings and in higher vertebrates ventricle is completely divided into two chamber by means of *interventricular septum*.

Heart valves (Fig. 2.6) : The heart valves are formed by cusps of fibrous tissue attached to the fibrous ring and covered on both sides by endocardium. They have no blood vessels. The most constant valves of the heart in the vertebrate series are the auriculo-ventricular valves found between auricles and ventricles and are under the control of *chorda tendeneae*. Actually in double heart as in man, there are five valves, two between the auricle and ventricle of the left side (bicuspid valves) and three (tricuspid valves) on the right side. The biscuspid valves are also called the *Mitral valves*.

At the base of *carotico-systemic* and *pulmonary* arches there are *semilunar valves*. These are cup like and block the passage-way when the blood attempts to retreat.

In man, the right auricle receive blood from a precaval and a post caval. The opening of post caval into atrium is guarded by the *Eustachian valves*.

The tissues of heart itself receive blood through the small *coronary artery*. Deoxygenated coronary blood is returned through several vessels which converge to enter the right atrium through the *coronary sinus* guarded by the *valve of Thebesius*.

Pace Maker

Pace maker region on or associated with heart, in which excitation originates and subsequently spreads over the cardiac muscles. Rhythmicity is one of the characteristic feature of all hearts. On the basis of rhythm and the nature of pace maker system hearts are divided into two types.

A. Neurogenic

B. Myogenic Heart

A. Neurogenic Heart

When the heart beat originates in ganglion cells and subsequently spreads over cardiac muscles, such a heart is called *neurogenic*. Pace maker system in this case is in the form of extracardiac nerve ganglions, which are situated in or close to the heart. In almost all invertebrates except molluscs the heart is neurogenic. In *Limulus*, the pace maker is mainly the large ganglionic mass which is made up of the multipolar nerve cells present in mid-dorsal region of heart (Fig. 2.7).

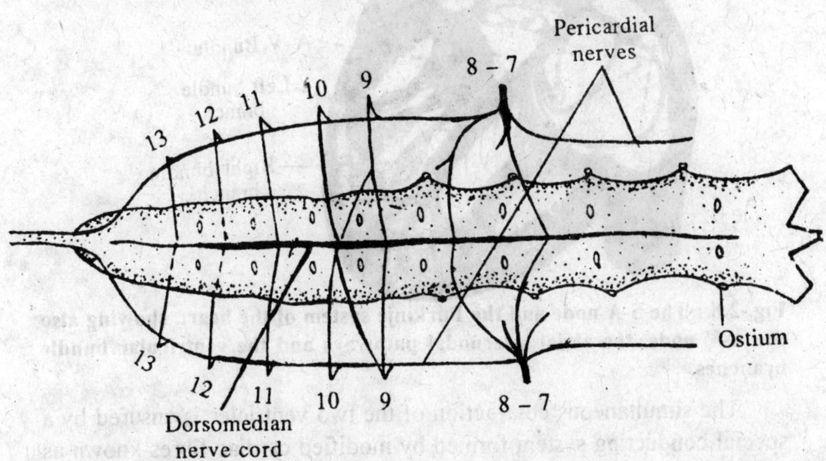

Fig. 2.7 : Neurogenic heart of Limulus showing internal structure of heart and its valves.

In neurogenic heart acetylcholine has accelerating effect on the rate of heart beats.

B. Myogenic Heart

The rhythmic activity of the heart is due to inherent power of muscles, in other words heart beat is initiated and controlled by a special group of modified heart muscles known as *sinus node or pace maker*. In fishes and frog, the rhythm starts at the sinus venosus and spreads over auricles and ventricles. As evolution proceeds,, in higher vertebrates the sinus venosus is disappeared and as represented as a specialized cardiac tissue called sinu-auricular node (S-A node) situated at the side of entrance of left precaval vein.

The beat originates spontaneously at the S-A node and spreads like rippler relatively slowly at a rate of 1 meter/sec along the whole auricular muscles. As a result the two auricles contract.

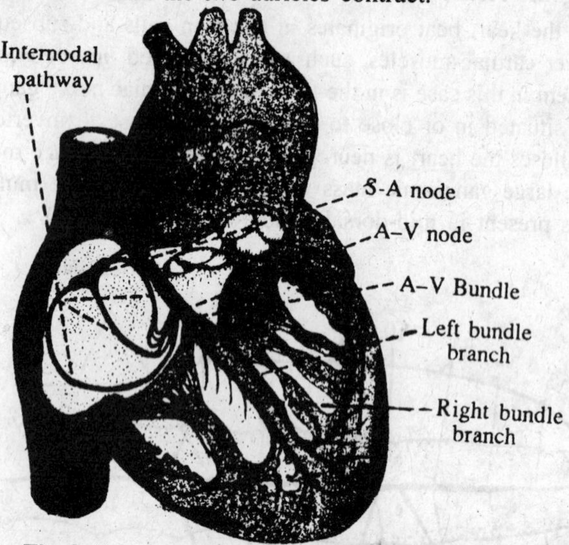

Fig. 2.8 : The S-A node and the Purkinje system of the heart, showing also the A-V node, the atrial internodal pathways and the ventricular bundle branches.

The simultaneous contraction of the two ventricles is ensured by a special conducting system formed by modified cardiac fibres-known as *Bundle of His* and *Purkinje tissue*. The Bundle of *His* originates from the *auriculo-ventricular node* or (A-V node) situated at the base of auriculo-ventricular septum and consists of histologically specialized cardiac muscle fibres, from this Purkinje fibres stem out spreading all over the muscular walls of the ventricle.

There is no special band of connecting tissue between S-A and A-V nodes. The impulse from S-A node acts as stimulus for A-V node. Which in turn stimulates rest of the system *i.e.,* Bundle of *His* and *Purkinje* fibres, as a result, ventricles undergo contraction.

Like neurons, the pacemaker cells also exhibit Donnan equilibrium and the membrane is always polarized, +ve from outside and –ve from inside. As an inherent property, these cells automatically generate change in the membrane potentials with subsequent depolarizations ultimately leading to the generation of an impulse. The impulse once generated causes depolarization and subsequent discharge of adjacent cells. In effect a wave of +ve charges passes over the whole system. Thus generation and transmission of impulses through the pace maker system involves an electrical chain reaction.

CARDIAC CYCLE

Cardiac cycle consists of two phases : the *systole* and the *diastole.* Systole is the contraction of heart whereas the diastole is the relaxation of heart. The rhythmic contraction and relaxation of the cardiac muscles is known as *heart beat.* Such series of events performed in quick succession by the heart during one complete heart-beat is called as *cardiac cycle.*

The contraction of the two auricles takes place simultaneously and constitutes the auricular systole. This is followed by ventricular systole. After each systole the auricles and ventricles enter the diastole in the same order. The detail process of diastole and systole is completed in following manner.

Auricular diastole : Blood from the large veins enter into the auricles as pressure within them is much less than those in the veins. The contraction of the ventricles augments the filling up of auricles by pulling the auricular base. Due to filling, pressure within the auricles becomes greater than the ventricles. Auriculo-ventricular valves open and sets the next event.

Auricular systole : Auricles by their contraction empty themselves into the ventricles. The contraction commences at the entrance of great veins and passes towards the valves.

Ventricular diastole : Ventricles are relaxed during whole of the auricular systole and last part of auricular diastole. Dilatation of ventricles is due to elasticity and pressure of the venous blood.

Ventricular systole : This contraction of ventricles takes more time than the auricular systole. Auriculo-ventricular valves close and prevent regurgitation of blood into the auricles. When the systolic phase reaches its climax, pressure within the ventricles exceeds the arteries. Semilunar valves at the base of the arteries open and ventricles drive their contents into aorta and pulmonary artery.

In human being the complete cycle takes about 0.8 second. The time for auricular systole is 0.1 sec. and that for auricular diastole is 0.7sec. Ventricular systole, which consists of the compression period (0.1 sec) and the expression period (0.2 sec) take 0.3 sec and ventricular diastole 0.5 sec. Hence the total systole occupies 0.4 sec and joint diastole-0.4 sec. so that the time for one complete cardiac cycle is 0.8 sec. The heart beat consists of systole and diastole. The human heart normally beats 72 times per minute; 100,000 times per day or about 40,000,000 times per year or about 2,800,000,000-times upto the age of 70 years. The newly born child has 120 or above heart beats per minute. In old age it slows down to 60 per minute.

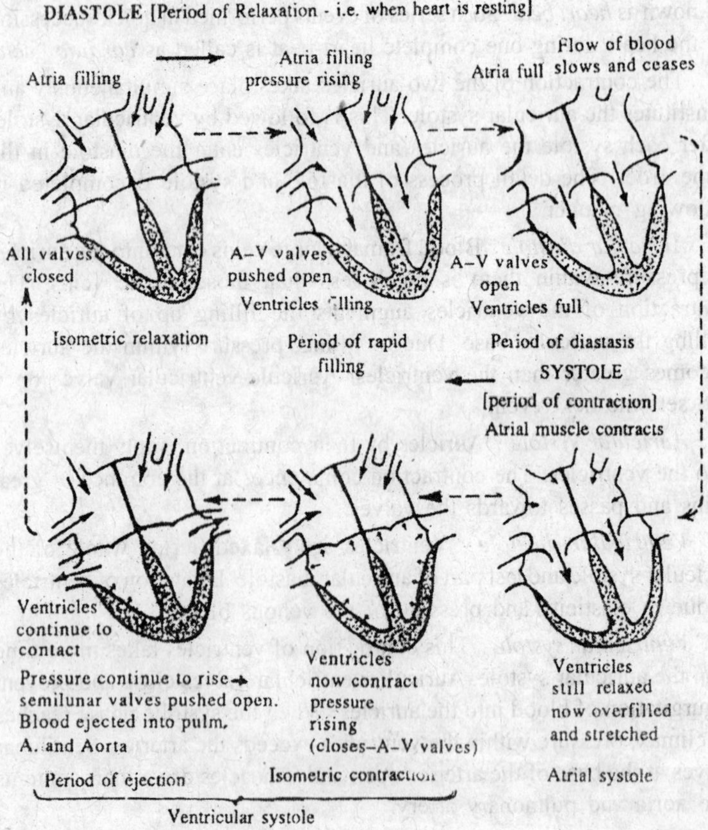

Fig. 2.9 : Diagrammatic representation of the sequence of event in the heart during one heart beat.

The total cycle of events takes about 0.8 second when heart is beating 75 times per minute

Heart Sounds

Because of its mechanical activity the heart vibrates over a wide range of frequencies. Some of these vibrations are in the range of human hearing and result in the *heart sounds*. By using a *stethoscope*, heart sounds can easily be heard in normal humans. The first sound, which can be described as a *lubb* sound, is a long booming sound. It is created by the closure of the atrioventricular valves soon after ventricular systole begins. The *second sound*, which is heard as a short, sharp sound, can be described as a *dubb* sound. It is created by the closure of semilunar valves of aorta and pulmonary artery.

Cardiac Output

Cardiac output is the quantity of blood pumped into the aorta each minute by the heart. This is also .quantity of blood that flows through the circulation and is responsible for transporting substances to and from the tissues. Therefore, cardiac output is perhaps the most important factor that we have to consider in relation to the circulation. The cardiac output is dependent on the volume of blood ejected at each contraction (stroke volume) and the rate of pulsation per minute. Volume of blood ejected per minute is the minute volume.

In a healthy young man this cardiac output amounts to about 5-6 litres/min or 80 ml/kg/min (minute volume). For women, this value is 10 to 20 per cent less. In 1870, a German physiologist, *A.fick*, described a simple method of estimating cardiac output from measurements of the oxygen consumption (or carbon dioxide production) and the difference between the oxygen (or carbon dioxide) contents of blood entering and leaving the heart. Thus

Cardiac output (litres/min)

$$= \frac{O_2 \text{ absorbed by lungs (ml/min)}}{\text{arteriovenous } O_2 \text{ difference (ml/liter blood)}}$$

If blood entering the right atrium contains 160 ml O_2/litre while that leaving the left ventricle holds 200 ml/litre, if follows that 40 ml O_2 has been picked up by each litre of blood which circulated through the heart and lungs. If oxygen is being removed from the inspired air at the rate of 200 ml/min, then it is obvious that 5 litres of blood must have been pumped through the heart and lungs to do the job. Several kinds of flow meters are also available but most of the measurements recorded in the literature are based on Pick's Principle or some modification of it.

The cardiac output usually remains almost proportional to the overall metabolism of body. That is, the greater the degree of activity of the muscles and other organs, the greater also will be cardiac output. During exercise the output may be increased 5 to 6 times more, due to augmented stroke volume and increased cardiac frequency. Anxiety may be accompanied by 10 to 20% rise above the normal level. Cardiac output is about 10% lowered during sleep. In severe anaemia the arterio-venous difference in O_2 content is very low to the extent of 2 ml per 100 ml; due to which cardiac output is increased to the extent of 12 litres per minute. In such cases the cardiac output is accompanied by a high pressure in the right atrium.

Cardiac Index

Because the cardiac output changes markedly with body size, it has been important to find out some means by which the cardiac outputs of different sized persons can be compared with each other. Generally cardiac output increases approximately in proportion to the surface area of the body. Therefore, it is frequently stated in terms of the *cardiac index*, which is the *cardiac output per square meter of body surface area.* The normal human being weighing 70 kg has a body surface area of approximately 1.7 square meters, which means that the normal average cardiac index for adults is approximately 3.0 litres per minute per square metre.

Electrocardiogram (ECG)

The wave of excitation spreading through the heart wall is accompanied by electrical changes (like nerve and skeletal muscle, active cardiac muscle is electrically negative relative to resting cardiac muscle ahead, of the zone of excitation). The electrical currents produced are conducted to the surface of the body and can be picked up, amplified and recorded by a special instrument-the electrocardiograph; and a graphic record of the electrical variation produced by the beating of heart is called as electrocardiogram (ECG). First complete recording of ECG was made by *waller* in 1887.

Electrocardiograph for a mammalian heart shows a complex wave pattern with PQRST waves (Fig. 2.10). There are two isoelectric periods, the shorter one between P and Q ; the longer one between S and T. The upward deflection are P, R and T ; while Q and S are downward waves

The waves are therefore alternately up and down tracings.

Analysis of Electrocardiograph

P–represents upward deflection recorded as a result of origin and spread of action current over auricular muscles. Its average duration is about 0.6 to 0.11 sec. The action current arrives at the A-V node, at about the summit of P. A normal P thus indicates:

1. The generation of action current at the S-A node;
2. Its subsequent spread over the auricle;
3. No defect in the conduction;
4. Auricular musculature and nutritional state is normal.

Q : As soon as a sweeping action current arrives at the muscular part of the septum, latter contracts producing the first wave Q. Hence

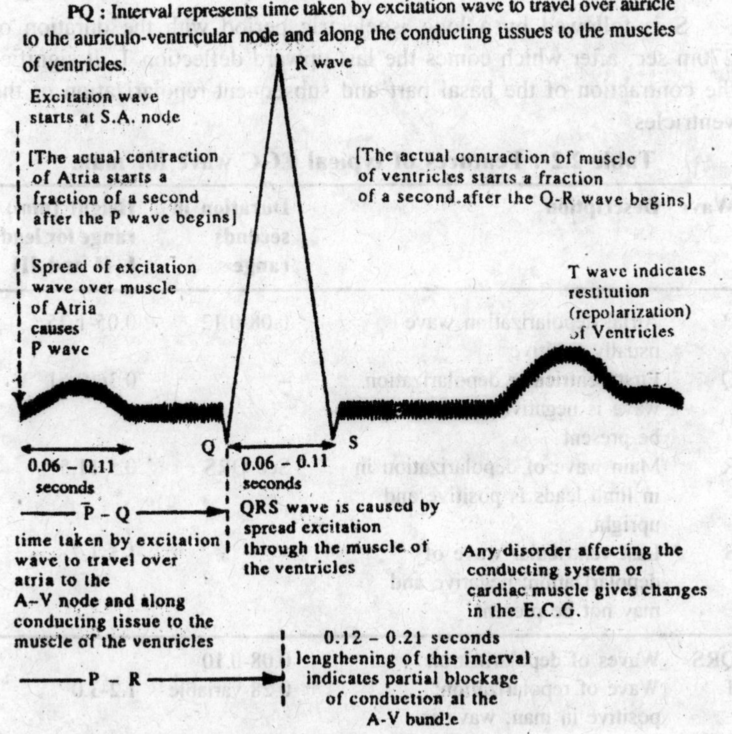

Fig: 2.10 : Showing normal EGC.

Q represents activity of the septum. It is small, downward and often inconspicuous deflection.

PQ : Interval represents time taken by excitation wave to travel over auricle to the auriculo-ventricular node and along the conducting tissues to the muscles of ventricles.

QRS : wave is caused by excitation through the muscles of ventricle. It is most constant and conspicuous wave having the tallest amplitude and duration of 0.06 to 0.11 sec. It follows immediately upon Q; S is the next downward deflection. In the record R represents activity of right ventricle and S that of left ventricle. The actual contraction of ventricular muscles starts a fraction of a second after Q-R wave begins.

P– R interval measures the conduction of the impulse from S-A node to the venricle. Normally its duration varies between 0.12-0.21 sec. Lengthening of this interval indicates partial blockage of conduction at the A-V bundle.

S is followed by a long isoelectric period with the duration of 270m sec; after which comes the last upward deflection T. It signifies the contraction of the basal part and subsequent repolarization of the ventricles.

Table 2.2 : Features of typical EGC wave for man.

Wave	Description	Duration in seconds range	Height (mm) range for leads I, II and III
P	Atrial depolarization wave usually positive	0.08-0.12	0.05-1.25
Q	First ventricular depolarization wave is negative and may not be present	–	0.36-0.61
R	Main wave of depolarization in in limb leads is positive and upright.	See QRS	0.5-11.5
S	Last ventricular wave of depolarization; negative and may not be present.	–	1.5-1.7
QRS	Waves of depolarization	0.08-0.10	–
T	Wave of repolarization; positive in man; wave is upright.	0.28-variable	1.2-3.0

Features of wave intervals

Wave	Intervals	Time
P-R	From beginning of P to beginning of P or Q, whichever is first.	0.18-0.20
QRS	From beginning of Q or R (whichever is first) to end of S or R if S is absent.	0.08
Q-T	From beginning of Q to end of T represents depolarization and repolarization of ventricle.	0.38-0.31
S-T	From end of S to beginning of T segment.	–

A very small period is lapsed between two ECG recordings during which ventricular surface becomes repolarized and excitability is restored.

The ECG may be used to detect cardiac abnormalities *Arrhythmias* are disruptions of the normal heart rate; when the heart rate is below normal, the condition is *brady cardia*; when the heart rate is faster than normal, the condition is the *tachycardia.* In *mitral stenosis* enlargement of P-wave indicates the enlargement of the atrium. The lengthening of P-R interval indicates the *arteriosclerotic heart disease* and *rheumatic* fever. An enlarged Q wave may indicate a *myocardial infraction.*

1. CONTROL OF HEART BEAT

Although, the heart beating is inherent, but the rate and strength of the beat is varied with remarkable precision by out side controls. Some of the outside controls affecting the heart beat are as follows:

1. *Nervous control :* By far the most important part of the autonomic nervous system for regulation of the circulation is the *sympathetic nervous* system. However, the parasympathetic nervous system is also important for its regulation of heart function. These systems have antagonistic influence to keep the heart rate within normal range.
2. *Sympathetic control:* Spinal cardio-accelerator centres are situated in the lateral horns of the upper thoracic segments in the spinal cord. The excitor cells are situated in the superior, middle and inferior cervical ganglia from where the postganglionic or excitatory fibres take origin and pass directly to the heart. The fibres from right side end in the S-A node and from the left side to the A-V node and Bundle of *His*. Fibres also carry vasodilator fibres to the caronary vessels. On stimulation, sympathetic nerves release adrenaline. The action of adrenaline as a whole increases

the frequency of heart rate, force of contraction (augmentor). Similarly there is an increase in the excitability and irritability of myocardium and bundle of His. On the whole, as a result of sympathetic stimulation cardiac Muscles and augumentation is brought about.

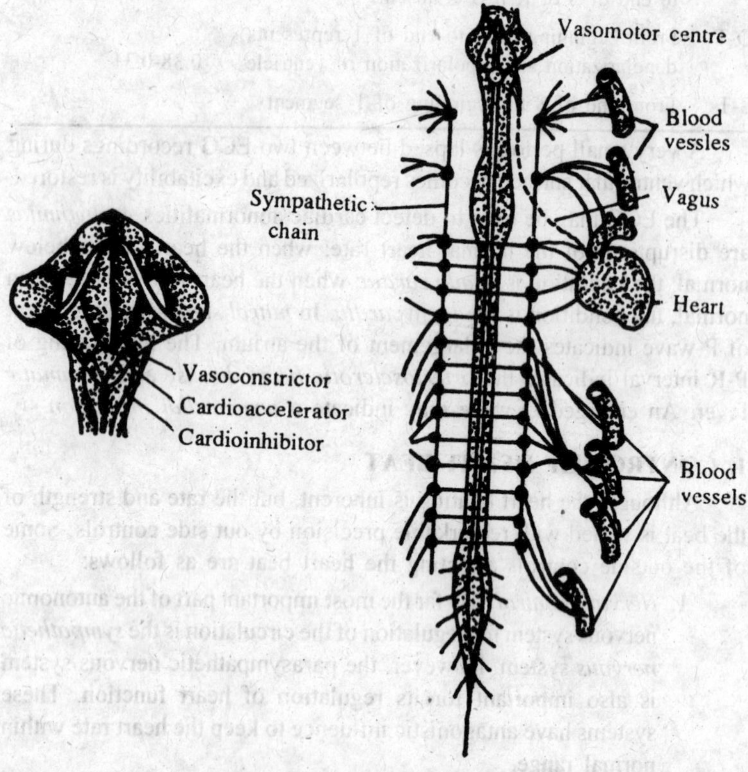

Fig. 2.11 : The vasomotor center and its control of the circulatory system through the sympathetic nerves and through the vagus nerves to the heart which are part of the parasympathetic system.

3. *Parasympathetic control :* Heart receives .nerve fibres from vagus, 10th cranial nerve. Right vagus sends branches to the S-A node while left vagus innervates A-V node in a similar manner from here, post ganglionic fibres arise and supply to the nodes, the bundle, the auricles and ventricles. They also supply contractor fibres to the caronary vessels.

This vagus exerts a *tonic inhibitory* control over all parts of heart. On stimulation acetylcholine is released from the post ganglionic fibres. Acetylcholine brings about cardiac inhibition as follows:

(a) The heart rate is slow down.

(b) The conductivity of the bundle is reduced thus producing various degrees of the heart block.

(c) The force of contraction is diminished.

(d) The duration of systole is diminished.

(e) Refractory period, during which muscular excitability is restored, is diminished.

Additionally, heart rate and blood pressure are under the influence of higher brain centres as well. Emotions have a pronounced effect. By the activity of cerebral neurones concerned with mental state, impulses are sent to the cardiac centre in the medulla oblongata. Some emotional states accelerate the heart-rate while some that are painful and disagreeable may cause inhibition to the point of fainting. It is through the hypothalamus that these impulses reach the cardiac centre.

2. HORMONAL CONTROL

Vasoconstrictor agents : Epinephrine and norepinephrine. Medulla of adrenal gland secretes these two hormones. Both has vasoconstrictor effect in almost all vascular beds of the body.

Angiotensin : It is one of the most powerful vasoconstrictor substance. When there is decrease in arterial pressure, the kidneys secrete a substance called *renin* substrate, which gives vasoactive peptide *angiotensin*. Angiotensin in turn has a number of important effects on the circulation related to arterial pressure control, but most importantly to constrict the blood vessels everywhere in the body. As little as one ten-millionth of a gram of angiotensin can increase the arterial pressure of a human being as much as 10 to 20 mm Hg.

Vassopressin : Also called *antidiuretic hormone*, is formed in the hypothalamus but is transported down the centre of nerve axons to the posterior pituitary gland, where it is eventually secreted into the blood. It is even more powerful than angiotensin as a vasoconstrictor.

Vasodilator Agents

Bradykinin : Several substances called *kinins* (small polypeptides that are split away from α_2-globulins in the plasma or tissue fluids) can cause vasodilation. One of the these substances is *bradykinin*. This once formed persists for only a few minutes, because it is digested by the enzyme *carboxypeptidase* or by converting enzyme. Bradykinin causes very powerful *arteriolar dilation* and also *increased capillary permeability.*

Serotonin : (5-hydroxy tryptamine) is present in large concentration in the chromaffin tissue of the intestine and other abdominal structures; and also in the platelets. Serotonin can have either a vasodilator or vasoconstrictor effect, depending on the condition or the area of the circulation.

Histamine : Histamine is released in essentially every tissue of the body whenever it becomes damaged. Probably it is derived from mast cells in the damaged cells and from basophills in the blood. It has a powerful vasodilator effect on the arterioles, and has ability to increase capillary porosity, allowing leakage of both fluid and plasma protein into the tissues.

Prostaglandins : Almost all tissue of the body under physiological and pathological conditions, contain several chemically related substances called prostaglandins. These have both vasoconstriction and vasodilatory effects.

3. EFFECTS OF DIFFERENT IONS AND OTHER CHEMICAL FACTORS ON VASCULAR CONTROL

Rate and force of contraction of the heart is subjected to chemical influence of the extracellular fluid in which the heart is bathed or with which it is perfused. Though the roles of these substances in the overall *regulation* of the circulation generally are not known, their specific effects can be listed as follows:

An increase in calcium ion concentration causes vasoconstriction because it stimulate smooth muscle contraction. An increase in *potassium* ion concentration causes vasodilation. Thus results from the ability of potassium ions to inhibit smooth muscle contraction. An increase in *magnesium ion* concentration causes powerful vasodilation, for magnesium ions inhibit smooth muscle generally.

Increased *sodium ion* concentration causes arteriolar dilatation. This results mainly from an increase in osmolality of the fluids rather than from a specific effect of sodium ion itself. *Increased osmolality* of the blood caused by increased quantities of *glucose* or other non-vasoactive substances, also causes arteriolar dilatation. Decreased osmolality causes arteriolar constriction.

The only anions to have significant effects on blood vessels are *acetate* and *citrate*, both of which cause mild degrees of vasodilation.

An increase in *hydrogen ion concentration* (decrease in pH) causes dilatation of the arterioles. A *slight* decrease *in hydrogen ion* concentration causes arteriolar constriction, but an intense decrease causes dilation, which is the same effect as that which occurs with increased hydrogen ion concentration.

An increase in CO_2 concentration causes moderate vasodilation in most tissues and marked vasodilation in the brain.. However, CO_2, acting on the vasomotor centre, has an extremely powerful indirect vasoconstrictor effect that is transmitted through the sympathetic vasoconstrictor system.

4. THERMAL CONTROL

Generally rise in temperature brings about an increase in the rate of heart beat. This is true both in poikilothems and homeotherms. Q_{10} is a measure (see thermoregulation) of such an increase in beats per 10°C rise in temperature. It has been found that generally the heart rate doubles by 10°C rise in temperature. Rise in temperature acts directly on S-A node and indirectly via the temperature regulating centres in the hypothalamus which relay excitatory impulses to the cardio-accelerating centre.

3

RESPIRATION

Voluntary and involuntary activities of body needs a continuous and steady supply of energy. This energy is obtained from the oxidation of food substances. When such energy is liberated, two poisonous substances CO_2 and H are produced as a by-product. It is essential to expel out these bi-products of oxidation, the poisonous H is immediately combined with oxygen to produce H_2O which is non-poisonous and which gets incorporated into the body fluid, CO_2 is produced not directly from the combination of carbon with oxygen but from the oxidative decarboxylation of keto acids in the citric acid cycles. In this way the body is constantly in need of oxygen. *This cellular process of oxygen use; energy liberation and carbon dioxide release is called respiration.*

In a simple language, the respiration can be said as the gas exchange between an organism and its environment *i.e.,* Oxygen is taken in and CO_2 is expelled out of the body. In many lower animals such as protozoans, coelenterates, flatworms etc. the gas exchanges is not a complex problem. These animals are capable of obtaining oxygen from air or water by simple diffusion through moist body surface. In higher animals, supply of oxygen to every cell is not so simple, it is done by a special system of tubules and sacs which is called *respiratory system*, which involves the gas exchange first between the blood and the air (external respiration) and second between the blood and the individual cell (internal respiration).

Kinds of Respiration

Respiration is a general process taking place in the presence or absence of oxygen. On the basis of presence or absence of oxygen it can be classified in two types.

1. *Aerobic respiration* : Most of the animals from protozoans to mammals including man .respire in the presence of oxygen. They take oxygen from their environment whether it is water or air. In the oxidation oxygen unites with carbon and hydrogen, forming carbon dioxide and water, and sets free the energy. In chemical terms it can be expressed as :

$$C_6H_{12}O_6 + 6O_2 \rightarrow 6\,CO_2 + 6H_2O + \text{energy}$$

carbohydrate oxygen carbondioxide water

2. *Anaerobic respiration* : It occurs in the absence of oxygen, but CO_2 is given out. Here the oxidation of carbohydrates, and possibly of fats is incomplete, only part of the energy is released and certain intermediate compounds are formed. It occurs in certain bacteria, yeast cells and in the parasitic worms like *Ascaris* and *Taenia solium*.

(I) *Respiratory organs* : In many simple animals such as protozoans, coelenterates and worms the gaseous exchange occurs directly through the body surfaces by diffusion, they have no special respiratory organs. Two conditions may be found in such animals–

1. Lack of a circulatory system and the distance between the internal cells and the body surfaces is not too much, simple diffusion fulfils the respiratory needs, examples, protozoans, coelenterates, etc.
2. A circulatory system is present and the oxygen absorbed from the body surfaces dissolves in the transport medium of circulatory system and is carried to the distantly located .cells. In the second situation, body surface or the integument acts as a respiratory organs. In some animals, certains parts of the body wall become specially respiratory. The gills of arthropods, molluscs, fishes and tadpoles, etc., are in a way special integumentary parts.

For atmospheric respiration, the terrestrial animals possess *tracheae* (insects etc.) and lungs (vertebrates, land molluscs etc.). However, from point of view of physiology following are the different respiratory organs..

Cutaneous Respiration

Gases move very slowly through the protoplasm. It has been estimated that diffusion alone cannot fulfil the respiratory needs of the organisms with diameter of more than 1 mm. The precise size limits depend not only on the rate of metabolism but also on the shape of the animal, any departure from the spherical will increase the surface area relative to the mass. Thus, a number of smaller metazoans and the larvae of much larger ones exceed the 1 mm diameter range. Giant land planerians (Terricola) are large and flat, the flatness lead to increase in surface area. In spite of their large size the coelenterates and sponges are able to manage respiration without having any special respiratory organs their metabolic needs are small and the oxygen diffusion distance is short on account of thin body walls. Besides, these organism have a variety of water circulatory devices like canals and spaces which help to increase the oxygen diffusion.

Principally, the occurrence of an efficient circulatory system in the body increases the rate of gaseous exchange through the skin and specially when the circulating fluid (blood) contain some respiratory pigment. The cutaneous respiration occurs in many annelids generally and in amphibians and fishes as a supplementary method. The *Chaetopterus* (annelid) possesses modified parapodia to move water over the skin for respiration. In frog, even when it is on land a sufficient amount of oxygen-carbon dioxide diffusion occurs through the skin. Relatively, very little respiration occurs in the buccal cavity of frog, because the capillary surface is very little. In many species the lungs and skin have almost the same capillary area and they contribute differently in respiration, for example, in the dry skin forms (toads) the cutaneous respiration is 20% or even less, where as in the aquatic form like *Triturus alpestris* it is nearly 76%.

Cutaneous respiration can-only be successful when the surfaces are thin, wet and well vascularized, soft covering are vulnerable to predators and prone to abrasion. A more permeable surface presents greater problems of transport of electrolytes and of water-balance. The terrestrial animals have to face a grave danger of the, drying of skin or the consequent loss of water leading to a substantial fall in gas exchange. Skin-respiring crustaceans generally have thin chitinous cuticle, ordinarily possess only small body size. In the eel fishes, 60% of the O_2 requirement is filled up through skin.

Gill or Branchial Respiration

Any body-appendage which serves for gaseous exchange through the aquatic medium, is termed a gill. Typically gills are filamentous structures richly supplied with blood capillaries. The size of the gills depends upon the amount of oxygen in water where such organisms are living. When they five in highly oxygenated water, their gills grow very slowly and when they live in water poor in oxygen the gills grow very large. The amount of gill surface is related to the habits of the organisms, sluggish bottom dwelling organisms have less surface area than rapidly moving organisms. The gills are of various types which differ widely.

External gills : They can be defined as the specialised areas or the skin where the external surface is folded and covered by thin vascular and permeable skin. External gills are normally branched but may be filamentous.

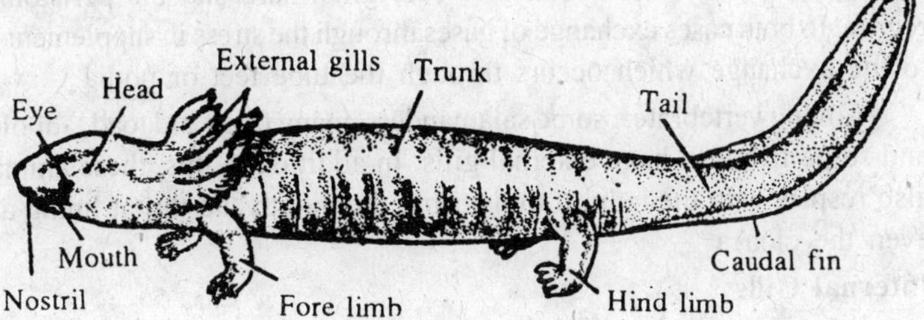

Fig. 3.1 : Necturus.

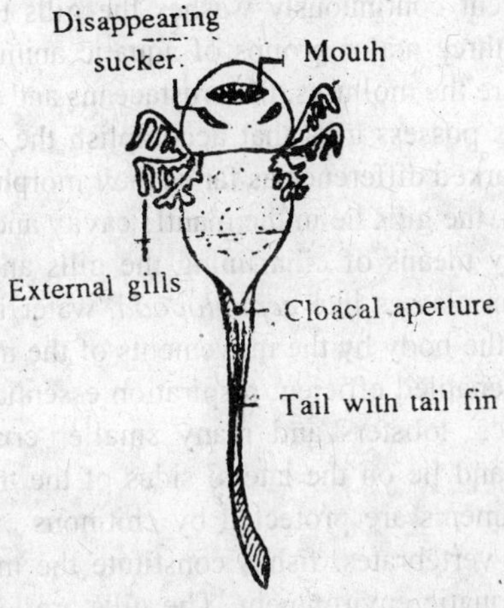

Fig. 3.2 : Tadpole showing external gills.

Polychaetes represent the best example of animals possessing external gills. These animals secrete or consolidate around their bodies hard, protective tubes through which gaseous exchange cannot occur. Many of these worms have fine, thread like gill filaments that project outside of the tube on and often to allow the gaseous exchange between the blood that flows through them and the respiratory medium. Others have shorter appendages that serves as gills. Filamentous gills are especially common among some of the marine worms that live in muddy layers at the bottom of the ocean where oxygen is often very less or totally absent due to the bacterial activity. In this case, the gills extend above the mud into oxygenated water to enable efficient gaseous exchange. In echinoderms (asteroid) body is rather uniformly clothed with hollow, papillate, body wall extensions from the coelom (papulae), while in most echinoids five pairs of small branched structures (the gills) surround the peristomial region. In both cases exchange of gases through the stress in supplementary to the exchange which occurs through the tube feet or podia.

Among vertebrates, some salamanders, many frogs and toad tadpoles, and some fish also have external gills. In addition to this, these animals also respire with the help of moist skin, the mouth and throat lining and even the cloaca.

Internal Gills

In active animals, gills have become internal to avoid the injury and attack of predators and parasites. The internal gills are located inside a cavity and usually contain a common protective flap, the *operculum*. The respiratory current continuously washes the gills to facilitate gaseous exchange. The three major groups of aquatic animals possessing such protected gills are the molluscs, the crustaceans and the fishes. Although the three groups possess gills that accomplish the same functions, but there exists a marked difference as far as their morphology is concerned.

In molluscs, the gills lie in the mantle cavity and water is circulated through them by means of cilia lining the gills and mantle cavity. In higher molluscan classes like *cephalopoda*, water is drawn inside and expelled out of the body by the movements of the muscular walls. This mechanism has enabled efficient respiration essential for an active life.

In crayfishes, lobsters and many smaller crustaceans, gills are relatively large and lie on the lateral sides of the thoracic region. The delicate gill filaments are protected by chitinous exoskeleton.

Among the vertebrates, fishes constitute the most dominant class inhabiting the aquatic environment. The gills are located on the edges of a series of lateral openings from the pharynx. There are often 4 to 5 openings or gill slits on each side of the pharynx. Anteriorly there may also be a pair of modified slits, the spiracles, one on each side, often specialized for water intake in bottom dwellers like rays. In sharks and rays the gill slits open directly to the outside, whereas in most of the bony fish, several gill slits open into an external chamber on each side lateral to the pharynx. The chamber in turn is protected by the operculum.

The rate of water-current flowing constantly over the internal gills, depend on the oxygen needs of the body. In these, the flow of water-current and the circulation of blood is in opposite direction (counter flow principle) and thus a maximum gradient is developed between the inner and outer environments.

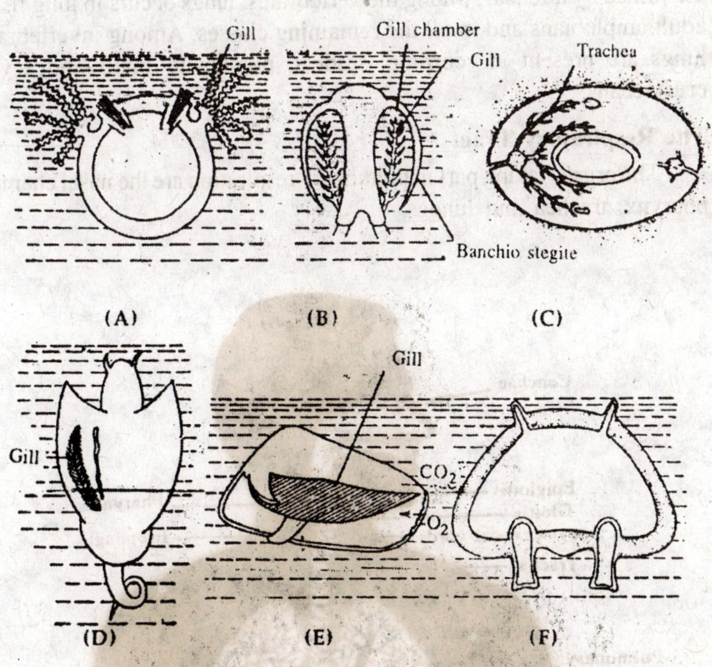

Fig. 3.3 : Invertebrate respiratory organs. A–T.S. of gill region of lungworm; B– T.S. of cephalothorax of cray fish; C-T.S. of an insect; D-A winkle removed from the shell and with mantle cavity opened to show gills; E- A mussel with one valve of the shell removed to show left gill; F-A starfish, T.S. of arm to show gills and tubefeet.

Lung or Pulmonary Respiration

Lungs are the internal vascularized cavities of air sacs where air and blood are brought together. They are the main breathing organs and function as aerial ventilators. Morphologically they consists of much elaborated respiration. Surface of maximum exposure within a minimum space, together with a system of noncollapsible passage way for admitting air from the outside, that passes over these respiration surfaces in intimate juxtra position with capillaries.

The lungs are highly elastic and capsulated in a double pleural sac, in the higher vertebrates. They are freely movable within the sac, except at the point of their attachment near the base of the bronchi, where they are joined by trachea. Among the vertebrates, lungs occurs in lung fishes, adult amphibians and in all the remaining classes. Among invertebrates, lungs are present in scorpion, spiders, pulmonate snails and several crustaceans.

The Respiratory Tract

The organs taking part in pulmonary respiration are the nasal chamber, pharynx, trachea and lungs.

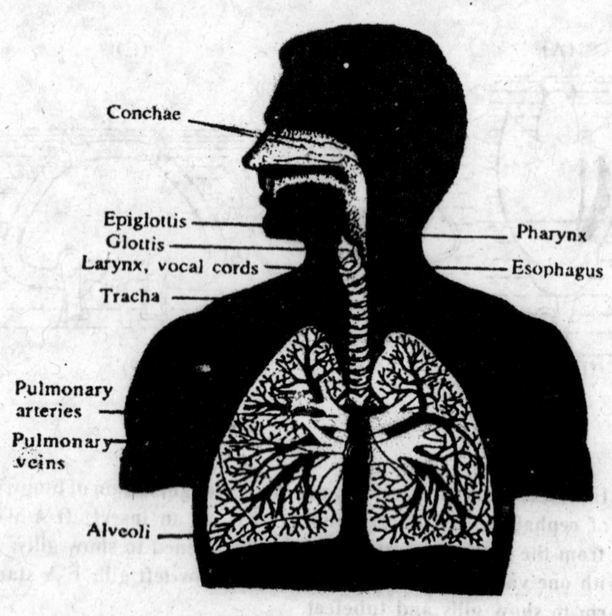

Fig. 3.4: The respiratory passages.

Nasal chamber : The space between external and internal nostrils is the *nasal chamber*. In most of the vertebrates external nostrils remain open. In mammals the nasal chamber is divided into right and left halves by a cartilage called *mesethmoid*.

The walls of the nasal chamber are variously enlarged in different vertebrates by scroll-like *turbinal bones*, which not only increases the moist vascular surface, but also prevent an easy entrance of undesirable objects by making the passage way tortuous. Each half of the nasal chamber is further differentiated into three regions.

(i) *Vestibular part* : This is anterior most region of the nasal chamber. It has hairs to remove dust and other foreign particles from air getting in.

(ii) *Respiratory part* : This is the air conditioning chamber. The tissues are richly supplied with capillaries thus providing moisture and certain degree of warmth for incoming air.

(iii) *Sensory or olfactory part* : In this the ethmoturbinal is covered with sensory membrane, the *Schneiderian membrane* that helps in the detection of smell.

Pharynx

Nasal chamber opens into pharynx. In human beings the respiratory channel in the roof is separated from the food channel by the development of *palate*. In this the respiratory and food passage cross each other forming *pharyngeal chiasma*; also to prevent food entry into respiratory tube, epiglottis is developed in the sound box.

Larynx

In most of the vertebrates larynx is the sound producing organ that is why also known *as sound box*. In man the larynx is known as *Adam's*

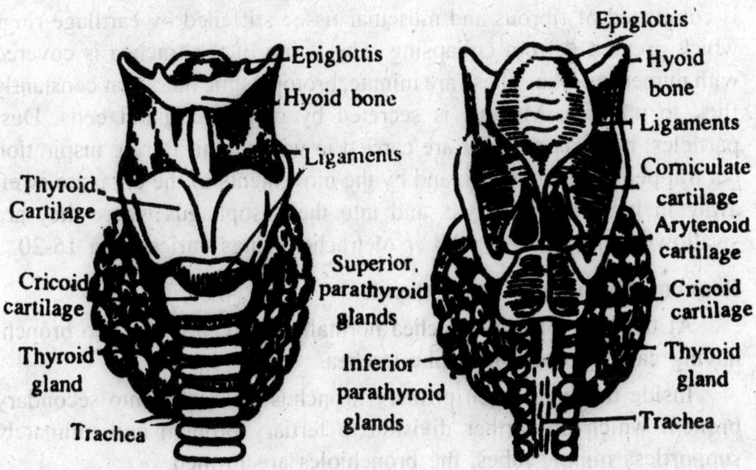

Fig. 3.5 : Larynx showing anterior and posterior view.

apple (Pomum Adami) and is supported by four cartilages, the largest one is *thyroid cartilage*, and is located on ventral side of the larynx, a ring like *cricoid cartilage* and a pair of *arytenoid cartilages*. The Free ends of arytenoid develop into cartilage of *santorini.* In some mammals small *corniculate* and *cuneiform* cartilages are arranged in close association with the arytenoid cartilages. Mammals have two parts of vocal cords between thyroid cartilage and arytenoid cartilage. Anterior pair of vocal cords is the *false vocal cords*, while posterior one is the pair of true *vocal cords*. False vocal cords connect the anterior part of arytenoid with the anterior part of thyroid cartilage, while the true vocal cords connect the posterior part of arytenoid with the anterior part of thyroid cartilage.

Each of the true vocal cords consists of a band like fold of yellow elastic tissue. They are covered by a thin layer of mucous membrane with a stratified squamous epithelium. The portion of the larynx in front of the true vocal cords is called the *vestibule*.

In human males, the larynx increases considerably in size and becomes much larger than that of the females. The enlarged vocal cords are responsible for the lower pitch of the musculine voice.

Trachea

It is also known as *wind pipe*. It is a rigid tube. The wall of trachea is composed of fibrous and muscular tissue stiffened by cartilage rings which prevent it from collapsing. The lining of the trachea is covered with numerous cilia. These are minute, protoplasmic hairs that constantly flick to and fro. Mucous is secreted by columnar gland cells. Dust particles, bacteria etc. that are carried in with the air during inspiration get trapped in mucous film and by the movements of the cilia, are sweft away in it up to the larynx and into the oesophagus where they are swallowed. In man the number of tracheal rings varies from 16-20.

Bronchi, Bronchioles and Alveoli

At the base of neck, trachea normally bifurcates into two bronchi having cartilagenous rings like trachea.

Inside the lungs each primary bronchus bifurcates into secondary bronchi which on further division to tertiary bronchi and ultimately supportless minute tubes, the bronchioles are formed.

Each bronchiole terminates in alveolar sac. Air sacs have exceedingly thin delicate highly elastic walls over the outside of which extends a closely woven maze of capillaries. Each alveolus is approximately 0.1 mm in diameter and has a thin wall 0.5 μ in thickness. In human beings lungs have about 750,000,000 alveoli covering the total area 100sq. metre which is 50 times than the surface area of skin.

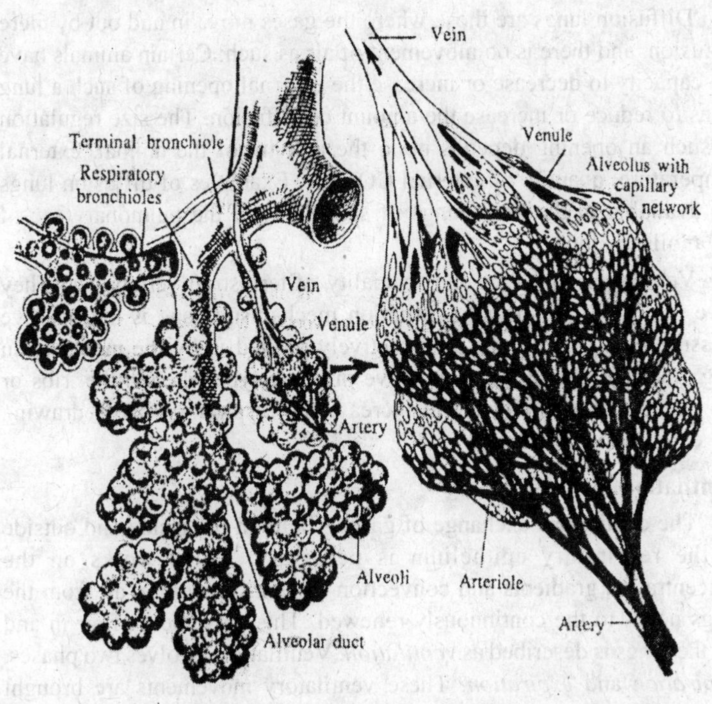

Fig. 3.6 : Structure of the mammalian lung.

The alveoli of the lung are analogous to connected soap bubbles, and because they are of different size, it might be expected that in their unstable condition they would collapse. It has been discovered that this does not happen because of the presence of substance called *pulmonary surfactant* in the fluid lining of the alveoli forming thin molecular layer over the surface. Surfactant is secreted by a special cell type in the respiratory epithelium; it is a phospholipoprotein containing dipalmitoyl lecithin. A unique feature of surfactant is that its surface tension increases as the lungs expand; when the lungs collapse, the surface tension is very low. If this did not happen it would be extremely difficult or impossible to refill a collapsed lung-as is the case in a few newborn babies who produce insufficient surfactant.

The lungs can be of two types.

(1) Diffusion lungs and (2) ventilation lungs

Diffusion lungs are those where the gases move in and out by mere diffusion, and there is no movement of air as such. Certain animals have the capacity to decrease or increase the external opening of such a lung so as to reduce or increase the amount of diffusion. The size regulation of such an opening depends upon the activity of the animal, external temperature, quantity of external CO_2, etc. Examples of diffusion lungs are available in the book-lungs of scorpion and the pulmonary sac of the molluscs lung.

Ventilation lungs are the speciality of terrestrial vertebrates. They have two kinds of special ventilation mechanisms, one is the positive pressure type wherein the air is actively pushed in by the mouth as in frog, and the second is the negative pressure type wherein the .ribs or the diaphragm, or both, act to increase the respiratory cavity drawing the external air passively.

Ventilation

The continuous exchange of gases - both on the inside and outside of the respiratory epithelium is necessary; which works on the concentration gradients and convection current. Therefore, air from the lungs needs to the continuously renewed. This movement of air in and out the lungs is described as *ventilation.* Ventilation involves two phases, *inspiration* and *expiration.* These ventilatory movements are brought about by special muscles.

Mechanism of Ventilation

The thoracic cavity is a closed box supported by mid-dorsally by vertebral column, midventrally by the mobile sternum and laterally by the ribs. It is separated from the abdominal cavity by a muscular diaphragm. The lungs themselves are enclosed by a double serous membrane known as *pleura.* Out of these; the inner *visceral pleura* invests the lungs and the outer parietal pleura lines the thoracic wall. These two layers are separated by a thin cavity filled with lymph. At the root of the lungs the two layers are however continuous with one another.

In the early development lungs completely fill the thoracic cavity but later thorax increases in volume than the lungs, as a result lungs are stretched away from the thoracic box. This results in lowering the intrapleural pressure within the pleural cavity to an extent of 3 to 4 mm Hg less than atmospheric air pressure. This negative intrapleural pressure prevents excess collapse of the lungs. Collapsing power of the lungs equals to 3 to 4 mm Hg pressure only.

Mechanism of ventilation

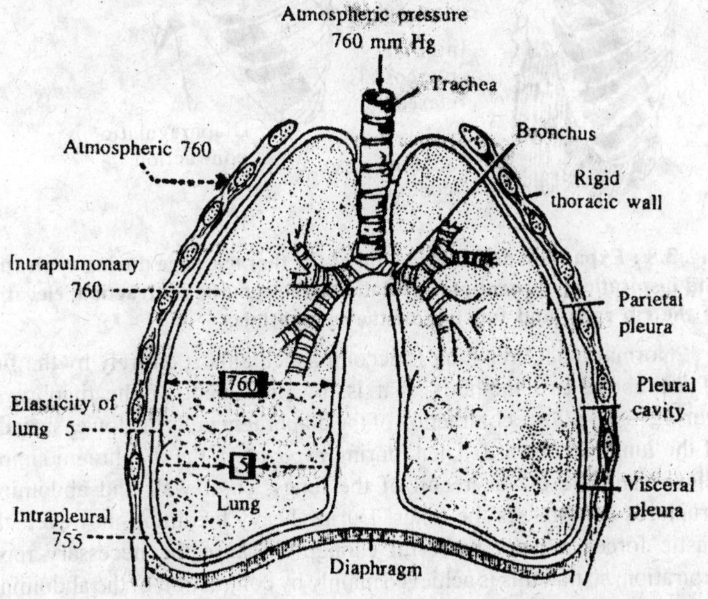

Fig. 3.7: Diagram of the structures of thoracic cavity, showing intrapulmonary and intra-pleural pressures with in resting position.

Breathing is simply the mechanical process of taking air into the lungs (inspiration) and letting it out again (expiration). To carry out this process expansion and contraction of lung is essential and this can be done in two ways:

1. by downward and upward movement of the diaphragm to lengthen or shorten the chest cavity, and
2. by elevation and depression of the ribs to increase and decrease the anteroposterior diameter of the chest cavity.

Fig. 3.8 illustrates these two methods.

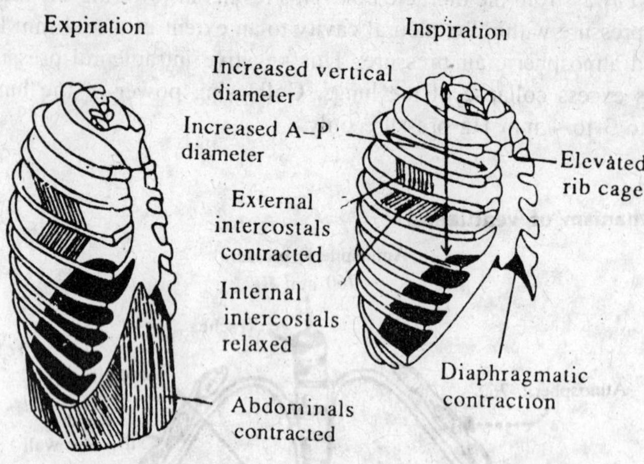

Fig. 3.8 : Expansion and contraction of the thoracic cage during expiration and inspiration, illustrating especially diaphragmatic contraction, elevation of the rib cage, and function of the intercostals.

Normal quiet breathing is accomplished almost entirely by the first of the above two methods, that is, by movement of the diaphragm. During *inspiration*., contraction of the diaphragm pulls the lower surfaces of the lungs downward. Then, during *expiration*, the diaphragm simply relaxes and the elastic recoil of the lungs, chest wall and abdominal structures compresses the lungs. During heavy breathing, however, the elastic forces are not powerful enough to cause the necessary rapid expiration, so that this is achieved mainly by contraction of the abdominal muscles, which forces the abdominal contents upward against the bottom of the diaphragm.

The second method for expanding the lungs is to raise the rib cage. This expands the lungs because, in the natural resting position, the ribs slant downward, thus allowing the sternum to fall backward toward the spinal column. But, when the rib cage is elevated, the ribs project directly forward so that the sternum now also moves forward away from the spine, making the anteroposterior thickness of the chest about 20% greater during maximum inspiration than during expiration. Therefore, those muscles that elevate the chest cage can be classified as muscles of inspiration and those muscles that depress the chest cage, as muscles of expiration. The muscles that raise the rib cage include;

(1) the *sternocleidomastoid* muscle that lift upward on the sternum;

(2) the *anterior serrati* that lift many of the ribs,

(3) the *scaleni* that lift the first two ribs, and the *external intercostals*.

The muscles that pull the rib cage downward during expiration are:

1. The *abdominal recti*, which have the powerful effect of pulling downward on the lower ribs at the same time that they and the other abdominal muscles also compress the abdominal contents upward toward the diaphragm; and 2. the *internal intercostals*.

Fig. 3.8 illustrates the mechanism by which the external and internal intercostals act to cause inspiration and expiration. To the left, the ribs during expiration are angled downward and the external intercostals are elongated in a forward and downward direction. As they contract, they pull the upper ribs forward in relation to the lower ribs and this causes leverage on the ribs to raise them upward. Conversely, in the inspiratory position, the internal intercostals are elongated, and their contraction pulls the upper ribs backward in relation to the lower ribs. This causes leverage in opposite direction and lowers the chest cage.

Respiratory Pressures

The respiratory muscles cause pulmonary ventilation by alternatively compressing and distending the lungs, which inturn causes the pressure in the alveoli to rise and fall. During inspiration the intra-alveolar pressure becomes slightly negative with respect to atmospheric pressure, normally slightly less than –1 mm Hg, and this causes air to flow inward through the respiratory passage ways. During normal expiration, on the other hand, the intra-alveolar pressure rises to slightly less than + 1 mm Hg, which causes air to flow outward through the respiratory passage ways. Means, how little pressure is required to move the air into and out of the normal lung.

During maximum expiratory effort with the glottis closed and the intra- alveolar pressure can be increased to as much as 140mm Hg in the strong, healthy man, and during maximum inspiratory effort it can be reduced to as low as-100 mm Hg.

In general, during inspiration, the alveolar pressure falls below the atmospheric one so air rushes in and during expiration, alveolar pressure goes above the atmospheric pressure and thus air goes out. Thus, the normal breathing is of negative pressure breathing. But if the atmospheric pressure is raised above the normal alveolar pressure, then the maintenance of respiration is of positive pressure breathing.

The Pulmonary Volumes

The average healthy adult has 14 to 18 breathes a minute. During every breathe the lungs exchange volumes of air with the atmosphere. The apparatus commonly used to measure the amount of air exchanged during breathing is referred to as and *spirometer* or *respirometer*.

In Fig. 3.9 are listed four different pulmonary lung "volumes" which, when added together, equal the maximum volume to which the lungs can be expanded. These are as follows:

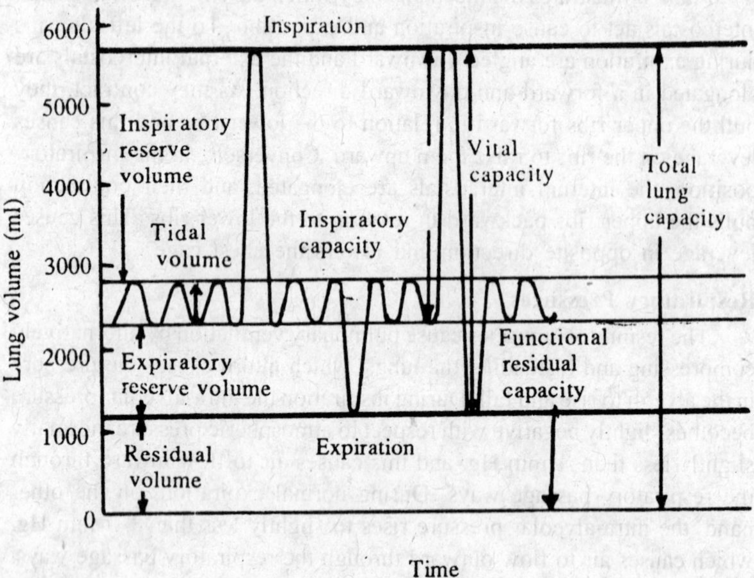

Fig. 3.9 : Showing different pulmonary lung volumes and pulmonary capacities.

1. The *tidal volume* is the volume of air inspired or expired with each normal breath, and it amounts to about 500 ml in the average young adult man.
2. The *inspiratory reserve volume* is the extra volume of air that can be inspired over and beyond the normal tidal volume, and if is usually equal to approximately 3000 mls.
3. The expiratory reserve volume is the amount of air that can still be expired by forceful expiration after the end of a normal tidal expiration; this normally amounts to about 1100 mls.

4. The *residual volume* is the volume of air still remaining in the lungs after the most forceful expiration. This volume averages about 1200 mls.

The Pulmonary "Capacities"

1. The *inspiratory capacity* equals the *tidal volume* plus the *inspiratory reserve volume.* This is the amount of air (about 3500 ml) that a person can breathe beginning at the normal expiratory level and distending the lungs to the maximum amount.
2. The *functional residual capacity* equals the expiratory *reserve volume* plus the *residual volume.* This is the amount of air remaining in the lungs at the end of normal expiration (about 2300ml),
3. The *vital capacity* equals the inspiratory *reserve volume* plus the *tidal volume* plus the expiratory reserve volume. This is the maximum amount of air that a person can expel from the lungs after first filling the lungs to their maximum extent and then expiring to the maximum extent (about 4600ml).
4. The *total lung capacity* is the maximum volume to which the lungs can be expanded with the greatest possible inspiratory effort (about 5800ml); it is equal to the vital capacity plus the *residual volume.*

All pulmonary volumes and capacities are about 20 to 25 per cent less in women than in men, and they obviously are greater in large and athletic persons than in small and asthenic persons.

Respiratory Rate

The respiratory rate varies as per the age. Man breathes about 500 ml of tidal air at every breath. The rate is 20 times a minute. Thus the *minute volume* or the amount of fresh air taken into the lungs is about 10 litres/minute (500 × 20 = 10,000). It is also called as pulmonary ventilation rate. In exercise the rate can increase to as much as 125 litres/minute. The respiratory rate is increased by following factors:

1. **Temperature :** As is seen during fever;
2. **Oxygen lack** : As one goes to high altitude where there is low oxygen concentration in the air;
3. **Carbon dioxide excess :** As occurs during exercise.

REGULATION OF RESPIRATION

The rate of respiration is determined both by nervous and chemical control.

Nervous control : In mammals, four centres have been localised in the medulla oblongata that are involved in the regulation of breathing, they are as follows:

1. Inspiratory centres,
2. Expiratory centres
3. Apneustic centre and
4. Pneumotaxic centre.

Inspiratory centre which send stimuli to muscles of thorax and diaphragm resulting in the expansion of the thoracic cage followed by inspiration. Such impulses are sent rhythmically to maintain the rate and force of respiration constant.

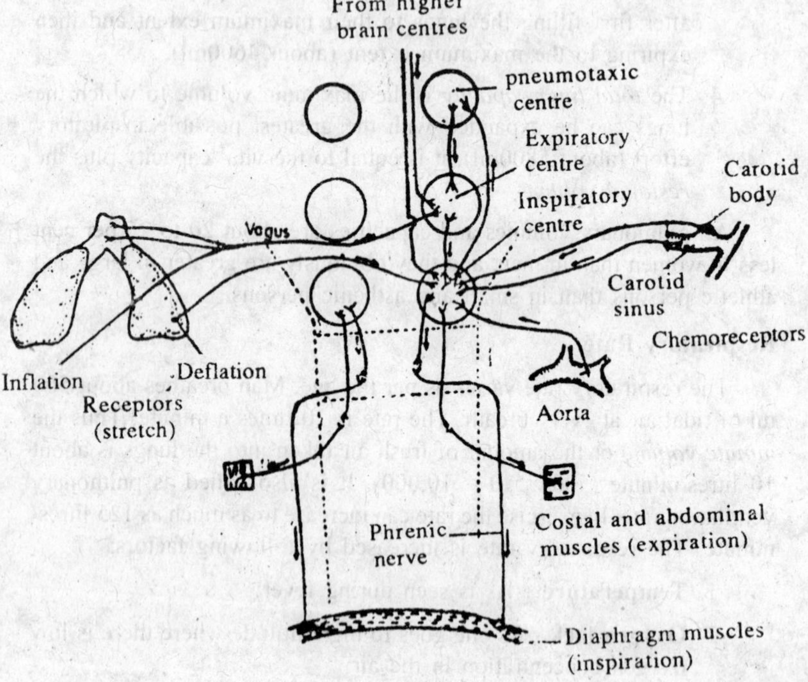

Fig. 3.10 : Reflex regulation of ventilation.

When the rate of breathing increases above the required level, expiratory centres are stimulated which in turn inhibit the inspiratory centres. The overriding influence of expiratory centres results in an interruption in the excitation to the inspiratory muscles of the thorax and diaphragm and passive exhalation follows. Ordinarily, exhalation requires no input of energy, rather the potential energy acquired by the stretched tissue during inhalation is sufficient for it.

Activities of inspiratory and expiratory centres are .superimposed by the *apneustic* and pneumotaxic centres in medulla. Messages from the apneustic centre bring about prolonged inhalation while those of the pneumotaxic centres inhibit the apneustic type of breathing, thus accelerating ventilation in accordance with different physiological states.

Vagal control (Hearing–Breuer reflex) : There are special stretch or inflation receptors in the lung tissue, these are innervated by afferent fibres of vagus nerve. When both vagi are cut, respiration becomes slow and deep. If, then, the central end of the cut vagus be stimulated, respiration becomes more or less normal in rate and depth. Since action of vagi slows down inhibit respiration and since stimulation of the central cut ends makes the respiration normal, it is likely that during normal respiratory movements some sensory impulses pass up the vagi and help to make the rate and depth of respiration normal. This inhibition of respiration by lung inflation was first described by Hearing and Breuer in 1868, so called Hearing-Breuer Reflex.

Reflex effects : The following factors adjust respiration by affecting respiratory centres reflexly.

(a) *Cough reflex* : Cough is a sudden forcible expiratory act. It is a protecting reflex. Irritation of the laryngeal mucous membrane produces cough. Its purpose is to drive out irritants and foreign bodies.

(b) Sneezing : Irritation of nasal mucosa produces this reflex.

(c) Swallowing reflex

(d) *Reflexes from carotid sinus and aortic arch* : Carotid and aortic bodies are the chemoreceptors and detectors of blood CO_2 and O_2 levels. They are small nodules of vascular and neurosensory tissue. Each one is about 2-5 mm in diameter. The carotid bodies are located bilaterally in the bifurcations of the common carotid arteries and aortic bodies are located along the arch of the aorta. They are supplied by carotid blood and receive fibres from cervical sympathetic, the glossopharyngeal and vagus nerves.

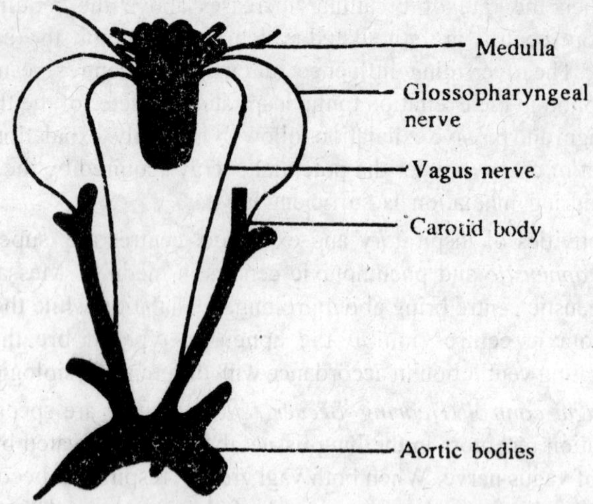

Fig. 3.11 : Respiratory control by the carotid and aortic bodies.

Carotid body is most sensitive to the O_2 content of the blood, and if the O_2 level falls, these chemoreceptors initiate impulses which are conducted to the respiratory centre where they stimulate the inspiratory cells. This stimulation can result in increased rate of respiration. Thus either an increased concentration of CO_2 or a decreased level of O_2 in blood will increase the ventilation of the lungs.

Chemical Regulation

The respiratory centre is highly sensitive to alterations in chemical composition of blood. Changes of CO_2 tension, O_2 tension and H-ion concentration alter pulmonary ventilation profoundly. In any case, the main purpose is to adjust respiration in such a way that it may be able to meet the demands of the body adequately.

1. **Effect of alteration of CO_2 tension :** Respiratory centre is extremely sensitive to slight alteration in CO_2 tension. A slight rise in CO_2 tension in the inspired air increases respiration enormously. In other words, breathing air containing upto 5.0% CO_2 will not do any harm, although respiration will be stimulated. But if CO_2 content is raised further, the alveolar CO_2 will rise. This will lead to accumulation of CO_2 in the blood and thereby cause the toxic effects of acidosis. CO_2 acts on the respiratory centre both directly as well as reflexly through *sino-aortic bodies*. Excess CO_2 stimulates and reduced CO_2 depresses respiration.

2. **Effect of Changes of O_2 tension**

(a) *Effects of O_2 lacks* : The results of O_2 lack will vary according to the rapidity and the severity with which the lack is produced. If severe O_2 lack is produced very rapidly, the results will be disastrous (*anoxia*). In the gradual reduction of O_2 pressure, it is seen that O_2 tension in the inspired air can be reduced to 13% without any appreciable change of respiration and any discomfort on the part of the subject. But with the further reduction, respiration starts rising with a feeling of uneasiness. This shows that the respiration apparatus is much less sensitive to O_2 lack than CO_2 excess.

(b) *Effects of O_2 excess* : 60% O_2 mixture can be breathed continuously for any length of time without any distress. 75% O_2 mixture can be tolerated for several days, after which ill effects appear and the animal dies. Pure O_2 at one atmosphere pressure can be breathed for a few hours without any ill-effect. When the O_2 pressure is raised to several atmosphere, the animal develops convolutions and dies rapidly. Human beings develop bad effects in less than one hour (fainting, low blood pressure etc.), if they are exposed to O_2 at four atmospheric pressure.

3. **Effect of H ion concentration :** Blood has a definite ratio of OH and H ions *i.e.*, 20% which represents the acid-base balance and equals pH 7.4. Increase in CO_2 content of the blood decreases the ratio of OH and H ions and pH is lowered ($H_2O + CO_2 = H_2CO_3$, $H_2CO_3 = H + HCO_3$). This condition is called as *acidosis*. This acidosis produced, stimulates the respiratory centres and the acidity of urine and excretion of ammonia salts is also increased. Thus, normal pH is attained. High degree of acidosis leads in Coma, while blood pH below 6-9 proves fatal.

If larger volume of CO_2 is expelled, a opposite effect called *alkalosis* will be produced. Decrease in H_2CO_3 increases the pH of blood. Lack of stimulation (less CO_2 content) induces ceasation of respiration till sufficient amount of CO_2 is formed and retained in the body to lower the pH to its normal value of 7.4. Severe alkalosis is accompanied by tetany and increased expulsion of alkaline salts.

Additionally, *emotions* which are due to intense activity of the cerebral cells have a depressing effect on the respiratory centre resulting in shallow and slow breathing. This adds to accumulation of CO_2 content of the blood which washes out the inhibitory influences from cerebral hemispheres. A deep inspiration is then followed by deep audible expiration the *sigh.* Influence of emotions can be marked in laughing, crying etc.

Respiratory Pigments

Four different respiratory pigments are recognized, haemoglobin, chlorocruorin, hemocyanin and haemerythrin. They are quite different biochemically. Even in the same phylum there may be several distinct pigments, and more than one pigment may exist in the same animal (Fig. 3.12). One can only generalize by saying that they are coloured proteins (chromoproteins) that contain a metallic element in their constitution and have the property of forming loose combinations with oxygen and sometimes with carbon dioxide. Table 3.1 lists the four pigments with their distribution and some of their properties.

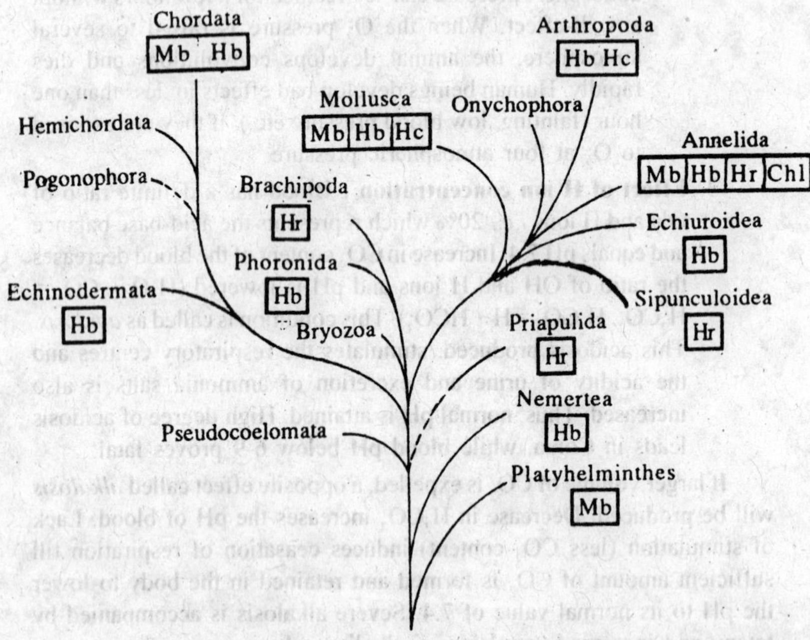

Fig. 3.12 : Distribution of the respiratory pigments in the animal kingdom, Chl, chlorocruorin; Hb, haemoglobin; Hc; hemocyanin; Hr, haemerythrin; Mb, myoglobin.

Haemoglobin : This is the most familiar, the most widespread, and the most efficient of the respiratory pigments. It is familiar because of its presence in human blood, but it occurs also in the plant world, in some protozoans, and in most of the major animal phyla. As indicated in Table 3.1, the most efficient haemoglobins combine with far greater amounts of oxygen than any of the other pigments.

Table 3.1 : Oxygen Capacities of Some Different Bloods (Values for usual Physiological and Environmental Conditions).

Pigment	Color	Site	Animal	Oxygen (volume per cent)	Molecular weight
Haemoglobin	Red	Corpuscles	Mammals	15-30	6.8×10^4
			Birds	10-25	
			Reptiles	7-12	
			Amphibians	6-13	
			Fishes (gnathostoma)	1-16	
			Cyclostomes	1-2	1.7×10^4
		Plasma	Annelids	5-15	3.0×10^6
			Molluscs	1-6	1.5×10^6
Hemocyanin	Blue	Plasma	Molluscs		
			Gastropods (Helix)	1-3	6.8×10^6
			Cephalopods	3-5	3×10^6
			Crustaceans	1-4	4.8×10^5
Chlorocruorin	Green	Plasma	Annelids	9	3.4×10^6
Haemerythrin	Red	Corpuscles	Annelids	2	6.6×10^4

Haemoglobin is made up of an iron porphyrin compound, HAEME, associated with a protein GLOBIN. Haeme is a metalloporphyrin. It is composed of four pyrrole rings linked by methenyl bridges to form a super-ring with an atom of ferrous iron in the center attached to the pyrrole nitrogens (Fig. 3.13). The cyclic tetrapyrrole structure is a PORPHYRIN. Porphyrins appeared early in biopoiesis and assumed critical roles in photosynthesis (chlorophyll), in enzymes (catalase), in electron transport (cytochrome), in gas transport (haemoglobin), and in many pigments (feathers, urine). Metabolically, the most important of the porphyrins are the METALLOPORPHYRINS, with an atom of metal chelated between four pyrrole nitrogen atoms (Figs. 3.13); haeme with its atom of ferrous iron and chlorophyll with magnesium are familiar examples.

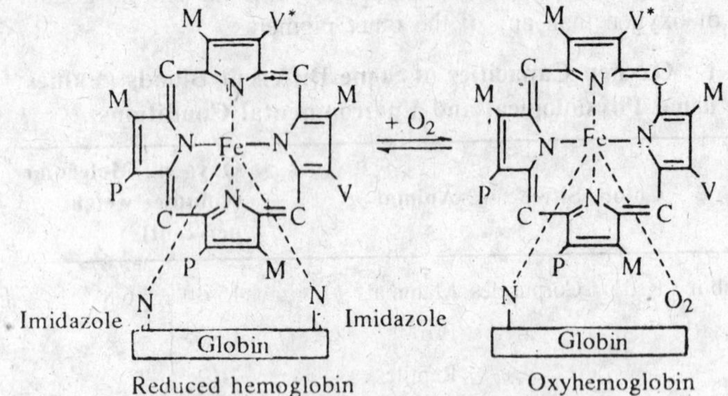

Imidazole conjugation in hemoglobin

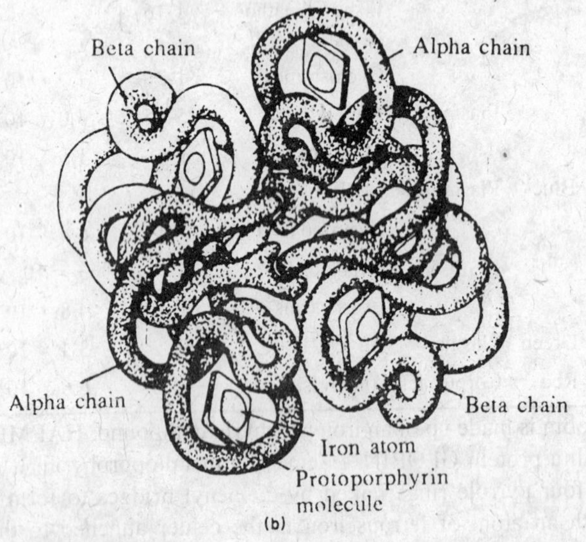

(b)

Fig. 3.13 : Structure of haemoglobin. (a) Structure of haeme, which is constant in all haemoglobins, with the attachment of a highly variable globin (protein) part of the molecule. M methyl group—CH_3; V, vinyl group—$CH = CH_2$; P, propionic group— CH_2—CH_2—COOH. In chlorocruorin, position 2 (asterisk) is filled by the formyl group O = CH. (b) Schematic representation of a molecule of human haemoglobin.

The haeme component is a constant structural feature of all haemoglobins, but the globin portion varies in different species. In addition, varying numbers of haemoglobin units unite to form polymers of different sizes. For example, the muscle haemoglobin of all vertebrates (myoglobin) and blood oxyhaemoglobin of cyclostomes correspond to one unit with a molecular weight of 16,500 to 17,000. Two basic units (mole, wt. 34,000) are united in some haemoglobins of the polychaete worms *Glycera* and *Notomastus*, several bivalves (Noetia, cardita), and the insect *Gastrophilus*. The molecular weight of the vascular haemoglobin of most vertebrates corresponds to four units (mol. wt. of about 68,000), while in some of the annelids (*Arenicola and Lumbricus*) the molecule may correspond to 180 units or a weight of 3,000,000.

The many different haemoglobins vary in oxygen-combining capacities (Table 3.1). This variation in oxygen capacity is a property of the total molecule and does not depend on structural differences or changes in the metalloporphyrin component. In all cases the atom of ferrous iron (haeme unit) is associated with one molecule of oxygen to form oxyhaemoglobin. The reaction is readily reversible; the unoxygenated compound is referred to as deoxyhaemoglobin or less accurately as reduced haemoglobin. These are not enzymatic reactions; whether or not the haeme unit combines with oxygen depends not only on the availability of the oxygen but on the pH and, ionic content of the solution as well as on the structure of the total haemoglobin molecule.

In man there are four different peptide chains in the vascular haemoglobins. In the adult human, 90% consists two α-chains combined with two β-chains to form single tetrameric molecules (called haemoglobin A). In normal human 100 ml of blood contains 14 to 15 gm of haemoglobin. One gram of haemoglobin combines with 3.4 ml of oxygen when fully saturated.

Chlorocruorin (chlorohaemoglobin) : This is a beautiful green pigment, biochemically allied to haemoglobin and the cytochromes. The metalloporphyrin group of the molecule, referred to as chlorohaeme, differs from protohaeme of haemoglobin only in the substitution of a formyl group for the vinyl group at position 2 in the porphyrin ring (Fig. 3.13). Chlorocruorin is confined to four families of polychaete worms and occurs only in the plasma (never intracellularly). It has high molecular weight (about 30,00,000) and an oxygen capacity similar to the more active of the invertebrate haemoglobins (Table 3.1). As anticipated from its molecular structure, many of its physiological properties are similar to those of haemoglobin; capacity to combine readily with carbon monoxide a sigmoid equilibrium curve, and a strong Bohr effect.

The distribution of Chlorocruorin and haemoglobin in the polychaete worms suggests a close phylogenetic history. Within the same family of worms (Sabellidae, Serpulidae and Ampharetidae) some species have Chlorocruorin while others have haemoglobin. Further in one genus *Serpula* both pigments are present in the blood, and the relative amounts vary with the age; younger individuals have more of the haemoglobin. In the sabellid *Potamilla*, chlorocruorin is the blood pigment but the muscles contain haemoglobin. These various facts suggest that a genetic mutation produced the chlorocruorin molecule in a world where haemoglobin already existed and that the mutation was, for some reason, preserved.

Haemerythrin : The third iron-containing chromoprotein was first discovered in the ancient brachiopod *Lingula* and is evidently confined to a very small number of marine invertebrates; all sipunculans, two priapulids, two branchiopods, and one polychaete. Like the low-molecular-weight haemoglobins, it is found only in the blood cells and occurs in multiple forms. Although the prefix "haeme" implies the presence of an iron-porphyrin ring the haemerythrin molecule is a twisted protein chain in which the active iron centre bears no resemblance to that of haemoglobin.

The molecular weight is about 100,000. Each molecule contains several iron atoms. One oxygen molecule combines with 2 or 3 iron atoms. Much have not been investigated about this pigments but it is well known fact, that this pigment has the less oxygen carrying capacity in comparison to haemoglobin and chlorocruorin.

Haemocyanin : Out of these four respiratory blood pigments, haemocyanin ranks next in importance to haemoglobin. It is a well known substance. Chemically it has a copper in its prosthetic group rather than iron. Its molecular weight ranges from 1 million to 7 million. It is never found contained in the cells but always is suspension in the blood. In oxygenated state, it is blue. The haemocyanin is present in certain higher crustaceans, in few arachnids such as *Limulus* and scorpions, in few gastropods such as *Buccinium,* and *Busycon* and in cephalopods such as *Loligo*, *Sepia* and *Octopus*. *Redfield* pointed out that this pigment occurs in two forms, the oxidised form and .the reduced form. As regards its carrying capacity of oxygen is concerned, it is much less efficient than haemoglobin. The two atoms of copper are necessary to carry one molecule of oxygen.

Haemoglobin as an Oxygen Carrier

Haemoglobin possesses a unique power of combining with oxygen to form an easily dissociable compound the oxyhaemoglobin. The reaction in which haemoglobin unites with O_2 to form oxyhaemoglobin behaves in same ways like a true chemical reaction and in others like a physical process. Its similarity to chemical reaction is found in the observation that when haemoglobin is thoroughly exposed to oxygen rich air, it is completely converted into oxyhaemoglobin so that further exposure to pure oxygen under high pressure does not further increase the amount of O_2 in combination with haemoglobin. In other words, haemoglobin reaches what is called its *saturation point*. Moreover, the amount of O_2 taken up by haemoglobin at its saturation point is just equal to that which represent two atoms of O_2 for every one atom of iron in haemoglobin. On the assumption that haemoglobin contains one atom of iron in its molecule, one molecule of O_2 combines with one molecule of the haemoglobin.

DISSOCIATION CURVE

As it is known that, one of the unique property of blood is that, it reversibly binds with oxygen with the help of haemoglobin molecule. This binding can be written as:

$$Hb + O_2 \rightleftarrows HbO_2$$

At high oxygen concentration the haemoglobin (Hb) combines with oxygen to form oxyhaemoglobin (HbO_2) and the reaction goes to the right. At low concentration, oxygen is given up again and the reaction proceeds to the left. If the oxygen concentration is reduced to zero, the haemoglobin gives up all the oxygen it carries.

The deoxygenated solution of respiratory pigment, when exposed to a gradually increasing oxygen tension, the gas is absorbed rapidly at first but after a time, the rate of absorption becomes progressively slower, and approaches the level 100 per cent saturation asymptotically. This relationship between oxygen tension and it's absorption by the pigment produces a characteristically shaped graph known as the oxygen dissociation curve or oxygen equilibrium curve (Fig. 3.14). However, the term oxygen equilibrium should be preferred, because the term dissociation refers only to the unloading of oxygen by the pigment, whereas the graph also describes how it takes up oxygen or the process of association.

The widely differing equilibrium curve of three pigments has been chosen to illustrate the extent to which the oxygen capacity of a blood pigment of the same basic type-in this case haemoglobin may vary between species. It is quite clear from the figure that the equilibrium curve of *Arenicola, haemoglobin* rises rapidly to become 95 per cent saturated at about 13 mm. Hg oxygen tension. The equilibrium curve for the pigeon represents the other extreme, since it never reaches 95 per cent saturation at the highest level as shown in the graph. The equilibrium curve for *Homo* falls between these two extremes.

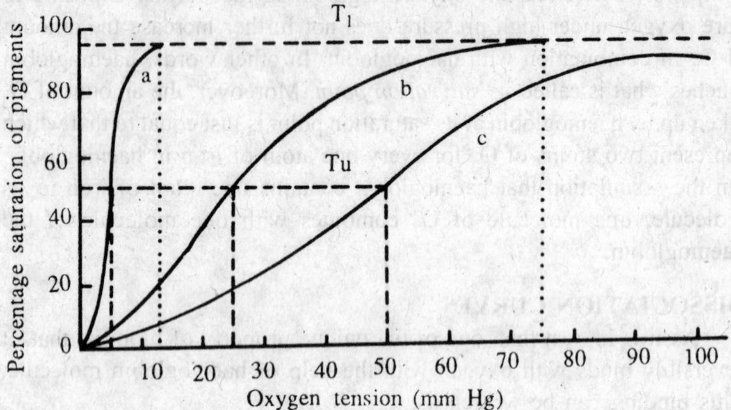

Fig. 3.14: Oxygen equilibrium curves of the (a) lung-worm (b) man (c) the pigeon.

Further, it is also clear from the graph that, the limit of 100 mm Hg oxygen, represents very nearly the maximum tension to which respiratory pigment will be subjected in a terrestrial animal. This is due to the fact that the respiratory organs have been placed inside the body and as such a dead space has created, through which the inspired air must pass before it teaches the actual respiratory surface. On expiration some of the expired gas remain in the dead space to mingle with the air taken in during the next inspiration. As a result of this, the oxygen tension in contrast to respiratory surface is about 100 Hg at the most in contrast to a pressure of 159 mm Hg in air. This is the situation in mammals such as man. Further the large air sacs of bird would be expected to increase the volume of the dead space compared with man, and this means that the haemoglobin can never reach loading tension.

It is also very clear from the equilibrium curve that the shape of the curve might have adaptive significance. At the Tu of the pigeon haemoglobin, the pigment will be unloading to a considerable extent, when the *Arenicola haemoglobin* is unloading hardly at all at Tu. Moreover, the much of the oxygen contained in *Arenicola haemoglobin* is unloaded at saturation level between 80 per cent and 95 per cent. The total amount which it will take up is small in comparison to the pigeon, but it is absorbed very rapidly. It is, however, clear that the pigment like that of Arenicola is a value to an animals that live in low oxygen tension, whereas one like that of pigeon is of value in high oxygen tension.

Dissociation Curve of foetal Blood

In many mammals, including man, the dissociation curve of foetal blood is located to the left of that of maternal blood. This is related to how the foetus obtains its oxygen by diffusion from the maternal blood. Because, foetal blood has a higher affinity for oxygen than maternal blood, so it can take up oxygen more readily. This facilitates the uptake of oxygen by foetal blood in the placenta. The difference in dissociation curve between foetal and maternal blood is due to two reasons, firstly, the foetal haemoglobin is slightly different from maternal haemoglobin, and secondly, the difference in the organic phosphate within the red cell. After birth foetal haemoglobin gradually disappears and is replaced by adult-type haemoglobin.

There are several factors which affect the equilibrium curve. These factors are as follows:

(i) *Effect of CO_2* : The effect of CO_2 on equilibrium curve is shown in Fig. 3.15. The top curve 'A' shows the percentage saturation of haemoglobin with oxygen at various, oxygen tensions ranging from 0 to 100 mm where the CO_2 tension is 0. The lower curve is for the carbon dioxide tension of 40 mm. At 100 mm of oxygen tension haemoglobin, in the absence of carbon dioxide is completely saturated with oxygen; but at 40 mm of CO_2 tension it is nearly saturated. At 40 mm of Oxygen tension the haemoglobin in the absence of carbon dioxide is 96% saturated; a 40 mm of CO_2 tension it is only 72% saturated. In this way it is apparent from the above observations and curves, *that the presence of carbon dioxide depresses the ability of haemoglobin to bind* oxygen, especially at the oxygen tension present in the venous blood. Therefore, in the tissues oxyhaemoglobin releases some of its oxygen. The curve also shows that the ability of haemoglobin to bind oxygen is dependent on the oxygen tension to which it is exposed.

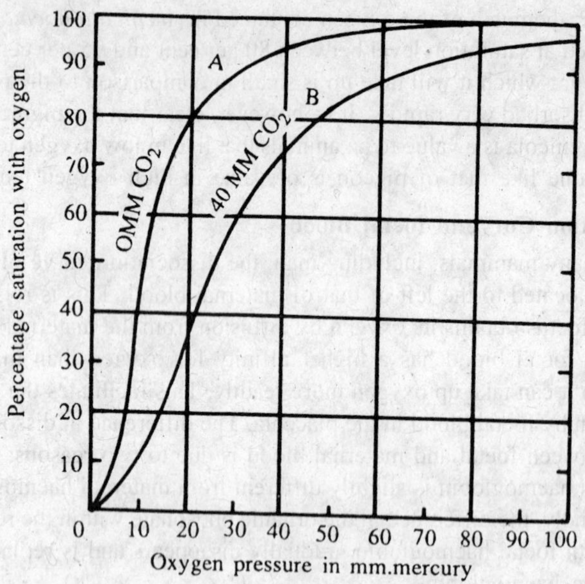

Fig. 3.15 : Percentage saturation of human blood with oxygen when exposed to different oxygen and carbon dioxide pressures.

(ii) *Temperature :* The temperature also affects the equilibrium curve of Oxyhaemoglobin. *The higher the temperature, the less is the amount of oxygen combined with haemoglobin at any given oxygen tension.* In other words, it can be said that the rise of temperature throws the reaction in the backward direction (right to left).

(iii) *Electrolytes :* The presence of electrolytes also effects the equilibrium curve of oxyhaemoglobin. *At the lower oxygen tension, oxyhaemoglobin dissociates more completely in the presence of electrolytes (salts) than it does in* their absence. This has however, the significance for the oxygenation of body tissues. As the blood passes through systemic capillaries where oxygen tension is very tow, the electrolytes of the blood favour to release the oxygen for tissue utilization.

(iv) *Acids :* Acid also affect the equilibrium curve. Increase in *hydrogen-*ion *concentration favours the dissociation of oxyhaemoglobin.* This effect is mainly studied in relation to carbon dioxide, the most abundant acid substance in the body. It however, affect through the formation of carbonic acid as $H_2O + CO_2 \rightarrow H_2CO_3$. The effect of CO_2 has already been discussed before.

Transport of Respiratory Gases

The movement of gases between environmental medium and the blood is in accord with the gas laws and is purely a physical phenomenon of diffusion. Exchange of gases occurs at different sites in the body.

(A) Exchange of Gases between Lung and Plasma

Carriage of oxygen : Gaseous exchange between the alveolar air and blood is described as *external respiration.* The uptake of O_2 from alveolar air and release of CO_2 from the blood capillaries into the alveoli of lungs is brought about by a process of diffusion due to differential pressures of these gases.

The partial pressure of oxygen in the alveolar air is about equivalent to 101mm of Hg whereas the venous blood coming from tissues to the lungs has got a partial pressure of about 40 to 50 mm of Hg. Oxygen, therefore, diffuses in the direction of pressure gradient *i.e.,* from alveolar air to blood, till the PO_2 is brought upto about 100 mm Hg. About 98% of the oxygen is carried in combination with haemoglobin and the rest is dissolved in the plasma in simple physical solution

Oxygen in the Form of Oxyhaemoglobin

As, stated earlier that haemoglobin carries about 98% of the total O_2 transported through blood. This mode of O_2 transport is of great importance. Haemoglobin of the RBC combines with the O_2 and forms *oxyhaemoglobin.* Each molecule of haemoglobin contains 4 molecules of haemoglobin. Since, each molecule of haeme can combine with one molecule of O_2, hence molecule of haemoglobin can maximally combine with 4 molecules of O_2. The formation of oxyhaemoglobin takes place in lungs and other respiratory organs. Hence the blood leaving the tissues contains largely haemoglobin, whereas that leaving the alveoli contains primarily oxyhaemoglobin. The colour difference in these two explains why systemic veins are dull red in colour and arteries are scarlet.

The amount of oxyhaemoglobin formed depends upon the partial pressure of O_2 in the blood. The greater is the PO_2, the greater is found the quantity of oxyhaemoglobin formed. In addition to partial pressure of O_2, the oxygen carrying capacity is also affected by partial pressure of O_2. It has been observed that the presence of CO_2 tends to reduce the amount of O_2 carrier. This effect of CO_2 on O_2 carrying capacity of blood is called as Bohr effect. Myoglobin and foetal haemoglobin, however, show no Bohr effect.

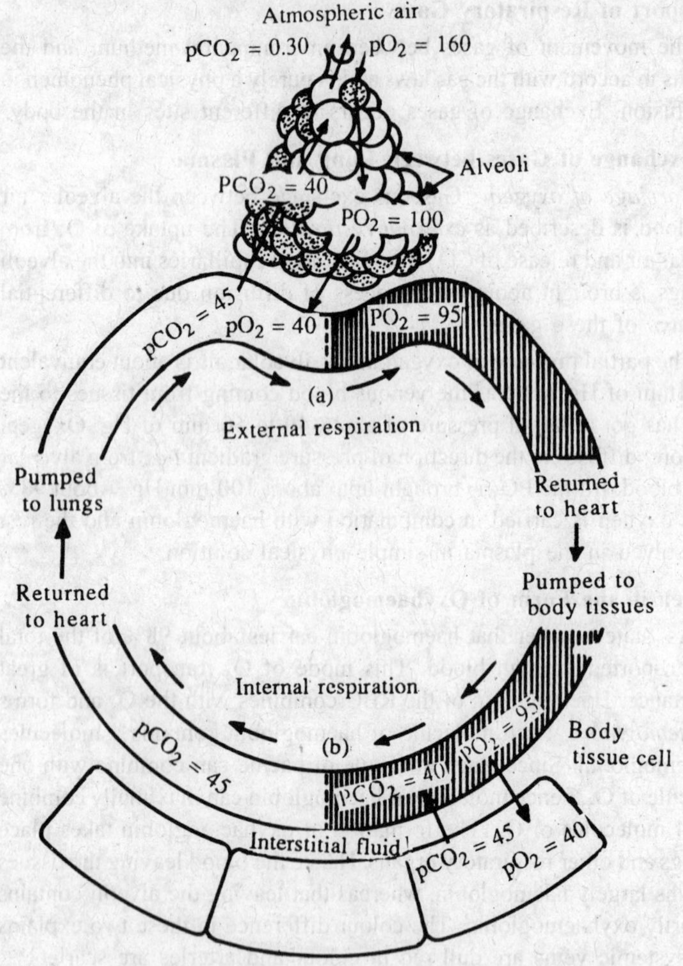

Fig. 3.16 : Partial pressure involved in respiration.

In tissues the oxyhaemoglobin is dissociated into haemoglobin and oxygen. The O_2 dissociation is governed by some factors like temperature, pH, electrolytes etc. (already discussed).

Oxygen in Physical Solution

Very little amount of O_2 is carried in the form of physical solution in plasma. The amount of O_2 carried in physical solutions; directly proportional to the partial pressure of O_2 in blood. The amount of O_2 transported by this means is of negligible importance as far as the total O_2 supply to the tissues under physiological condition is concerned.

(B) Exchange of Gases Between Blood and Plasma

Gaseous exchange between blood and extracellular fluid surrounding the tissues is effected on the same diffusion gradient principle as in external respiration.

Carriage of Carbon Dioxide

The various metabolic reactions in the cells results the release of CO_2 which diffuses into blood. The total amount of CO_2 in venous blood is about 60ml per 100 ml blood and the arterial blood contains about 50 ml total CO_2 per 100 ml. There is a clear cut difference in CO_2 concentration between tissue and blood, and CO_2 flows in the direction of this gradient *i.e.,* from tissues to the blood. About 4 ml of CO_2 per 100 ml of blood is given off by the tissues which is carried to the lungs. In lungs, a tension gradient is established and CO_2 flows from blood to the alveolar air. If, however, the alveoli become unable to eliminate CO_2 as in disease (pneumonia), the carbonic acid will build up in the blood which will then become more acid than usual, resulting in a condition called *acidosis*. Tissues cannot tolerate this acid condition and will soon die.

Both plasma and red blood corpuscles transport CO_2. Plasma transports about one third and corpuscles remaining two-thirds of the total CO_2. CO_2 is carried in the following forms:

1. *In physical solution by the plasma :* Under normal conditions of temperature and pressure, only about 2.7 cc of CO_2 is carried in physical solution as (H_2CO_3) in 100 cc of venous blood. Since this represents very small part of total CO_2 carried.

$$H_2O + CO_2 \rightleftharpoons \underset{\text{carbonic acid}}{H_2CO_3}$$

2. *As chemical compounds :* Two types of compounds are formed with CO_2 in blood.

   (a) *Bicarbonates :* (i) $NaHCO_3$ in plasma (arterial blood 33%, venous blood – 35.2%).

(ii) $KHCO_3$ in erythrocytes (atrerial blood – 9.8%, venous blood 10.5%).

(b) *Carbamino compounds* : (i) Carbamino haemoglobin in erythrocytes. (arterial blood – 2%, venous blood – 2.6%).

(ii) Carbamino proteins (with plasma proteins) in the plasma (arterial blood 1%; venous blood – 1.1%).

(c) *Carriage of CO_2 as bicarbonate* : About 85% of the total CO_2 is carried in both plasma and red blood cells in the form of bicarbonates. The CO_2 produced inside the cells diffuses freely into the plasma and a major fraction of it diffuses from plasma into RBC's. The red blood cells are rich in an enzyme *carbonic unhydrase* which can actively and reversibly convert CO_2 into carbonic acid.

$$H_2O + CO_2 \rightleftharpoons H_2CO_3$$

Inside the RBC the carbonic acid dissociates into H^+ and HCO_3^- ions.

$$H_2CO_3 \rightleftharpoons H^+ + HCO_3^-$$

Sodium ions are plentiful in plasma and potassium ion in RBC's. Some of the bicarbonates ions are bound by K^+ ions present therein forming $KHCO_3$, whereas the remaining bicarbonate ions diffuse out of RBC into the plasma due to concentration gradient and combine with sodium to form $NaHCO_3$.

In the corpuscles, haemoglobin remains combined with K and forms bicarbonates in the following ways.

$$KHb + H_2CO_3 \rightarrow HHb + KHCO_3$$

Potassium haemoglobinate   Carbonic acid

In the plasma alkaline phosphate combine with H_2CO_2 and forms sodium bicarbonate

$$Na_2HPO_4 + H_2CO_3 \rightarrow NaH_2PO_4 + NaHCO_3$$

The plasma proteins mostly remains combined with sodium (to be represented as NaPr) and form bicarbonate in the following way.

$$NaPr + H_2CO_3 \rightarrow HPr + NaHCO_3$$

Chloride Shift or Hamburger's Phenomenon

When whole blood is saturated with CO_2, the following changes are seen :

1. The bicarbonate content of plasma and corpuscles is increased.
2. The chloride content of plasma is diminished and that of the cell (erythrocytes) is increased.
3. The total base (cations) of both plasma and corpuscles remains unchanged.
4. The water content and the volume of corpuscles are increased.

When CO_2 is removed from a sample of blood, reverse changes are seen. From these observations, it is evident that, when CO_2 enters blood, chlorine from plasma enters the red cells, while the base (Na) is left behind. When CO_2 escapes from blood, chlorine leaves the cells, enters plasma and combines with the base sodium again. This movement of chlorine ion is called as *chloride shift* or *Hamburger's phenomenon.* This phenomenon can be explained with the help of Fig. 3.17 and following lines.

The membrane of red cell is not permeable to basic ions (K^+, Na^+, etc.), but is permeable to anions (HCO_3^-, Cl^- etc.). When CO_2 enters the blood stream in the tissue capillaries, H_2CO_3 is formed very largely in corpuscles and little in plasma because red cells are rich in carbonic anhydrase which is absent in plasma. H_2CO_3 formed reacts with KHb (haemoglobin in red cell is in combination with the base K) in the red cells producing $KHCO_3$ and HHb. Thus, the bicarbonate content of the red cell increases and thereby the reaction of the cells tend to become alkaline. To maintain a constant pH, either the alkali ion (K) is to get out of the cell or an acid ion from the plasma should enter the cell. Since, the red cell membrane is not permeable to alkali ion, K cannot come out. Consequently, the acid ion Cl^- of NaCl from the plasma enters the red cells and combines with $KHCO_3$ forming KCl and HCO_3^- ions. The free HCO_3 ion now tends to make the cell reaction acidic. This is prevented by the migration of HCO_3^- ion now tends to make the cell reaction acidic. This is prevented by the migration of HCO_3^- ion from the cell into the plasma. It combines with Na of NaCl, which is left free by the shift of chlorine (Cl^-) ion and forms $NaHCO_3$ in the plasma. All these change take place in the tissue capillaries. Owing to this reaction a large amount of Na of NaCl of plasma is made available for CO_2 carriage.

In the lungs, these changes are reversed. Chlorine comes out of the cells, reacts with $NaHCO_3$ of plasma, forming NaCl and carbonic acid. Carbonic acid, thus, liberated passes out through the lungs. In the tissue capillaries, chlorine shifts from plasma to cells. Thereby the osmotic pressure of the cell will rise, water will be drawn in and cell volume will increase. In the pulmonary capillaries, chloride-shifts from the cells back to the plasma, and this will reduce the osmotic pressure of the cell and cell volume will shrink.

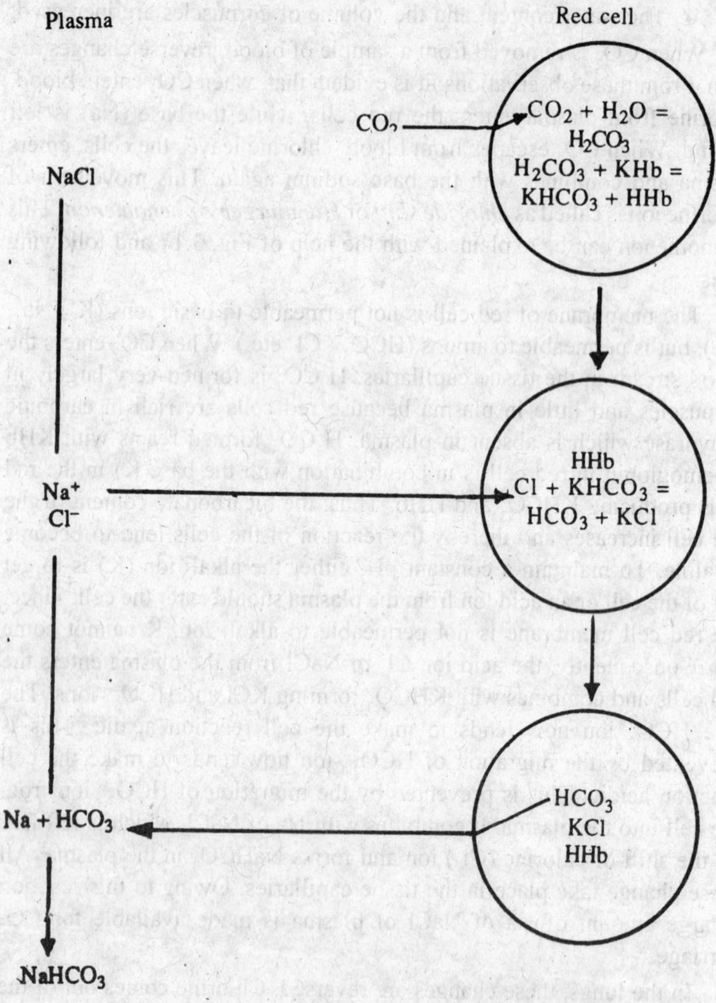

Fig. 3.17 : Showing the steps of chloride shift.

(b) *Carriage of CO_2 as carbamino-compounds* : About 10 % of the CO_2 is given out in the combined form with haemoglobin. The combination occurs at the free — NH_2 groups of the globin part of the haemoglobin, which results in the formation of neutral carbamino haemoglobin which is a reversible reaction. It does not require the help of carbonic anhydrase. Thus,

$$CO_2 + Hb.NH_2 \rightleftharpoons Hb.NH.COOH \text{ (carbo haemoglobin)}$$

At the lung surface all the above reactions are reversed and the free carbon dioxide then diffuse in the alveolar space to be expired out.

Respiratory Quotient

The ratio of the amount of oxygen (volume) used up and the amount of CO_2 (volume) produced simultaneously during respiration in any animal is called the respiratory quotient (R.Q.)

$$R.Q. = \frac{\text{Volume of } Co_2 \text{ given out in time t}}{\text{Volume of oxygen absorbed in time t}}$$

This ratio is different for the oxidation of different food substances. When hexose sugar is being oxidised the amount of O_2 consumed and the amount, of CO_2 produced are equal.

$$C_6H_{12}O_6 + 6CO = 6CO_2 + 6H_2O$$

Hence the R.Q. of hexose sugar is,

$$\frac{\text{Volume of } CO_2 \text{ formed}}{\text{Volume of } O_2 \text{ utilized}} = \frac{6}{6} = 1$$

Different from this, the oxidation of fat such as triolein the reaction proceeds as follows:

$$C_{57} + H_{104}O_6 + 80\ O_2 \rightarrow 57\ CO_2 + 52\ H_2O$$

and the R.Q. here is, 57/80 *i.e.,* 0.71. The RQ of an average protein is less than one (0.802) because protein consists of amino acids which require more O_2 for their complete oxidation than carbohydrate.

The RQ of an individual taking an ordinary mixed diet denotes the oxidation of a mixture of carbohydrate, fat and protein, and it is nearly 0.85. It is, therefore possible to make a rough estimate of the food of an organism by measuring its RQ. Sometimes RQ is more than 1, which indicates that the carbohydrates would be transforming into fats and just contrary to this, if the RQ is less than 0.7 it indicates that carbohydrate are being formed from the fats.

Basal Metabolic Rate (BMR)

The basal metabolic rate means the rate of energy utilization in the body during absolute rest but while the person is awake. The following basal conditions are necessary for measuring the basal metabolic rate in human beings.

1. The person must not have eaten any food for at least 12 hours because of the specific dynamic action of food.
2. The BMR is determined after a night of restful sleep, for rest reduces the activities of the sympathetic nervous system and other metabolic excitants to their minimal level.
3. No strenous exercise is performed after the night of restful sleep, and the person must remain at complete rest in a reclining position for at least 30 minutes prior to actual determination of BMR.
4. All psychic and physical factors that come excitement must be eliminated and the subject must be made as comfortable as possible.
5. The temperature of the air must be comfortable, and be some where between the limits of 68° and 80° F.

The commonest way of expressing BMR is in terms of heat production and is measured in kcal. Heat produced is normally calculated from the oxygen consumption. In relation to body weight BMR in a man between 20 to 50 years is 1 cal/kg of body weight per hour. Rate of BMR is affected by age, sex, body weight, health and internal secretions of body.

Table 3.2 : Normal Standards of BMR.

Age in years	BMR (Male)	BMR (Female)
6	53.0	53.6
7	52.5	49.1
8	51.8	47.0
$8\frac{1}{2}$	51.2	46.5
9	50.5	45.9
$9\frac{1}{2}$	49.4	45.9
10	48.5	45.9
$10\frac{1}{2}$	47.7	45.6

Age in years	BMR (Male)	BMR (Female)
11	47.2	45.3
12	46.7	44.3
13–15	46.3	–
16	45.7	38.9
$16\frac{1}{2}$	45.3	38.3
17	44.8	37.8
$17\frac{1}{2}$	44.0	37.4
18	43.3	36.7
19	42.3	36.7
$19\frac{1}{2}$	42.0	–
20–21	41.4	36.2
22–23	40.8	36.2
24–27	40.2	35.7
28–29	39.8	35.7
30–34	39.3	35.7
35–39	38.7	35.7
40–44	38.0	35.7
45–49	37.7	34.9
50–54	36.7	34.0
55–59	36.1	33.2
60–64	35.5	32.6
65–69	34.8	32.3

4

PHYSIOLOGY OF AVIATION, HIGH ALTITUDE, SPACE AND DEEP-SEE DIVING

The word aviation in its modern usage refers generally to the art of flying. In a common use, it refers to the operations and usage of heavier-than-air flying machines, but it is also applied to operation of lighter-than-air equipment; *i.e.,* balloons and airships. In the present article, principal concern, however, will be with those classes of aircraft whose flight depends upon the dynamic reaction of lifting surfaces (or wings) and the atmospheric air flowing over and around them.

When human beings ascend above the sea-level, the pressure around them decreases tremendously. This exposes the blood in the lungs to extremely low alveolar pressure, a condition called *hypobarism* or *low oxygen pressure mechanism.* It is know that at see-level, the barometric pressure is 760 mm Hg; at 10,000 feet, only 523 mm Hg; and at 50,000 feet, 87 mm Hg. This decrease in barometric pressure is the basic cause of all the *hypoxia* problems in high-altitude physiology because, as the barometric pressure decreases, the atmospheric oxygen partial pressure decreases proportionately, remaining at all times slightly less than 21% of the total barometric pressure PO_2 at sea-level about 159 mm Hg but at 50,000 feet only 18 mm Hg.

Even at high altitudes, CO_2 is continually excreted from the pulmonary blood into the alveoli. Also, water vaporizes into the inspired air from the respiratory surfaces. Therefore, these two gases dilute the O_2 in the alveoli, thus reducing the O_2 concentration.

Water vapour pressure in the alveoli remains 47 mm Hg as long as the body temperature is normal, regardless of altitude. In the case of CO_2, during exposure to very high altitudes, the alveolar PCO_2 falls from the sea-level value of 40 mm Hg to lower values. In the *acclimatized* person, who increases his or her ventilation about fivefold, the decrease is to about 7 mm Hg because of increased respiration.

Now let us see how the pressures of these two gases affect the alveolar oxygen. For instance, assume that the barometric pressure falls from the normal value of 760 mm Hg to 253 mm Hg, which is the measured value at the top of 29, 028-Foot mount Everest forty-seven millimeters of mercury of this must be water vapour, leaving only 206 mm Hg for all the other gases. In the *acclimatized* person, 7 mm of the 206 mm Hg must be CO_2, leaving only 199 mm Hg. If there were no use of O_2 by the body, one fifth of this 199 mm Hg would be O_2 and four fifths would be nitrogen; or the PO_2 in the alveoli would be 40 mm Hg. However, some of this remaining alveolar O_2 would be absorbed into the blood, leaving about 35 mm Hg O_2 pressure in the alveoli. Therefore, at the summit of Mount Everest, only the best of acclimatized people can barely survive when breathing air.

A person remaining at high altitudes for days, weeks, or years becomes more and more acclimatized to the low PO_2, so that it causes fewer deleterious effects on the body and becomes possible for the person to work harder without hypoxic effects or to ascend to still higher altitudes. The principal means by which acclimatization comes about are (1) a great increase in pulmonary ventilation, (2) increased red blood cells, (3) increased diffusing capacity of the lungs, (4) increased vascularity of the tissues, and (5) increased ability of the tissue cells to use oxygen despite low PO_2.

On immediate exposure to very low PO_2, hypoxic stimulation of the arterial chemoreceptors increases alveolar ventilation to a maximum of about 1-65 times normal. This is an immediate compensation, within seconds, for the high altitude, and it alone allows the person to rise several thousand feet higher than would be possible without the increased ventilation. Then, if the person remains at a very high altitude for several days, the chemorecaptors increase ventilation gradually to about five times normal (400% above normal). The basic cause of this gradual ventilation increase is as follows: The immediate increase in pulmonary ventilation on rising to a high altitude blows, off large quantities of CO_2 reducing the PCO_2 and increasing the pH of the body fluids. Both these changes *inhibit the effect of low PO_2 to stimulate respiration by way of the peripheral arterial chemoreceptors in the carotid and aortic bodies*. But during the ensuing 2 to 5 days, this inhibition fades away, allowing the respiratory centre to respond with full force to the peripheral chemoreceptor stimuli resulting from hypoxia, and the new ventilation increases to about 5 times normal instead of only 1.65 times. The cause of this fading inhibition is believed to be mainly a reduction of bicarbonate ion concentration in the cerebrospinal fluid as well as in the brain tissues. This in turn decreases the pH in the fluids surrounding the chemosensitive neurons of the respiratory center, thus increasing the respiratory stimulatory activity of the centre.

In animals native to altitudes of 13,000 to 17,000 feet, cell mitochondria and cellular oxidative enzyme systems are slightly more plentiful than in sea-level inhabitants. Therefore, it is presumed that the tissue cells of acclimatized human beings as well as of these acclimatized animal can be O_2 more effectively than can their sea-level counterparts. Many native human beings in the Andes and in the Himalayas live at altitudes above 13,000 feet and above. Many of these natives are born at these altitudes live there all their lives. In all aspects of acclimatization, the natives are superior to even the best-acclimatized low lenders, even though the low-landers might also have lived at high altitudes for 10 more years. The acclimatization of the natives begins in infancy. The chest size, especially, is greatly increased, where as the body size is some what decreased, giving a high ratio of ventilatory capacity to body mass. In addition their hearts are considerably larger then the hearts of lowlanders.

ACUTE EFFECTS OF HYPOXIA

Generally to acute effects of hypoxia, beginning at an altitude of about 12,000 feet, are drowsiness, lassitude, mental and muscle fatigue, sometimes headache, occasionally nausea, and sometimes euphoria. These progress to a stage of twitchings or seizures above 18,000 feet and end, above 23,000 feet in the unacclimatized person, in coma, followed shortly by death.

One of the most important effects of hypoxia is decreased mental proficiency, which decreases judgment, memory, and the performance of discrete motor movements, for instance, if an unacclimatized aviator stays at 15,000 feet for 1 hour, mental proficiency ordinarily falls to about 50% or normal, and after 18 hours at this level it falls to about 20% of normal.

CHRONIC MOUNTAIN SICKNESS

Occasionally, a person who remains at high altitude too long develops *chromic* sickness, in which the following effects occur.

(1) The red cell mass and hematocrit become exceptionally high,

(2) The pulmonary arterial pressure becomes elevated even more than the normal elevation that occurs, during acclimatization,

(3) The right side of the heart becomes greatly enlarged,

(4) The peripheral arterial pressure begins to fall,

(5) Congestive heart failure ensues, and

(6) death often follows unless the person is removed to a lower altitude.

EFFECT OF ACCELERATORY FORCES ON THE BODY

Several types of acceleratory forces often affect the body during flight, because of rapid changes in velocity and direction of motion in airplanes and Spacecraft. There are three types of acceleratory forces act, first at the time of beginning of flight (simple linear Muscles); at the end of flight (deceleration); and at the time when vehicles turn (centrifugal Muscles).

CENTRIFUGAL ACCELERATORY FORCES

When an airplane makes a turn, the force of centrifugal Muscles is determined by the following relation:

$$f = \frac{mv^2}{r},$$

in which f is the centrifugal acceleratory force, m is the mass of the object, V is the velocity of the travel, and r is the radius of curvature of the turn. Formula indicates that as the velocity increases, the force of centrifugal Muscles increases in proportion to the square of the velocity. It is abo obvious that the force of Muscles is directly proportional to the sharpness of the turn (the less the radius).

MEASUREMENT OF ACCELERATORY FORCE "G"

When a man is simply sitting in his seat, the force with which he is pressing against the seat results from the pull of gravity and is equal to his weight. The intensity of this force is said to be + 1 G because it is equal to the pull of gravity. If the force with which he presses against the seat becomes five times his normal weight during pullout from a dive, the force acting on the seat is +5 G.

If the airplane goes through an outside loop so that the man is held down by his seat belt, *Negative G* is applied to his body; if the force with which he is thrown against his belt is equal to the weight of his body, the negative force is –1 G.

EFFECTS OF CENTRIFUGAL ACCELERATORY FORCES ON BODY POSITIVE G

The most important effect of centrifugal acceleration is on the circulatory system as blood is mobile and so translocated by centrifugal forces.

When a aviator is subjected to *positive G*, the blood is centrifuged toward the lowermost part of the body. Thus, if the centrifugal acceleratory force is +5 G and the person is in an immobilized standing position, the hydrostatic pressure in the veins of the feet becomes five times normal, or about 450 mm Hg; even in the siting position, this pressure becomes nearly 300 mm Hg. As the pressure in the vessels of the lower part of the body increases, the vessels passively dilate and a major proportion of the blood from the upper body is translocated into these lower vessels. Because the heart cannot pump unless blood returns to it, the greater the quantity of blood "pooled" in this way in the lower body, the less becomes cardiac output.

Acceleration greater than 4 to 6 G causes "blackout' of vision within a few seconds and unconsciousness shortly thereafter. If this degree of Muscles is continued, the person will die. Extremely high acceleratory forces for even a fraction of a second can fracture the vertebrae. The degree of positive acceleration that the average person can withstand in the sitting position before vertebral fracture is about 20 G.

NEGATIVE G

The effects of negative G on the body are less dramatic acutely but possibly more damaging permanently than the effects of positive G. An aviator can usually go through outside loops up to negative acceleratory forces of –4 to –5 G without causing permanent harm but still causing intense momentary hyperemia of the head. Occasionally, psychotic disturbances lasting for 15 to 20 minutes occur as a result of brain edema.

Occasionaliy, negative G forces can be so great (–20G, for instance) and centrifugation of the blood into the head is so great that the cerebral blood pressure reaches 300 to 400 mm Hg, sometimes causing small vessels on the surface of the head and in the brain to rupture.

EFFECTS OF LINEAR ACCELERATORY FORCES (SPACE TRAVEL)

Unlike an airplane, a spacecraft cannot make rapid turns; therefore, centrifugal acceleration is of little importance except when the spacecraft goes into abnormal gyrations. However, blast-off acceleration and landing deceleration can be tremendous; both of these are types of linear acceleration, one positive and the other negative.

Fig 4.1 shows an approximate profile of acceleration during blast-off in a three-stage spacecraft, demonstrating that the first-stage booster causes acceleration as high as 9 G and the second-stage booster, as high as 8 G. In the standing position, the human body could not withstand this much acceleration, but in a semireclining position transverse to the axis of acceleration, this amount of acceleration can be withstood with ease despite the fact that the acceleratory forces continue for as long as several minutes at a time. Therefore, we see the reason for the reclining seat used by astronauts.

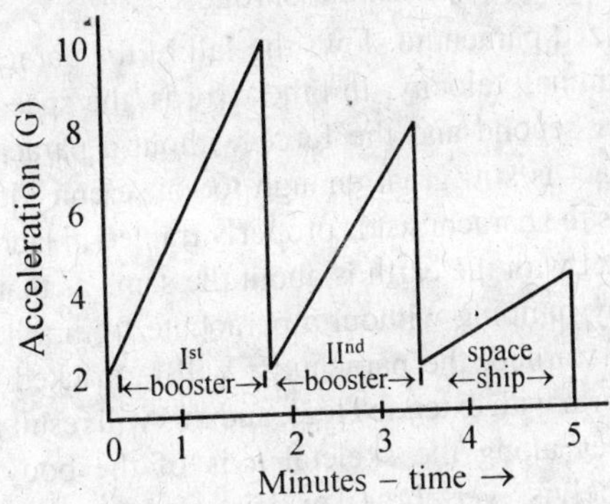

Fig. 4.1 : Acceleratory forces during the takeoff of a spacecraft.

Problems also occur during deceleration when the spacecraft reenters the atmosphere. A person travelling at Mach I (the speed of sound and of fast airplanes) can be safely decelerated in a distance of about 0.12 mile where as a person travelling at a speed of Mach 100 (a speed possible in interplenetary space travel) would require a distance of about 10,000 miles for safe deceleration. The principal reason for this difference is that the total amount of energy that must be dispelled during deceleration is proportional to the square of the velocity, which alone increases the required distance about 10,000-fold. But in additional to this, a human being withstand far less deceleration if the period of deceleration lasts for along time than for a short time. Therefore, deceleration must be accomplished much more slowly from high velocities than is necessary at lower velocities.

DECELERATORY FORCES ASSOCIATED WITH PARACHUTE JUMP:

When the parachuting aviator leaves the airplane, the velocity of fall is exactly O feet per second at first, however, because of the acceleratory force of gravity, within 1 second, the velocity of fall is 32 feet per second (if there is no air resistance); in 2 seconds it is 64 feet per second; and so on. As the velocity of fall increases, the air resistance tending to slow the fall also increases. Finally, the deceleratory force of the air resistance exactly balances the acceleratory force of gravity; so that after falling for about 12 seconds, the person will be falling at a "terminal velocity" of 109 to 119 miles per hour (175 feet per second).

If the parachutist has already reached the terminal velocity of fall before opening the parachute, an "opening shock load" of up to 1200 pounds can occur on the parachute shrouds.

The usual-sized parachute slows the fall of the parachutist to about one ninth the terminal velocity. In other words, the speed of landing is about 20 feet per second and the force without a parachute. Even so, the force of impact is still great enough to cause considerable damage to the body unless the parachutist is properly trained in landing. Actually, the force of impact with the earth is about the same as that which would be experienced by jumping without a parachute from a height of about 6 feet. Unless forwarned, the parachutist will be tricked by the senses into striking the earth with extended legs, and this will result in tremendous deceleratory forces along the skeletal axis of the body, resulting in fracture of the pelvis, vertebrae, or leg. Consequently, the trained parachutist strikes the earth with knees bent but muscles tact to cushion the shock of landing.

ARTIFICIAL CLIMATE IN THE SEALED SPACECRAFT

Because there is no atmosphere in outer space, an artificial atmosphere and climate must be produced. Most important, the oxygen concentration must remain high enough and the carbon dioxide concentration low enough to prevent suffocation. In some of the earlier space missions, a capsule atmosphere containing pure oxygen at about 260 mm Hg pressure was used, but in the space shuttle, gases about equal to those in normal air are used, with four times as much nitrogen as oxygen and a total pressure of 760 mm Hg the presence of nitrogen in the mixture greatly diminishes the likelihood of fire and explosion. It also protects against the development of local patches of lung at *electasis* that often occur when breathing pure oxygen because oxygen is absorbed rapidly when small bronchi temporarily blocked by mucous plugs, for space travel lasting more than several month, it will be impractical to carry along an adequate oxygen supply and enough carbon dioxide absorbent for this reason, recycling techniques have been proposed for use of the same oxygen over and over again. Some recycling processes depend on purely physical procedures, such as distillation and electrolysis of water, to release oxygen. Others depend on biological methods, such as use of algae with their large store of chlorophyll to generate foodstuffs and as the same time release oxygen from carbon dioxide by photosynthesis. A completely practical system for recycling is yet to be achieved.

WEIGHTLESSNESS IN SPACE

A person in an orbiting satellite or a nonpropelled spacecraft experiences weightlessness. That is, the person is not drawn toward the bottom, sides or top of the spacecraft but simply floats inside its chambers. The cause of this is not failure of gravity to pull on the body, because gravity from any nearby heavenly body is still active. However, the gravity is exactly balanced by the forces of gravity and other trajectory forces acting on both the spacecraft and the person at the same time so that both are pulled with exactly the same acceleratory forces and in the same direction for this reason the person simply is not attracted toward any specific wall of the spacecraft.

PHYSIOLOGIC PROBLEMS OF WEIGHTLESSNESS

Most of the problems that do occur are related to three effects (a) motion sickness during the few days of travel, (b) translocation of fluids within the body because of failure of gravity to cause hydrostatic pressure, and (c) diminished physical activity because no strength of muscle contraction is required to oppose the force of gravity.

Almost 50% of astronauts experience motion sickness, with nausea and sometimes vomiting, during the first 2 to 5 days of space travel.

The observed effects of a prolonged stay in space are the following: (1) decrease in blood volume, (2) decrease in red blood cell mass, (3) decrease in muscle strength and work capacity, (4) decrease in maximum cardiac output, and (5) loss of calcium and phosphate from the bones.

AVIATION MEDICINE

The science of preventing or treating illness and injuries that occur to aviators and those who work in the manufacture, maintenance and operation of aircraft and missiles. The practitioners of aviation medicine must be intimately acquainted with the science of flight, the characteristics of aircraft and the nature of the tumultuous atmosphere in which they are operated, french physiologist *Paul Bert* is generally regarded as the "father" of modern aviation medicine, he described his pioneer investigations of the physiological effects of air pressure, both above and below normal.

A primary function of aviation medicine has been to examine and determine the fitness of aviators and of candidates for flight training. It is universally recognised that the safety of a flight may be threatened if the pilot or other members of the flight crew possess inadequate sight, hearing, strength, coordination, intelligence, courage, equilibrium, emotional stability or lack ability to retain consciousness. Specialists in aviation medicine have sought to ensure that persons in whom these inadequacies are found or suspected are not permitted to operate aircraft. Aviation medicine specialists constantly study the hours crews spend per month at the controls, their diet, their peace of mind and the physical and mental stresses to which they are subjected by low air and O_2 pressure, noise, vibration, air turbulence, poor visibility and heavy responsibility. In missile support operations the aviation medicine specialists must combine clinical knowledge and psychological understanding with a detailed knowledge of fuel toxicities, firing systems and ground and range safety to prevent human failures that can cause missile failures. Most remedies for motion sickness appeared during aviation, contain some form of sedative or quieting drug many of ;the antiallergic drugs lessen and tendency of the average person to succumb to motion sickness. Most of these drugs, however, have some sedative or other undesirable side effects.

DEEP-SEA DIVING

When human being descend beneath the sea, the pressure around them increases tremendously. To keep the lungs from collapsing, air must be supplied to inflate them, also under high pressure. This exposes the blood in the lungs to extremely high alveolar gas pressure, a condition called hyperbarism. Beyond certain limits, these high pressures can cause tremendous alterations in the body physiology and can be lethal.

There is always a relationship of sea depth to pressure. A column of seawter 33 feet deep exerts the same pressure at its bottom as all the atmosphere above the earth. Therefore, a person 33 feet beneath the ocean surface is exposed to a pressure of 2 atmospheres, one atmospheres of pressure caused by the air above the water and the second atmosphere by the weight of the water itself. At 66 feet the pressure is 3 atmospheres and so forth.

Another important effect of depth is the compression of gases to smaller and smaller volumes. A bell jar at sea level contains 1 liter of air. At 33 feet beneath the sea, where pressure is 2 atmosphere, the volume has been compressed to only one-half liter and 8 atmospheres

(233 feet) to one-eight liter. Thus, the volume to which a given quantity of gas is compressed is inversely proportional to the pressure. This is the principle of physics called *Boyle's law*, which is extremely important in diving because increased pressures can collapse air chambers of the diver's body, especially the lungs, and often cause serious damage.

The gases to which a liver breathing air is normally exposed are N_2, O_2 and CO_2, and each has its own effect on body.

EFFECT OF N_2

About 4/5th of the air is nitrogen. At sea-level pressure, the nitrogen has no known effect, but at high pressure it can cause varying degrees of *narcosis*. Nitrogen narcosis has characteristics similar to those of alcohol intoxication, reason behind it is that nitrogen dissolves freely in the fats of the body and then membranes of the neurons, and because of its physical effect on altering ionic conductance through the membranes, reduces neuronal excitability.

When the diver remains beneath the sea for an hour or more and is breathing compressed air, the depth at which the first symptoms of mild narcosis appear is about 120 feet, at which level the diver begins to exhibit joviality and to lose many of his or her cares. At 150 to 200 feet, the diver becomes drowsy. A 200 to 250 feet, his or her strength wanes considerably, and the diver often becomes too clumpsy to perform the work required. Beyond 250 feet, the diver usually becomes almost useless as a result of nitrogen narcosis if he or she remains at these depths too long,

EFFECT OF OXYGEN

When the PO_2 in the blood rises far above 100 mm Hg, the amount of O_2 dissolved in the water of the blood increases markedly. Because of the extremely high tissue PO_2 that occurs when O_2 is breathed at a very high alveolar pressure, one can readily understand that this can be detrimental to many of the body's tissues. This is especially true of the brain. In fact, exposure to 4 atmospheres pressure of O_2 (PO_2 = 3040 mm Hg) will cause *seizures* followed by coma in most people within 30 to 60 minutes. The seizures often occur without warning and, for obvious reasons, are likely to be lethal to divers submerged beneath the sea.

Other symptoms encountered in acute oxygen poisoning include *nausea, muscle twitching, dizziness, disturbances of vision, irritability*, and *disorientation*. Exercise greatly increases a diver's susceptibility to

O_2 toxicity, causing symptoms to appear much earlier and with for greater severity than in the resting person.

EFFECT OF CO_2

If the diving gear is properly designed and functions properly, the diver has no problem due to CO_2 toxicity because depth alone does not increase the CO_2 partial pressure in the alveoli. This is true because depth does not increase the rate of CO_2 production in the body; as long as the diver continues to breathe a normal tidal volume, he or she continues to expire the CO_2 as it is formed, maintaining alveolar CO_2 pressure at a normal value.

In certain types of diving gear, however, such as the diving helmet and some types of rebreathing apparatuses, CO_2 can frequently build up in the dead space air of the apparatus and be rebreathed by the diver. Up to an alveolar CO_2 pressure (PCO_2) of about 80 mm Hg, twice that of normal alveoli, the diver usually tolerates this buildup by increasing the minute respiratory volume a maximum of 8– to 11– fold to compensate for the increased CO_2. Beyond the 80– mm Hg alveolar PCO_2 level, the situation becomes intolerable, and eventually the respiratory center begins to be depressed, rather than excited, because of the negative tissue metabolic effects of high PCO_2. The diver's respiration then begins to fail rather than to compensate. In addition, the diver develops severe respiratory acidosis, and varying degrees of lethargy, narcosis, and finally anaesthesia ensue.

DECOMPRESSION SICKNESS

When a person breathes air under high pressure for a long time, the amount of nitrogen dissolved in the body fluids becomes great. The reason for this is following. The blood flowing through the pulmonary capillaries becomes saturated with nitrogen to the same high pressure as that in the breathing mixture. Over several hours, enough nitrogen is carried to all the tissues of the body to saturate the tissues with dissolved nitrogen. Because nitrogen is not metabolized by the body, it remains dissolved until the nitrogen pressure in the lungs decreases, at which time the nitrogen can be removed by the reverse respiratory process; but this removal takes hours to occur, which is the source of multiple problems collectively called *decompression sickness.*

If a diver has been beneath the sea long enough that large amounts of nitrogen have dissolved in his or her body and the diver suddenly comes back to the surface of the sea, significant quantities of nitrogen bubbles can develop in the body fluids either intracellularly or extracellularly and cause minor or major and serious damage in almost any area of the body, depending on the number and sizes of bubbles formed; this is called *decompressing sickness.*

Decompression sickness has many synonyms like "Bends", compressed Air sickness, caisson Disease, Diver's paralysis, Dysbarism. At the first stage, only the smallest vessels are blocked by minute bubbles, but as the bubbles coalesce, progressively larger vessels are affected. Tissue ischemia and sometimes tissue death are the result. In most people, the symptoms are pain in the joints and musscles of the legs or arams, affecting 85 to 90% of those persons who develop decompression sicknes. The joint pain accounts for the term "bends" that is often applied to this candition.

In 5 to 10% of people with decompression ssickness, nervous system symptoms occur, ranging from dizziness in about 5% to paralysis or collapse and unconsciousness in as many as 3%. The paralysis may be temporary, but in some instances, the damage or part of the damage is permanent. Finally, about 2% of people with decompression sickness develop "the chokes", caused by massive numbers of microbubbles plugging the capillaries of the lungs; this is characterised by serious shortens of breath, often followed by severe pulmonary edema and, occasionally, death.

TREATMENT OF DECOMPRESSION SICKNESS

A widely used treatment for decompression sickness of professional divers is to put the diver in to a pressurised tank and then to lower the pressure gradually back to normal atmospheric pressure. About two thirds of the total nitrogen is eliminated in 1 hour and about 90% in 6 hours through lungs to prevent decompression sickness.

Tank decompression is even more important for treating people in whom symptoms of decompression sickness develop minutes or even hours after they have returned to the surface. In this case, the diver is recompressed immediately to a deep level. Then decompression is carried out over a period several times as long as the usual decompression period.

Decompression tables have been prepared by the V.S. Navy that detail procedures for safe decompression. To give the student an idea of the decompression process, a diver who has been breathing air and has been on the bottom for 60 minutes at a depth of 190 feet is decompresses according to the following schedule:

10 minutes at 50 feet depth
17 minutes at 40 feet depth,
19 minutes at 30 feet depth,
50 minutes at 20 feet depth,
84 minutes at 10 feet depth,

Thus, for a work period on the bottom of only 1 hour, the total time for decompresion is about 3 hours.

SATURATION DIVING AND USE OF HELIUM OXYGEN MIXTURES IN DEEP DIVES

When divers must work at very deep levels (250 feet and 1000 feet), they frequently live in a large compression tank for days or weeks at a times, remaining compressed at a pressure level near that at which they will be working. This keeps the tissues and fluids of the body saturated with the gases to which they will be exposed while diving. Then, when they return to the same tank after working, there are no significant changes in pressure, so decompression bubbles do not occur.

In very deep dives, especially during saturation diving, helium is usually used in the gas mixture instead of nitrogen, as it has 1/5 the narcotic effect of nitrogen; reducing the problem of decompression sickness and the low density of helium keeps the airway resistance for breathing at a minimum.

SCUBA DIVING

Before the 1940s, almost all diving was done using a diving helmet connected to a hose through which air was pumped to the diver from the surface. Then in 1943, *Jacques Cousteau* developed *Self-Contained Underwater Breathing Apparatus*, popularly known as the *SCUBA* apparatus; which is used in more than 99% of all sports and commercial diving.

This system consists of the following components:

(1) one or more tanks of compressed air or some other breathing mixture,
(2) a first-stage "reducing valve" for reducing the very high pressure from the tanks to low pressure level,
(3) a combination inhalation "demand" valve and exhalation valve that allows air to be pulled into the lungs with slight negative pressure of breathing and then to be exhausted into the sea at

a pressure level slightly positive to the surrounding water pressure, and

(4) a mask and tube system with small "dead space".

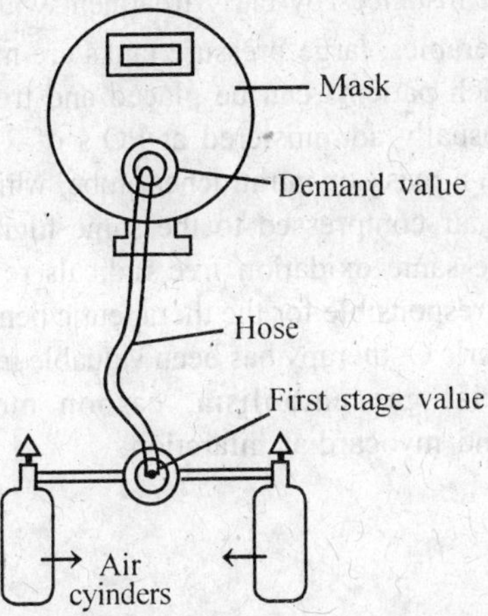

Fig. 4.2 : Open-circuit demand type *SCUBA* apparatus.

ESCAPE FROM SUBMARINES–A SPECIAL PHYSIOLOGICAL PROBLEM

One of the major problems of escape from submarines (300 to 600 feet) is prevention of air embolism. Is the person ascends, the gases in the lungs expand and sometimes rupture a pulmonary vessel, allowing the gases to enter the pulmonary vascular system and cause embolism of the circulation. Therefore, as the person ascends, he or she must consciously exhale continually.

Exhalation of the expanding gases from the lungs during ascent, even without breathing, is often rapid enough to blow off the accumulating CO_2 in the lungs. This keeps the concentration of CO_2 from building up in the blood and keep the person from having the desire to breathe for an extra long time during ascent.

HYPERBARIC O_2 THERAPY

Probably the most successful use of hyperbaric (high pressure O_2) oxygen has been in the treatment of *gas gangrene* and curing *leprosy*. The bacteria that cause this condition, *clostridial organisms* and leprosy *bacillus*, grow best under anaerobic condition and stop growing at oxygen pressures greater than 70 mm Hg. There fore, hyperbaric oxygenation of the tissues can frequently stop the infections process entirely and thus convert a condition that formerly was almost 100% fatal into one that is cured in most instances by early treatment with hyperbaric therapy.

For such therapies, large pressure tanks are made in many medical centres into which patients can be placed and treated with hyperbaric O_2. The O_2 is usually administered at PO_2s of 2 to 3 atmospheres of pressure through a mask or intratracheal tube, while the gas around the body is normal air compressed to the same high-pressure level. It is believed that the same oxidation free radicals responsible for oxygen toxicity are also responsible for the therapeutic benefits. Other condition in which hyperbaric O_2 therapy has been valuable include decompression sickness, arterial gas embolism, carbon monoxide poisoning, osteomyelitis, and myocardial infarction.

5

THERMOREGULATION

Survival and distribution of various forms of life on earth depend on temperature which is one of important environmental limiting factor. Activity of organism is the result of biochemical processes that take place in their body. All such processes are so much temperature sensitive that even a slight change in temperature alters the rate of these reactions. Therefore, there is need to maintain a specific body temperature for the life of an animal to be carried on in a perfect manner. The way in which the organisms maintain their body temperature within a certain limited range is called as *thermoregulation*.

The temperature range of universe is quite large from near absolute zero (–273°C) to about 6000°C around sun. On earth natural air temperature range only from –65°C in polar areas to + 60°C in devasting deserts; meaning range of environmental temperature is much greater; however, an active life is normally restricted to a narrow range of it from 0 to 40°C. Usually organisms can grow and remain metabolically active at range from –2 to 100°C, this range sometimes referred to as the "biokinetic zone".

Organisms generally occupy either aquatic or terrestrial or aerial habitat. Temperature within the water does not vary much because of the high specific heat of water and thus the effects of change of temperature on organisms as such not much. But the animals of terrestrial habitat are directly exposed to the radiant heat and also because of low specific heat of air, the temperature changes with the diurnal and seasonal variations, are much prominent. Thus, terrestrial animals have to face more changes in temperature as compared to aquatic animals.

The body of an organism in its environment continuously gains and loses heat from exogenous and endogenous routes. Inspite of such continuous turnover, the temperature of body precisely remains more or less matching with that of changing environment in Poikilotherms and constant in homeotherms. This temperature constancy or variation in relation to the environmental temperature in homeo and poikilotherms respectively is achieved by organisms due to certain thermal adaptations. Thus, the temperature adjustments are controlled by the physiological adjustments. Animals with a low rate of metabolism can not adjust themselves to extremes of temperature, but those with a high rate of metabolism are capable of manipulating the rate of metabolism so as to accord with the thermal changes taking place in the environment.

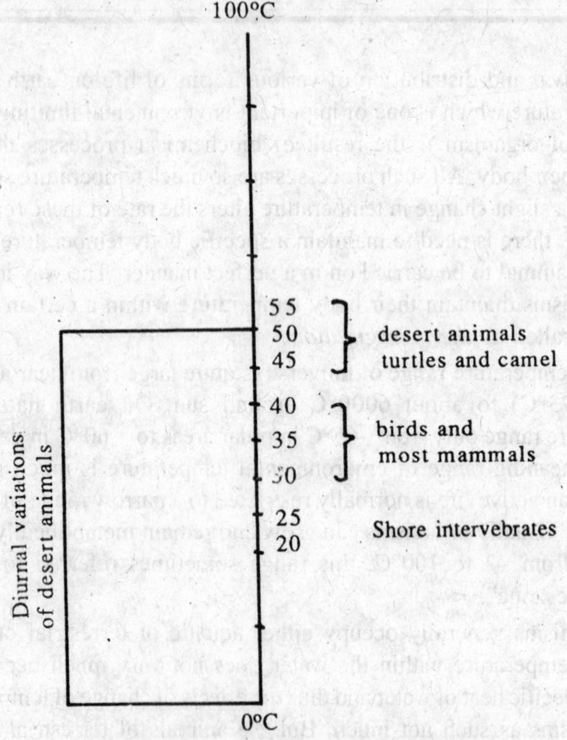

Fig. 5.1 : Temperature tolerance in animals.

Temperature Related Changes in Metabolism

From the foregoing discussion it can be stated that the physiological processes are highly temperature sensitive and are confined to very acute temperature measurements. Environmental temperature whether rising or falling manipulates, the rate of metabolic processes accordingly. The quantitative relationship between the temperature and the rate of a reaction was first pointed out by the *Jacobus Van't Hoff*. He stated that for every 10°C rise in temperature the rate of biochemical reactions becomes almost double. This is known as Q_{10} or *Temperature coefficient law* and is expressed as:

$$Q_{10} = \frac{(K_t + 10)}{K_t}$$

where K_t is the velocity constant at temperature t, and K_t + 10 is the velocity constant at 10°C temperature higher (t + 10).

In case of chemical reactions the values of Q_{10} are found to be quite constant. However, in case of enzymatic reactions this law is not applicable linearly. It is known that enzymes are proteins and beyond a temperature of about 40°C they undergo denaturation with a resultant loss in activity. After 40°C, a rise in temperature of 10°C accelerates the rate of denaturation not by two fold but a hundred-fold or even more. For this reason few organisms survive temperatures of 70°C and more. At low temperature the enzymes also become inactivated. This explains why bacteria generally grow faster at 37°C than at 20°C, why milk curdles rapidly in summer and why food keeps longer when refrigerated. So it is very much logical that under such circumstances they will not follow any such law. Therefore, in the case of enzymatic reactions the Q_{10} law is followed but in a very limited range Or temperatures between 0 and 50°C.

In case of poikilothermic animals, with change in environmental temperature the rate of metabolic processes change. Consequently the body temperature. But in homeothermic animals the change in the external temperature has no or very little effect on body temperature which remains almost constant and this is possible only because of certain temperature regulating mechanisms present in their tissues.

Types of Animals

On the basis of various aspects of temperature regulation, animals are classified in three groups, those are as follows:

1. Depending upon the body temperature the animals are grouped as warm blooded and cold blooded. But these terms are replaced by more authentic terms *i.e.,* homeotherms and poikilotherms. Animals which inspite of fluctuations or great variations in the atmospheric temperatures maintain a relatively constant body temperature are called as *homeotherms*, (G. homoios = similar), it includes birds and mammals. Whereas the animals whose body temperature varies with changes in environmental temperature come under the category of *poikilotherms*

(G, poikilos = variable), aquatic animals, invertebrates, amphibians are included in this group.

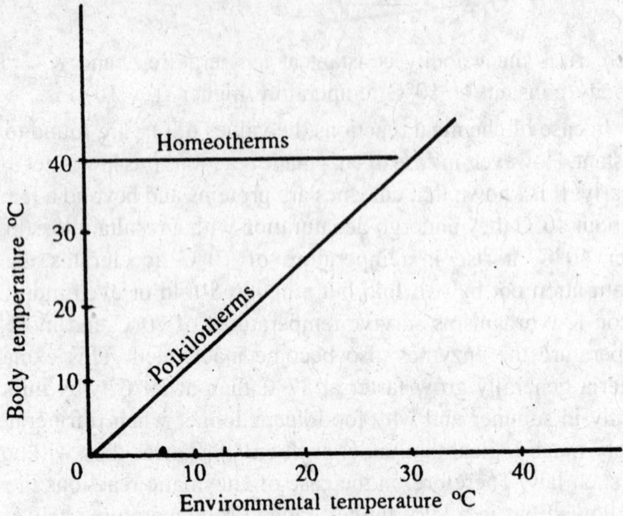

Fig. 5.2 : Relation of body temperature to environmental temperature in homeotherm and poikilotherm.

2. Because of their own oxidative metabolism some animals are capable of producing sufficient heat to maintain a constant body temperature. These animals are termed as *endothermic* (G. endon = within) animals. Examples of endothermic animals are birds and mammals, while others have low production and high conduction of heat with the result they have to depend upon the atmospheric heat for maintaining their body temperature. Such animals are put together under the term *ectothermic* (G. ektos = outside) animals which include vast number of animals *e.g.*, the invertebrates, fishes, amphibians, reptiles etc.
3. There is a term *heterotherms* (G. heteros = one or other) or the *facultative endotherms*, is applied to those animals which show variable characteristics of being able to generate heat and maintain their body temperature themselves at times when they are active and being unable to do, so when they are at rest. So during the time of low metabolism they have to depend upon the atmospheric heat to regulate their body temperature like ectotherms and

when active they behave like endotherms, such animals, present just on the critical line, like monotremes, some marsupials, armadillos etc.

Effect of Low Temperature

There exists varied responses when animals are exposed to cold. A few of them migrate to avoid such unfavourable conditions while the others who face such low temperatures either adjust themselves accordingly or one sure to be effected adversely. The low temperature effects the animals not only by slowing down the fate of metabolism but also it causes ice formation in extracellular fluid. As a result the water comes out of the cells by osmosis and concentration of salts within the cells change. This produces lethal effects and the animals are forced to die if the same effect continues. This lethal temperature for different animals varies according to the dosage of exposure to low temperature and to the temperature in which the animal was living before its exposure to low temperature. Many invertebrates (poikilotherms) inhabiting extreme habitates have used the principal of *supercooling* to avoid the effects of extreme cold. In this phenomenon, temperature of a solution is lowered continuously without agitation *i.e.,* without disturbing the solutes suspended, water can be prevented from undergoing freezing. The ability of insects to survive in temperatures below freezing through the phenomenon of supercooling has been known. The body temperature of *Saturnia pyri*, for example, when exposed to an air temperature of –13.5°C, drops steadily to –9°C. Insects that supercool to temperature below - 40°C have all been found to have low freezing points because of high solute concentrations in their body fluid. In homeotherms all this is done by the temperature regulating mechanisms but it is found that as a result of severe cold, these mechanisms, if break down to operate, result in the death of the animals.

The second principle for avoiding protoplasmic freezing and subsequent cold death at extremely low temperature is done by *freezing point depression.* Generally, freezing point of a solution is always lower than pure solvent. In the winter hardening in insects and fishes osmolarity of die body fluids is high ultimately saving the animals during cooler environmental conditions.

Effect of High Temperature

The high temperatures are found to effect the life of animals and the effects of high temperature are much more severe than those of low temperature. The dependence of animals for temperature is based again on the exposure time and temperature of environment that the animal was inhabiting before the high temperature condition. Aquatic animals face less variations in temperature because of high specific heat of water and thus their lethal temperatures are lower as compared to those of land animals.

Various ways in which the high temperatures are found to effect the animals may be one or more or all of the following. After a certain limit, if the temperature rises the body activities cease down and the animals finally die. Protoplasm constituting the animals contains proteins and enzymes, coagulate and get denatured at high temperatures. Thus they effect the body activities in general and finally result in death. Also the excess of heat leads to an increased viscosity of cellular fluid, as a result vacuolation also takes place. Vacuolation lead to release of Ca^{++} ions within the cells and the Ca^{++} ions so released have a disruptive influence on the cell by affecting the permeability of plasma membrane. All these factors combiningly or alone affect the organisms adversely. Effect of high temperature is opposite to that of low temperatures.

Regulation of Body Temperature

The "DU Bois Temperature Balance " has been shown in Fig. 5.3. It shows graphically how the physiological and metabolic reactions that produce heat must be matched against those that radiate or conduct it away in order to provide a constant body temperature. Except in a very-narrow "Thermally neutral zone", the maintenance of a constant body temperature makes a steady demand either on the chemical processes of heat production or on the physical devices for heat loss.

In most of mammals, body temperature lies somewhere between 36 and 38°C, birds however, maintain body temperature slightly higher between 39 to 42°C. This constancy of body temperature permits a steady high level of both metabolic and locomotary activities. In general 35 to 40°C is the thermal range preferred by homeotherms.

Body temperature is the balance between heat loss and heat gain conditioned by heat production which is proportional to the metabolic rate. For a typical mammal, even to date, the Du Bois temperature balance accounting for heat loss and heat gain is applicable. The relationship between energy metabolism in terms of oxygen consumption and ambient temperature can be studied by considering a case of hypothetical homeotherm (Fig. 5.4). Over some range of temperature (27 to 35°C) O_2 consumption is minimal and virtually independent of temperature. This minimum O_2 consumption zone is called as the *thermal neutral zone*. Two ends of this zone are lower critical temperature and upper critical temperature. Below the *lower critical temperature*, O_2 consumption increases linearly as temperature decreases. Above the upper critical temperature zone O_2 consumption increases rapidly as ambient temperature rises, but the rate of increase is not usually linear.

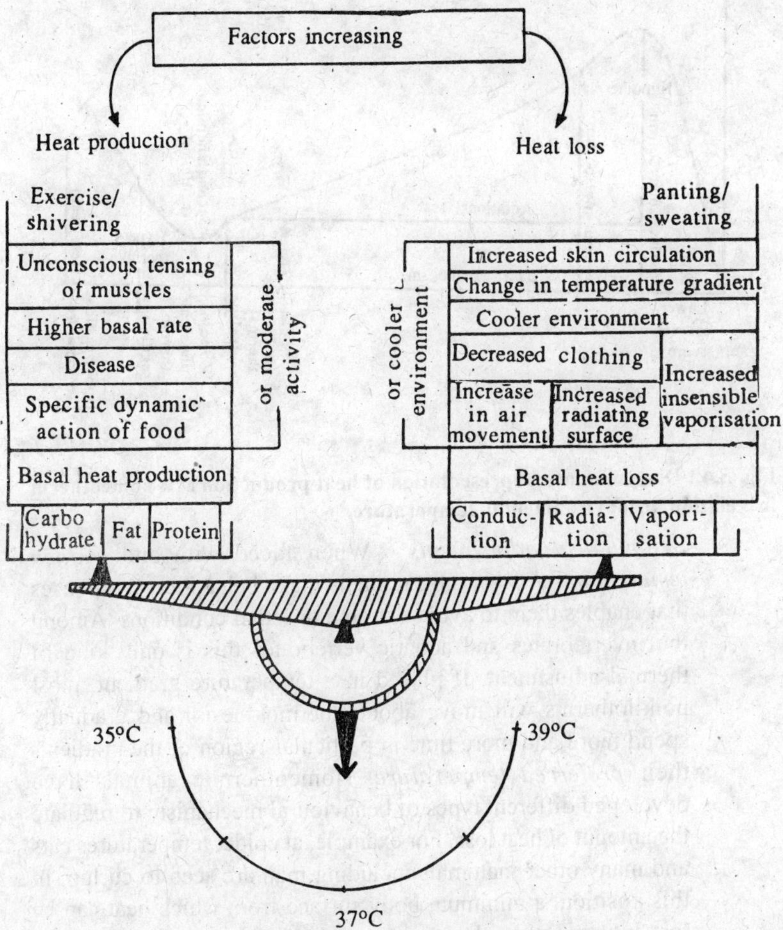

Fig. 5.3 : The Du Bois temperature balance.

Thus, in the thermal neutral zone, animal is expending a minimum amount of energy on thermoregulation, and neither physical nor chemical mechanisms for controlling heat production or heat loss need to employed.

Again, above and below critical temperatures, animal will have to do additional metabolic work in order to maintain body temperature constant, so needs physical adaptations and chemical mechanisms and those are as follows:

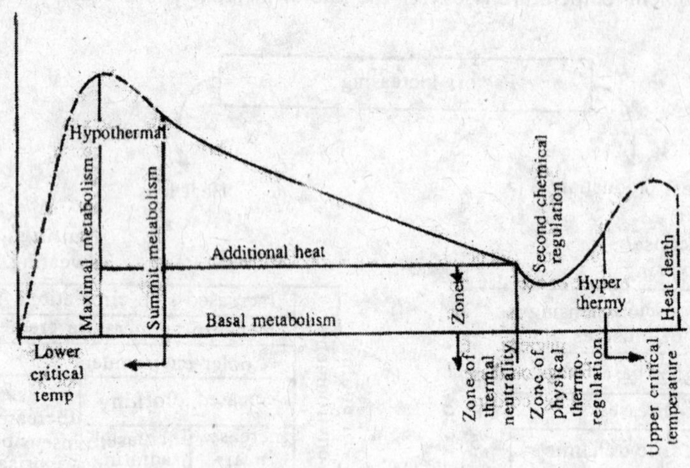

Fig. 5.4 : Diagrammatic representation of heat production of a homeotherm in relation to environmental temperature.

1. *Behavioural adjustments* : When faced with and *sudden temperature change*, most animals make behavioural responses that enables them to avoid extreme or lethal conditions. Among the invertebrates and aquatic vertebrates this is only kind of thermal adjustment. If placed in a temperature gradient, most poikilotherms will move about (thermokinesis) and gradually spend more and more time in particular region of the gradient-their *preferred temperature*. Homeothermic animals have developed different types of behavioural mechanism to regulate the amount of heat loss. For example, at colder temperatures cats and many other mammals including man are seen to curlup. In this position, a minimum body surface from which heat can be lost is exposed to the environment. Under warmer conditions such animals may stretch out, thus a greater surface for heat loss is provided. Hudding or crowding together is evident in the new born and naked pups, rats etc. Behavioural mechanisms also

include avoidance of cold situations, exposure to sun, migration from a thermally hostile environment, construction of burrows etc.

It is interesting to see various thermoregulatory devices employed by human beings on these lines. Man is basically a tropical species and for him withstanding colder conditions is both morphologically difficult and metabolically expensive. The success in inhabiting thermally adverse habitates goes almost entirely to behavioural capacities operating through intellect. In addition to physiological and behavioural adaptations he has also developed sufficient technology to create artificially an environment that he can tolerate comfortably (clothing, artificial cooling and warming devices, ingestion of thermally appropriate foods etc.)

2. *Pelage :* Different groups of homeotherms inhabiting variety of colder environment have evolved different (insulating devices). For example, animals inhabiting polar regions are covered with thick fur, similarly from colder climates with feathers and hairs. Such hairy covering of a mammal is called *pelage*.

   When such furred or hairy animal suddenly exposed to cold stress, reflexly make their hair stand more or less erect with the help of piloerecter muscles. Due to piloerection there is increase in thickness and depth of insulating layer and air trapped in it. This morphological situation help in reducing the amount of heat lost. The growth, quantity and insulative quality of pelage dependent on time exposed. Animals exposed continuously to intense cold possess a thick fur coat. The arctic fox who is insulated in this way can easily survive in snow at –40°C. If, cold occur in regular cycle, heavy fur is grown for that period only. Such thick fur is seen in porcupine, squirrel, rabbit, dog etc. In summer, such thick pelage is sheded proportionately thereby increasing their surface conductance and heat dissipation.

3. *Subcutaneous fat :* Special insulative qualities have been claimed for fat. The fatty layer tends to be thicker in animals acclimatized cold and particularly so in bare skinned animals. The selective deposition of more fluid fats (lower melting point) in colder environments; and in more exposed tissues such as those in the extremities of the Arctic animal. The semiaquatic polar bear, is

provided with thick layer of subcutaneous fat or blubber, whose thickness however varies in different parts of its body (about 60 to 110 mm thick on abdominal region).

Aquatic mammals inhabiting cold seas are provided with negligible pelage. (Whale, porpoise, walrus and several seals) but there is a uniformly thick layer of subcutaneous fat or blubber; which being a poor conductor forms an insulating coat around visceral organs. Blubber constitutes about 40-50% of body substance in porpoise, 20 to 45% in various whales and 30-40% in seal.

4. *Brown fat* : All organs produce heat as a by product of metabolism but the mammals, and only the mammals, have a special thermogenic organ Or tissue known as *Brown fat* or *Brown Adipose tissue*. This tissue is most conspicuously developed and active in many newborn mammals (including the human), in hibernating animals at the time of arousal and in cold acclimated mammals. In this animals brown fat serves as a "chemical furnace" –an oil burner, to it respond to cold stress with a large burst of heat. The tissue is strategically localized in the neck and thoracic regions in relation to major blood vessels so that its heat is quickly transported to those organs (brain and heart) whose continuous high temperature are vital to the operation of a homeotherm.

Brown fat was first described in hibernating mormots (a rabbit like rodent), *Muris alpinus*. Brown fat also occurs in the young ones of hamster. rat, cat, dog, macaques, rabbit, man etc.

Histologically, it is an extremely vascular tissue with high concentration of myoglobin, cytochromes and flavin compounds, this given it a pale buff to dark brown colour. Cytologically, the cells are smaller, polygonal, with central nuclei and numerous fat droplets, which are dispersed (multilocular) rather than concentrated in a single vacuole (unilocular), mitochondria are small, numerous and closely associated with the fat droplets. Biochemically, it consists of high concentration of water, protein, phospholipid, cholesterol and certain mitochondrial enzymes. The metabolic pathways in this tissue generate heat probably by way of uncoupled oxidative phosphorylation rather than ATP. Heat production is mainly by oxidation of fatty acids. This tissue can be thought of as a rapidly firing furnace that warms some mammals up quickly in an emergency, without muscular activity or shivering.

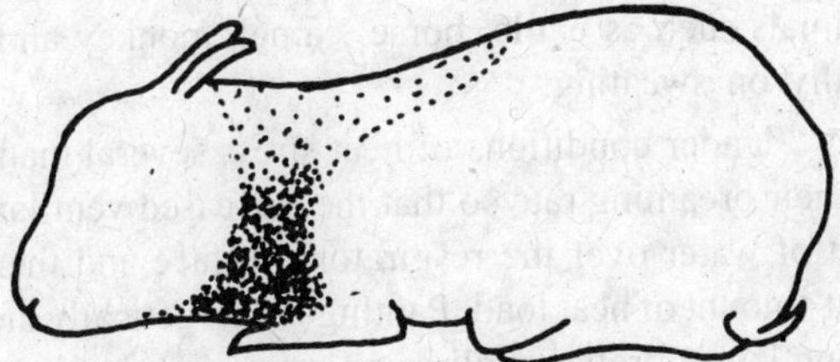

Fig. 5.5 : Distribution of brown-fat (shaded area) in new-born rabbit.

The physiological mediator for the stimulation of brown adipose tissue (BAT) is nor adrenaline. According to present concept, noradrenaline released in brown fat during sympathetic stimulation.

5. *Evaporative cooling (sweating and panting)* : Evaporative cooling is the most efficient mechanism accounting for the heat loss whenever body temperature rises. In most of mammals like rabbit, cat, dog, along with man employ sweating and/or panting as active thermoregulatory devices under a heat stress. Some evaporation and, loss of water occurs through insensible perspiration that accounts one third of the total water loss, remainder is lost via skin. The water diffuse from dermal circulation over skin and evaporates before wetting the surface. Similarly, when environmental temperature rises the cutaneous blood supply is increased thereby increasing the supply of water for insensible perspiration. When a rise in body temperature exceeds physiological limit at higher environmental temperatures or during heavy muscular exercise, sweating starts.

Sweating : Sweating is an efficient mechanism for increasing heat loss particularly in those animals that possess less sweat glands. Sweating is under the control of hypothalamic thermostats responding to the changes in the core temperatures. The thermostat may detect the temperature changes as conveyed to it by receptors on the skin or from blood drained from peripheral circulation. The secretory activities of sweat glands with subsequent dilations or contraction are controlled by parasympathetic system through cholinergic nerves which have overriding influence of hypothalamic thermostats. Thus, the cooling processes by sweating are ultimately controlled by thermostats, which selectively switch on or off the thermogenetic and thermoregulatory processes. Sweat glands from certain regions like palm of the hand and sole of the foot are primarily controlled by emotions that influence the cerebral cortex. Animals such as cattle, horse, camel, monkey and man depend almost totally on sweating.

Panting : Under conditions of heat stress several mammals pant or accelerate their breathing rate so that the increased ventilation promotes evaporation of water over the respiratory surface and thereby removes a significant amount of heat load. Panting is energetically more expensive than sweating but is preferentially employed by animals such as rabbit, sheep, deer, cat, dog etc. Panting has one disadvantage in that the increased ventilation may lead to excessive loss of CO_2 from the lungs, which can result in severe alkolosis. This tendency to develop alkalosis can in part be counteracted by shifting to a more shallow respiration (smaller tidal volume) at an increased frequency, so that the increased ventilation takes place mostly in the dead space of the upper respiratory tract. Thus respiratory rate of these animals increases with increasing temperature. At higher temperatures they hold their mouth open and breath deeply. This evaporative water loss through buccal mucosa and from the respiratory system lowers down the body temperature, when it rises above the tolerable range.

6. *Shivering and nonshivering* : The most conspicuous mechanism by which a homeotherm increases heat production is by increase in muscular activity. One of such effective thermogenic activity is *shivering*. This involves rapid, involuntary and thythmic contraction of the muscles and occurs when the body is at rest. Sudden exposure to cold generally results in shivering. This activity may commence either by a slight fall in core or skin, temperature. Shivering need not be visible for it to increase heat production. Muscle tremors too small to be evident can be visualised instrumentally. Exercise avoids shivering.

   In several mammals, heat production can be augmented metabolically but without increased muscular activity or muscle tones, this type of thermogenesis is called non shivering. During cold stress, acclimated rats produce as much as 65 percent of their heat from thermogenesis that is not accompanied by an increase in the electrical activity of muscles.

7. *Regional heterothermy and counter current heat exchangers* : Some low grade mammals like *Echidna*; *Oppossum*, *Ornithorhynchus* etc., are not very much efficient in maintaining a constant body temperature and large fluctuations of temperature

is observed in them. To some extent their body temperature changes with that of environment. It is also mechanically impossible to insulate all parts of the body with an equal effectiveness. The legs, tail, ears, eyes and muzzle of mammals and the legs, wings, beak and eyes of the birds obviously cannot have insulation as effective as that of the other body parts. Such terminal portions exhibit regional heterothermy (variable body temperature) and these localized regions are capable of effective functioning in spite of great thermal differences between core temperature and these parts. In Alaskan sled dog, whose leg shows a steep thermal gradient from 35°C at shoulder to 0°C, the temperature of sole. The reindeer's leg may be at 8 to 10°C with a core body temperature of about 37°C.

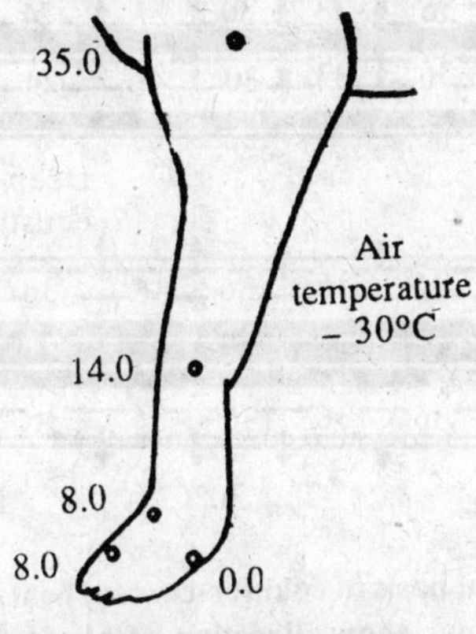

Fig. 5.6 : Regional heterothermy in the fore-leg of the Alaskan sled dog. (Figures are Subcutaneous temperatures in °C.

This type of heterothermy involves specialized physiological adaptations that maintain the region efficient even at low temperature. One of such physiological adaptations is *counter-current heat exchanger*. Counter current heat exchanger is termed so because thermal transfer occurs between closely associated vessels in whom the blood flow is in opposite direction. In aquatic mammals such as seal, porpoise and whale possess major arteries to the appendages which are located centrally and are closely invested by numerous thin walled veins when heat is to be conserved, the subcutaneous veins constrict and the warm arterial blood flowing into the limb transfers heat to the cool blood returning through the neighbouring veins (Fig. 5.7), the arterial blood is thus cooled and the venous blood warmed. When on the other hand, heat is to be unloaded, the animal responds in exactly the opposite way. Its deep veins constrict and the superficial veins dilate (Fig. 5.7). The warm arterial blood bypasses the heat exchanger and is returned through these dilated veins which unload the heat to the water through physical devices. The circulatory system of the extremities thus functions in both, heat conservation and dissipation.

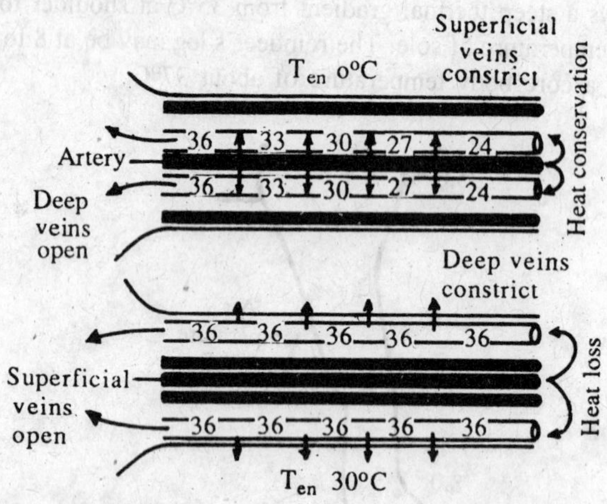

Fig. 5.7 : The anatomical basis of counter-current heat exchange (Constricted veins, solid black; arrows show direction of blood flow).

In many birds and mammals (sloth, armadillo, loris etc.) This vascular arrangement is elaborated into a multichanelled *Rete* (Retia mirabilia) made up of bundles of hundreds of intermingled arteries and veins. The tail, as well as the legs, often forms the site for these specialized vascular bundles.

8. *Modulation of peripheral blood flow* : Like sweating or panting another mechanism regulating heat loss is peripheral circulation. Skin surface, particularly man and other scantily haired mammals, serves as a large heat exchanging surface. Vasomotor activities like vasodilation and vasoconstriction are used to shunt blood to various regions of the body. Vasomotor activity in the skin arterioles determine the amount of blood passing through the

skin and therefore, determines the amount of heat that can be transferred from the blood to the environment. Increased vascular flow to the skin also brings about a greater volume of fluid available for evaporation from the skin after diffusion or secretion by the sweat glands.

At higher environmental temperatures or during periods of exercise. Skin venels dilate (vasodilation) and the flow of blood in the peripheral regions increases thus permitting greater heat loss. On the other hand, in cold conditions skin blood vessels constrict (vasoconstriction) thus cutting down the blood flow and subsequent heat loss from the skin. Stimuli controlling vasomotor activities may be sent by localized warm or cold receptors or even hypothalamus may be directly stimulated by the temperature of blood passing through it.

Types of Adaptive Hypothermia

Some animals show daily cycles of torpidity (sluggishness), whereas others show an annual period of dormancy, that depending upon the season is called either *hibernation or aestivation*. Still others show a partial torpidity associated with a degree of hypothermia, which is usually referred to as seasonal lethargy or partial hibernation.

(a) *Daily torpor* : Due to small size and aerial habit in many groups of birds and mammals (bats and rodents) strict homeothermy is metabolically expensive. This condition is still, acute for small insectivorous bats and humming bird because of limited stored food materials and period of feeding, night in bats and day in humming birds. Such groups of homeotherms undergo daily-period of torpidity. They generally maintain high body temperature during active periods which undergoes profound drop during resting stages. Homeothermy enables them to achieve a degree of functional freedom inspite of environmental temperature variations. While resting they are profited from the economy of energy conservation made possible by temporary adaptations of poikilothermy. Thus, due to daily torpor, they are able to exploit a variety of habitats that would not otherwise have become available to them.

Stimulus for daily torpor is, lowered environmental temperature. Studies on the California pocket mouse, *Perognathus californicus*, have shown that entry into torpor can occur at any temperature below the lower critical temperature (32.5°C). The essential events during preparation for torpor are, a cessation of thermoregulation and a reduction in the metabolism to the basal level. The thermostat is adjusted at lower level and thermal conduction is maximum. As a result, heat loss exceeds heat generation and the body temperature starts falling down. The falling body temperature at the end approximately matches the ambient temperature or even it remains slightly higher. During arousal from torpor, thermal conductance is minimized, the animal shivers violently and oxygen consumption becomes maximum. As heat production exceeds heat loss, body temperature rises at a rate of more than 0.5°C/min.

Adaptive hypothermia in the form of daily torpor thus enables energy conservation at least for endotherms for whom homeothermy, otherwise, would have been metabolically expensive. Such adaptive hypothermia is prominently seen in many mammals including monotremes, marsupials and placentals and in at least three groups of birds-the swifts, goat suckers and humming birds.

(b) *Hibernation (L. hiberna = winter) :* In areas where the low temperature of winter represent a regular and acute adaptive challenge, many medium and small sized mammals undergo prolonged period of hypothermia and dormancy called hibernation. It is a physiologically specialized state associated with the evolution of homeothermy in certain extreme habitats. Hibernation may be defined as a *regulated seasonal phenomenon in which body temperature and all physiological activities get readjusted to a new, lower level from which spontaneous or induced arousal to normal level is possible at all times.*

Hibernation is thus a cyclic phenomenon and before it, a *period* of *preparation* and adjustment usually observed. Many small rodents store large quantities of food in their burrows prior to entry into the hibernation. In nearly all species that experience periods of dormancy, enormous amounts of fat are deposited. Animals experience progressively increasing periods of lethargy and undergo a series of increasingly deep and prolonged periods of hypothermia.

During hibernation body temperature is allowed to fall upto, a limit and if it starts going below it, the hibenator starts arouses and thermogenetic processes are switched on thus bringing body temperature to normal level. Stimulus for such arousal is sent through the hypothalamus in which the thermostat is adjusted at its altered thermal range. Thus during hibernation although peripheral temperature falls down, a particular core temperature is always maintained with the help of thermostat adjusted on that range.

The stimulus that induces hibernation is a progressively lowering of the external temperature and after preceded by physiological and metabolic changes taking place during the summer. Hibernation is characterised by overall retardation in the vital activities. Thus, metabolic, respiratory and cardiac rates may fall to anywhere from a tenth to a hundredth of their normal values depending on the species, A normally active marmot produces heat at a rate of 2.8 kcal/kg/h, but this declines to 0.09 kcal/kg/h during hibernation. The respiratory quotient (R.Q.) in hibernation is about 0.7.

In mormots and squirrels (*e.g.*, the ground squirrel (*Itellus beecheyi*), is characterised by a series of gradually depending "test-drops" of body temperature with complete arousal between each hypothermic period. The decline in metabolism and body temperature occurs within a few days of cool weather and the extent of this fall depends upon the state of prepareness. When this is complete, results in winter sleep,

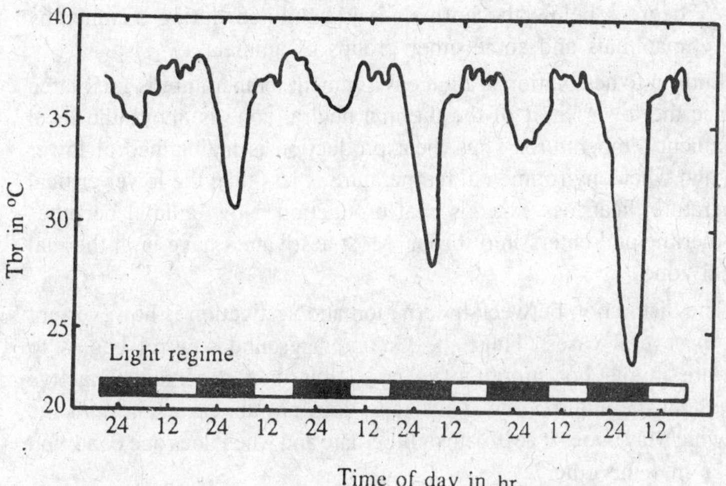

Fig. 5.8 : "Test-drops' in the brain temperature (Tbr) of the ground squirrel during preparation for hibernation.

During arousal, awaking from hibernation, the hibernator rapidly activates both heat generating and heat conserving mechanisms. Initial awakening includes an increase in respiratory rate and muscular activities followed by cardio Muscles. Both shivering and nonshivering thermogenesis is employed and in this process of endogenous thermogenesis heat production in the deposits of brown fat is quantitatively important, particularly during the early stages. Thus, during termination of hibernation core temperature is raised in the beginning and the heart and nervous systems are the first vital organs to achieve high temperature followed by rest of the body. In ground squirrel, during arousal the temperature rises from 4° to 35°C in 4 hrs. while the birchmouse warms at a rate of 1°C/min.

To summarise, hibernation is a specialized state of adaptive hypothermia, which is a solution to seasonally a regularly appearing colder conditions, also is a means of solving the annual problem of food scarcity, and other adverse conditions arising from extreme temperature changes and falling environmental temperature acts as the stimulus for it.

3. *Aestivation (L. aestas = summer) :* It is specialized adaptive mechanism developed to face the periods of drought, heat and any other prolonged and recurrent pattern of seasonal stress. The dormancy is characterized by the normal physiological levels of many activities although body temperature may be several degrees below the normal. It is exhibited during summer by mammals and some other groups of animals.

Entry into aestivation at high environment temperature is facilitated because the lower limit of the thermal neutral zone is above the level of ambient temperature. Thus, heat production is maintained at lower level and when environmental temperature is less than the lower critical temperature, heat loss exceeds heat production. Now, animal becomes hypothermic and enters into torpor. Most aestivators have high thermal neutral zone.

The distinction between hibernation and aestivation is however not easy in several cases. Thus, the Columbia ground squirrel begins to aestivate in the hot month of August, but then it remains inactive throughout the autumn and winter and does not appear again until the following May. Does it aestivate or hibernate and when does one condition change into the other?

Role of Temperature Regulating Centres in the Development of Homeothermy

The immediate responses to acute temperature changes are mediated through the central nervous system. Today it is conclusively proved that hypothalamus acts as the thermostat. Information regarding thermal states of the environment reaches to it either through nerve circuits or through the peripheral circulation. In response to these thermal changes the hypothalamus switches on or off various thermoregulatory responses related with the heat gain or loss. Hypothalamus has the ability to perceive and respond to temperature fluctuations as low as 0.01°C.

If the body needs more heat, the hypothalamus sends impulses to the muscles, causing increased tone and shivering. If the body requires cooling. impulses to the sweat glands induce sweat production. If the hypothalamus is cooled locally, shivering starts at once. It has been found that anterior region of the hypothalamus contains the neurons that respond to warmth whereas the posterior region of it contains the neurons responsible for reactions to cold. It is further evident from the fact that injury to the posterior region of hypothalamus leads to the failure of spontaneous eating, shivering, capacity of piloerection and normal posture-capacity of thermogenesis is completely lost. Thus, destruction of this region physiologically transforms a homeotherm into a poikilotherm.

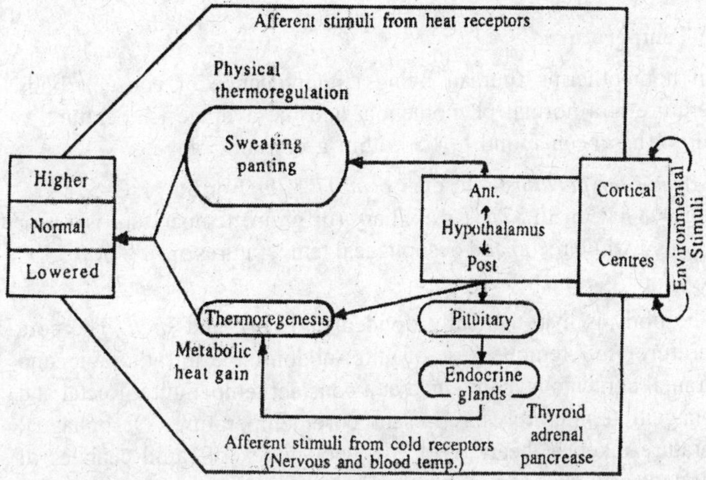

Fig. 5.9 : Role of hypothalamus in the thermoregulation in case of homeotherms.

Both central and peripheral thermoreceptors play an important role in temperature regulation. In this regard hypothalamus has two roles. It integrates all of the sensory information, *i.e.,* temperature conditions both internal and external of itself acts as a sensory mechanism for determining the core temperature. It also functions to integrate two homeostatic functions-osmoregulation and thermoregulation and also exerts influence on endocrine glands like thyroid, adrenal etc. engaged in the regulation of cellular metabolism in the process of thermogenesis.

There are two thermoreceptors which regulate body temperature in mammals skin and upper part of diagram tract contain *peripheral thermoreceptors*. These are heat sensitive nerve endings and respond variously to heat or cold. The scrotum of male mammals and udders (mammary glands) of the female are such highly sensitive thermosensory areas. These heat receptors activate the cooling response irrespective of the core temperature, such a local control is necessary for since sperms, for example develop normally only over a narrow temperature range which is slightly below that of the body.

The *central thermoreceptors* are also present deep in the body. These include the vana cava and rumen in sheep and the femoral vein in cat and man, however, the best known and principal central thermoreceptor is hypothalamus present on floor and sides of the posterior part of the forebrain (already discussed).

Body Temperature

In homeotherms (human beings) maintenance of constant body temperature is a normal phenomenon, and the average temperature as measured, has been found to lie within a constant range.

Normal temperature : In man *oral* 97°f–99°f or 36.11°C–37.22°C (average 98.4°f or 36.87°C). Auxiliary (or grain) temperature is 1°f or 0.55°C less, while rectal and oesophageal temperatures are 1°f or 0.55°C more.

The body is hypothetically divided into *core* and *shell*. The core temperature *i.e.*, temperature of intra-abdominal, intrathoracic and intracranial contents is maintained at a constant temperature. Rectal and oesophageal temperatures represent core temperature. Oesophageal temperature taken at heart level is a good index of rapid changes of cardiac and aortic blood temperatures (as during induction of hypothermia, rewarming from hypothermia), whereas rectal temperature gives a poor reflection of rapid change of blood temperature and may be misleading. Shell temperature *i.e.*, temperatures of the limbs and the surface layer of the trunk exhibits wide variation of the temperatures. Although, rectal and oesophageal temperatures are most reliable, yet, for practical advantage, oral temperatures is taken for routine clinical purposes.

Heat is continually being produced in the body as a by-product of metabolism and body heat is also continually being lost to the surroundings. When the rate of heat production is exactly equal to the rate of loss, the person is said to be in heat balance. But when the two are out of equilibrium, the body heat and the body temperature as well, will obviously be either increasing or decreasing.

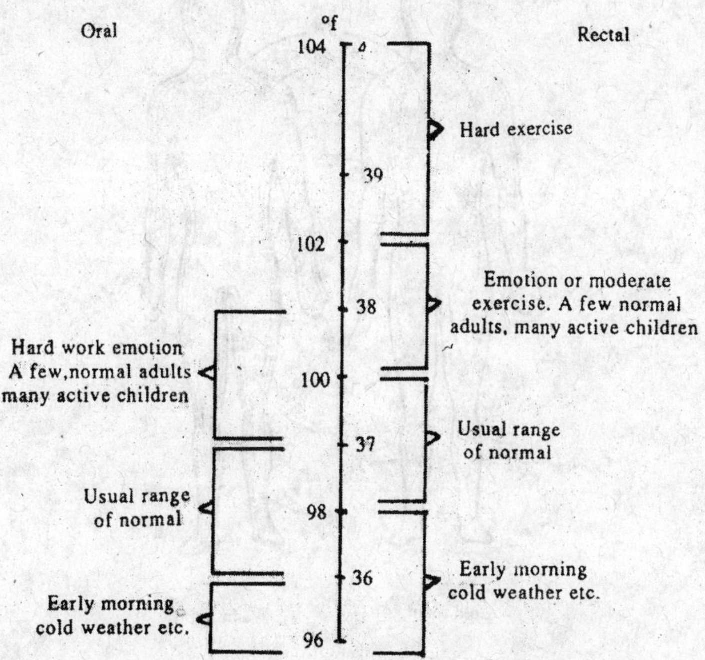

Fig. 5.10 : Estimated range of body temperature in normal person.

The important factors that play major role in determining the rate of heat production were :

1. Basal rate of metabolism of all the cells of body.
2. Increase in rate of metabolism caused by muscle activity, including that caused by shivering
3. Increase in metabolism caused by the effect of thyroxine on cells
4. Increase in metabolism caused by the effect of norepinephrine and sympathetic stimulation on cells and

5. Increase in metabolism caused by increased temperature of the body cells

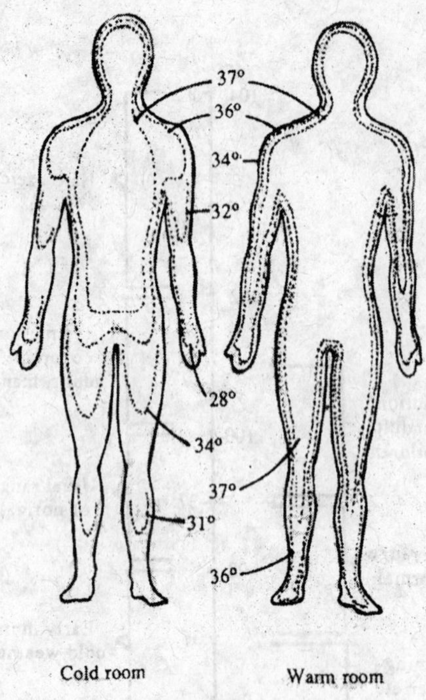

Fig. 5.11 : The temperature gradients (°C) forming a' core' and a' shell' in a man in warm and a cold environment.

Heat Loss

The various methods by which heat is lost from the body are pictured in Fig. 5.12. These include radiation (loss of heat in the form of infrared heat rays, a type of electromagnetic waves in all directions), *conduction* (loss of heat from surface of body to other objects, like a chair or a bed etc.), convection (loss of heat by air currents), evaporation (0.58 calories of heat is lost for each gram of water that evaporates from body surface). Water evaporates insensibly from the skin and lungs at a rate of about 600 ml per day.

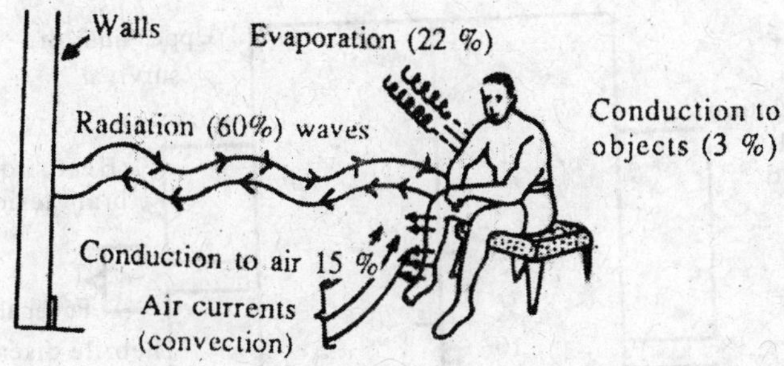

Fig. 5.12 : Mechanisms of heat loss from the body.

Heat Coma

From the foregoing discussion it is evident that biological activities are smooth at optimum temperature from 37°C or 98°f in the human beings. When the body temperature rises beyond a critical temperature *i.e.,* range of 106° to 108°f, the rate of biological reactions are get affected which results into damage of parenchyma of many cells in different organs, but especially in the brain. Unfortunately, once neuronal cells are destroyed, they can never be replaced. In such cases the person is likely to develop *heat coma* or *heat stroke.* The symptoms of heat coma includes dizziness, abdominal distress. Sometimes, exposure to erature may result in death. Heat coma may be recovered by placing the person in an ice water bath or sponge cooling of skin is likely to be more effective.

The limits of extreme heat that on can stand depend almost entirely on whether the heat is dry or wet. If the air is completely dry and sufficient convection air currents are flowing to promote rapid evaporation from the body. However, if the air is 100% humidified or if the body is in water, the body temperature begins to rise whenever the environmental temperature rises above approximately 94°f.

Fig. 5.13 shows that once the body temperature has fallen below 85°f, ability of the hypothalamus to regulate temperature is completely lost and it is greatly impaired even when the body temperature falls below approximately 94°f. Part of the reason for this loss of temperature is that the rate of heat production in each cell is greatly depressed by the low temperature. Also, sleepiness and even chill coma are likely to develop which depress the activity of the central nervous system heat-control mechanisms and prevent shivering. Body heat is best therapy to recover from chill coma.

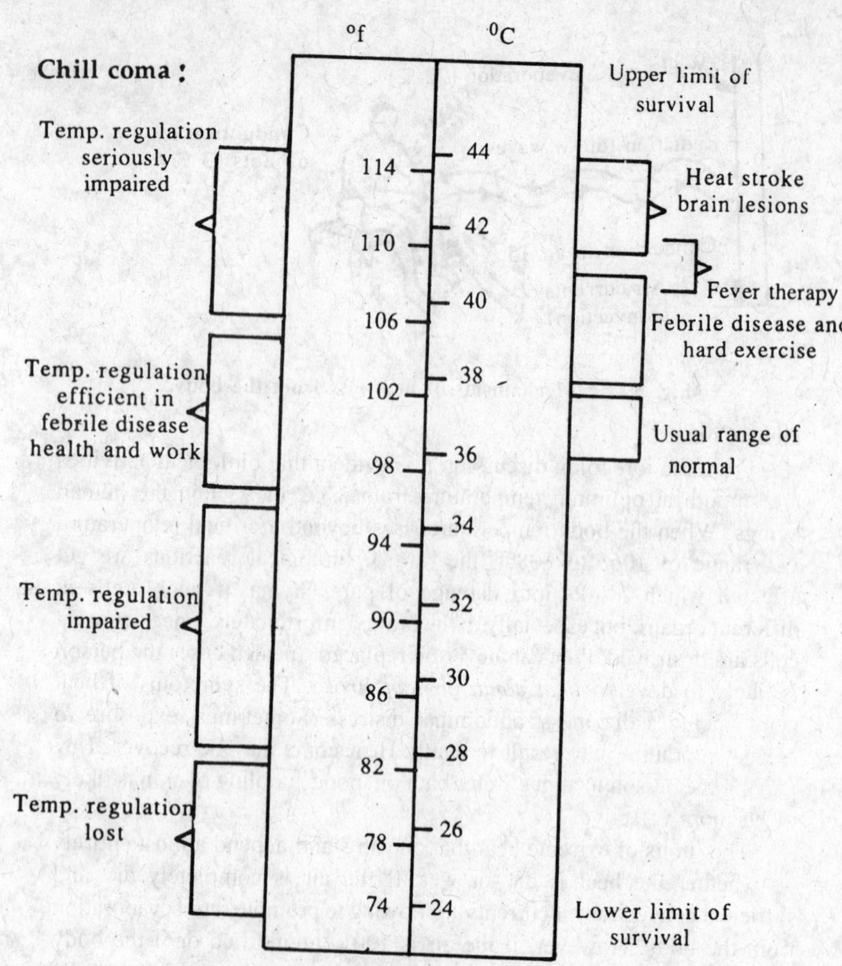

Fig. 5.13 : Body temperatures under different conditions.

Frost bite : When the body is exposed to extremely low temperatures, surface areas can actually freeze; the freezing is called *frost bite*. This occurs especially in the lobes of the ears and in the digits of the hands and feet. If the parts are thawed immediately, especially with water that is not above approximately 110°f, no permanent damage may result. On the other hand, prolonged freezing causes permanent circulatory impairment as well as local tissue damage. Often gangrene follows thawing, and the frostbitten areas are lost.

6

OSMOREGULATION

I. WATER

Water was undoubtedly the medium in which the life first appeared on the earth and still it remains to be the medium containing the greatest abundance and diversity of living forms today. Further among those animals that have adapted terrestrial mode of life, only some of the insects have completely escaped aquatic life; all the others, including mammals must spend at least the larval period immersed in water.

Animal body, in general, is composed of water to the extent of 60 to 70% by volume and this percentage is a constant feature. Water is the major component of the protoplasm and constitutes more than 60% of the total protoplasmic mass. However, it varies in different tissues of the same animal and the same tissues of different animals. For example, the enamel of tooth has only 2% water, where as in a nerve tissue it ranges upto 80%. Water is the most effective and universal solvent and furnishes a medium in which most biochemical reactions occur. Loss of 20% body water usually leads to death. The unique biological properties of water are a reflection of its exceptional physiochemical characteristics.

Chemical Nature and Properties

Water is formed from hydrogen and oxygen atoms with two covalent bonds, holding the two hydrogens to one oxygen and forming an angle of 104.5°. The length of each bond is 0.99 A°.

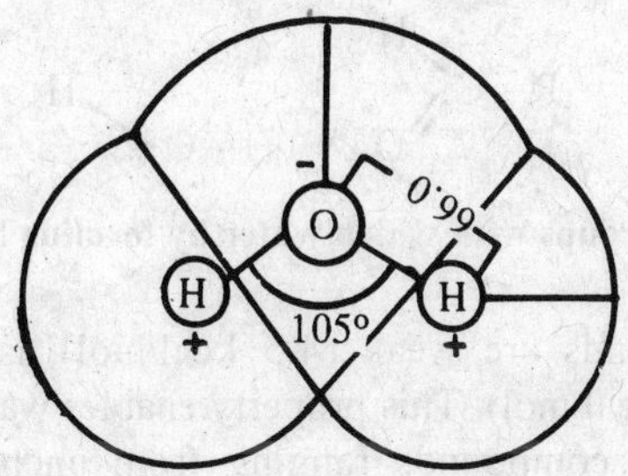

Fig. 6.1 : The structure of water molecule and its dipole nature.

Dipole movement of water : Water is a dipole, a particle with two charges of opposite sign. In a molecule of water the hydrogen (H) atoms are positively charged, whereas the oxygen (O) atom is negatively charged and the configuration of the bond angle makes electric charge on the molecule unevenly distributed. Therefore, it tends to orient itself as a dipole in an electric field.

Water as a solvent : The unequal distribution of charge on a water molecule enables it to form hydrogen bonds by electrostatic attraction (Fig. 6.2).

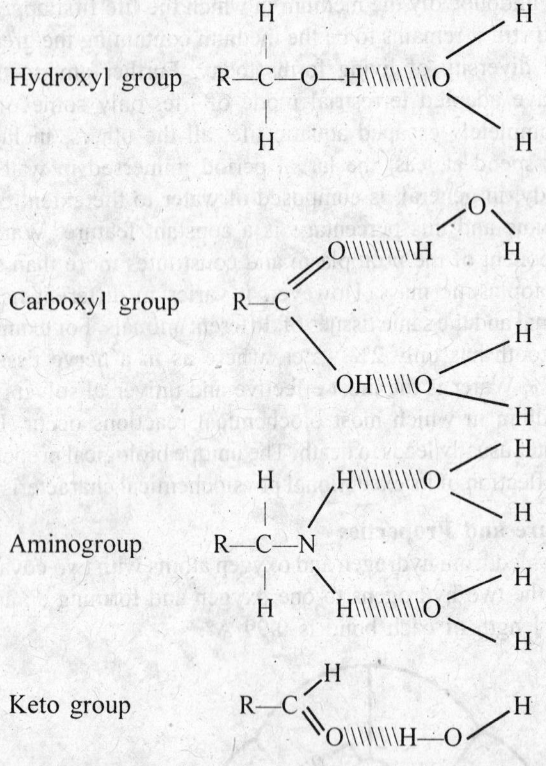

Hydroxyl group R—C(H)(H)—O—H\\\\\\\\\\O(H)(H)

Carboxyl group R—C(=O\\\\\\\\\\H—O—H)(—OH\\\\\\\\O(H)(H))

Aminogroup R—C(H)(H)—N(H\\\\\\\\\\O(H)(H))(H\\\\\\\\\\O(H)(H))

Keto group R—C(H)=O\\\\\\\\\\H—O—H

Fig. 6.2 : The organic groups with which water by forming hydrogen bonds enhances the solubility.

However, the bonds are weak (4.5 kcal/mol) as compared to covalent bonds (110 kcal/mol). This property enables water to act as an excellent solvent for compounds ranging from uncharged organic compounds to salts that are completely dissociated into ions even in solid, crystalline state.

High Surface Tension

The force with which the surface molecules are pulled towards the interior is known as *surface tension.* It is a measure of the energy required to expand a surface. Water has a high surface tension because its molecuies are more closely bound together at the interfaces between water and other media (Fig. 6.3). For this reason dissolved substances also tend to be concentrated at the surface under such conditions, chemical reactions between various dissolved substances occur more rapidly. This effect is much like the action of inorganic *catalysts* in promoting chemical reactions by holding reactants together in a reactive configuration. This property also is of great biological significance on it enables formation and maintenance of lipoprotein membranes of cell organelles in proper functional configuration.

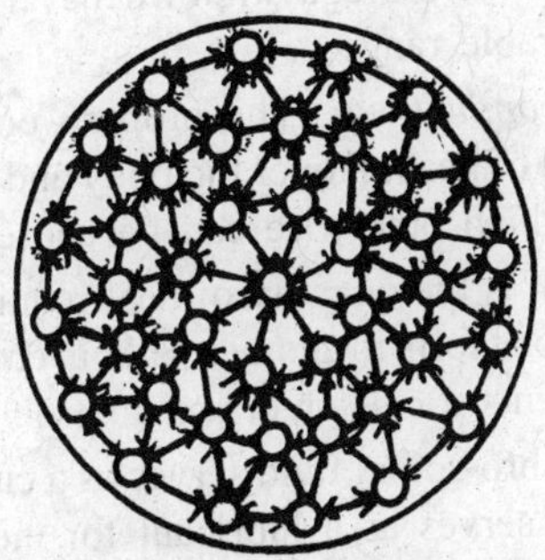

Fig. 6.3 : Surface tension.

Low viscosity : Viscocity is a measure of the ease or difficulty of flow of a liquid. Water has low viscosity and this property serves as an efficient vehicle for the transport of substances (nutrients, waste, hormones, gases etc.) inside a cell as well as through animal body. Low viscosity also enables the movement associated with the charges in the form that generally occur during muscle contraction, amoeboid movements etc.

Thermal properties of water : Water plays an important role in equalization of the body temperature as to maintain it at a fairly constant range. The following three physical properties enable it to act as a temperature regulator.

(a) *High specific heat :* It is the quantity of heat in calories or joules required to raise the temperature of one gram of substance through one degree celcius (one calorie = 4.185 joules). The higher the specific heat of substance the less is the change in temperature when the heat is gained by it. Thus, during metabolic reactions, as the temperature rises the hydrogen bonds of water molecules gradually break up by the absorption of heat energy. The higher specific heat enables heat gain without considerable rise in the temperature, thus helping thermal stabilization of the cells.

(b) *High heat of vaporization :* It is the amount of heat absorbed released when a substance is transformed from liquid into a gaseous state. The high heat of vaporization accounts for evaporative cooling that avoid overheating. Thus, a large amount of heat can be dissipated by vaporization of water. This principle operates in the process of sweating, a physiological mechanism employed in thermoregulation whenever body temperature rises above tolerable range.

(c) *High heat conductivity :* This property enables prompt and equal distribution of heat all over the body and thus prevents localized damages which otherwise can be caused by overheating.

Latent heat : It is the quantity of heat required to change the state of a substance from one form to another without change in the temperature. This property prevents a cell or organism from freezing.

Cushion : Cerebro-spinal fluid serves as a cushion for the brain and spinal cord. It also serves as a lubricant for moving surfaces such as joints, the heart and intestine.

Sense organs : Water plays an indispensable part in sense organs. Sound is conducted through inner ear by a liquid which is chiefly water. Sense of equilibrium depends on water present in the semicircular canals. The transparency of the media of the eye is maintained by water. Sense of taste and smell is revealed by chemical compounds in solution.

The Anomalous Density of Water

A continuous decrease in the temperature increases density of all substances. However, it has a limitation in case of water, if the temperature of water is continuously lowered down it follows this principle upto 4°C and with the farther downfall in temperature water density is reduced and it floats on the surface as an ice. This property, although is not directly related with the water of protoplasm, still has got wide application in the preservation of life at the polar regions where environmental temperature goes down below 4°C. Whenever environmental temperature goes below 4°C, water becomes ice and due to low density floats over the surface thus forming a layer (ice bergs). In these regions, below the layers of ice, animals live quite comfortably, as the liquid water below is effectively protected from further cooling.

II. BIOLOGICALLY IMPORTANT IONS

Minerals are those inorganic homogeneous materials found in the earth's crust. They play a very important role in some cells associated with particular organs and systems. They may occur in ionic forms or in combination with organic compounds and inorganic substances, in turn, forming salts and conjugated fats, proteins and carbohydrates. When salts ionize, cations and anions are formed which are important in maintaining osmotic pressure and acid base balance of body fluids as well as cells.

The occurrence of different minerals in different cells depends upon the physiological state of a cell in consideration. In case of man, the minerals required are calcium, chloride, magnesium, phosphorus, potassium and sodium and others so called *trace elements* like copper, iodine, iron, manganese and probably fluorine, molybdenum, selenium and zinc. Cobalt is also a part of vitamin B_{12} molecule Iron is associated with respiratory pigments, similarly iodine is essential for thyroxine synthesis. Ionized calcium, chloride, magnesium and sodium are essential for proper bone formation, nerve transmission etc. Similarly trace elements are associated with a number of enzymes as cofactors, phosphates in tissue fluids and blood are either in ionized form or are conjugated with some other compounds. They form an important buffering system of the cell, maintaining the pH of the medium in a physiological range. Tissue ions include sulphate $\left(SO_4^-\right)$, carbonate$\left(CO_3^-\right)$ and magnesium $\left(Mg^{++}\right)$. A proper balance of the ionic flux is essential for the normal functional state of a cell.

Transport Through the Cell Membrane

The fluid inside the cells of the body, called *intracellular* fluid, is very different from that outside the cells, called *extracellular fluid*. The extracellular fluid includes both the interstitial fluid that circulates in spaces between the cells and also fluids of the *blood plasma* that mixes freely with the interstitial fluid through the capillary walls. It is the extracellular fluid that supplies the cells with nutrients and other substances needed for cellular function. But before the cell can utilize these substances, they must also be transported through the cell membranes.

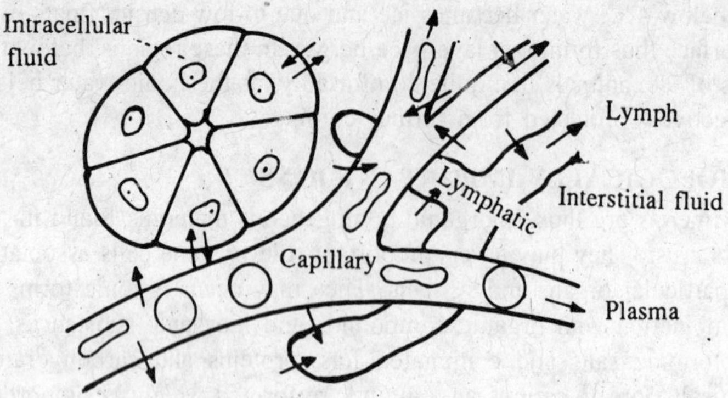

Fig. 6.4 : Main subdivisions of body fluids.

Fig. 6.5 gives the compositions of both the extracellular and intracellular fluids. Note that the extracellular fluid contains large quantities of *sodium* but small quantities of *potassium*. Exactly the opposite is true of the intracellular fluid. Also, the extracellular fluid contains large quantities of chloride, while the intracellular fluid contains very little. But the concentrations of phosphates, essentially all of which are organic metabolic intermediates and proteins in the intracellular fluid are considerably greater than in the extracellular fluid. These differences

	Extracellular fluid	Intracellular fluid
Na^+	142 mEq/L	10 mEq/L
K^+	4 mEq/L	140 mEq/L
Ca^{++}	5 mEq/L	1 mEq/L
Mg^{++}	3 mEq/L	58 mEq/L
Cl^-	103 mEq/L	4 mEq/L
HCO_3	28 mEq/L	10 mEq/L
Phosphates	4 mEq/L	75 mEq/L
SO_4^-	1 mEq/L	2 mEq/L
Glucose	90 mgm %	0 to 20 mgm %
Amino acids	30 mgm %	200 mgm % ?
Cholesterol, phospholipids, Neutral fat	0.5 gm %	2 to 95 gm %
PO_2	35 mm Hg	20 mm Hg ?
PCO_2	46 mm Hg	50 mm Hg ?
pH	7.4	7.0
Proteins	2 gm % (5 mEq/1)	16 gm % (40 mEq/L)

Fig. 6.5 : Chemical compositions of extracellular and intracellular fluids.

between the components of the intracellular and extracellular fluids are extremely important to the life of the cell.

Substances are transported through the cell membrane by three major processes,

1. Diffusion or passive transport.
2. Osmosis movement of water across cell membrane.
3. Active or metabolically linked transport.

1. *Diffusion :* Diffusion is the simplest type of exchange mechanism meaning thereby, the transport of substances in response to concentration gradient, *i.e.,* from higher concentration to lower concentration. There are a number of examples where this mechanism accounts for the transport of various substances for example, the intestinal absorption of different hexoses and amino acids to some extent is accompanied by passive transport. In this case, as the concentration of hexoses, amino acids, fatty acids and other products of digestion is higher in the lumen of intestine than in the epithelial cells, these substances will pass passively from lumen to epithelial cells and in turn, from epithelial cells into the circulation. Same principle of diffusion will be followed in the process of gaseous exchange also.

Energy Considerations of Passive Transport

Any movement in the space involves an expenditure of energy, however, when we consider the energy change on the part of membrane during passive transport, it goes on in response to existing concentration gradient and does not involve an expenditure of energy. Thus, during passive transport membrane system practically offers no resistance. Moreover, the molecules undergoing diffusion possess sufficient amount of kinetic energy required for crossing membrane barrier.

2. *Osmosis : Transport of water through the cell membrane :* Plasma membrane is readily permeable to the water and it moves in and out through membrane at all times. However, such movements are not demonstrable if the solute concentration is the same on both sides of the membranes. Further, the movements become evident only when the solute concentration inside and outside of the plasma membrane varies. In such conditions, the movement of water will always take such a direction which will favour equalization of concentration on both the sides. Thus, *diffusion of water through the plasma membrane (semipermeable*

membrane) against concentration gradient i.e., from lower concentration to the higher concentration is termed as osmosis. In osmosis, the solute concentration, inside and outside, conditions the direction of movement of water through the plasma membrane.

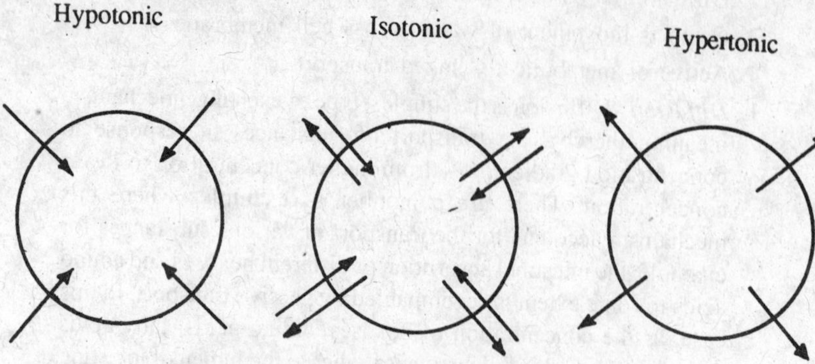

Hypotonic Isotonic Hypertonic

Fig. 6.6 : Conditions of osmosis.

Generally, three terms are used to define conditions for osmosis, they are : Hypotonic, Isotonic and Hypertonic (Fig. 6.6). In relation to cellular fluid concentration, when the surrounding medium is less concentrated (low tonicity), it is said to be *hypotonic* (hypo–below, tonic–concentration), when the concentration is equal it is called as isotonic and when the concentration is more it is said to be hypertonic.

A simple experiment can illustrate the concept of osmosis: if two different solutions of glucose, A and B of different concentration 2 M and 1 M respectively, are separated by a semipermeable membrane which allows movements of only water molecules ; water from dilute medium (B) migrates to concentrated solution (A), till an equilibrium is restored *i.e.,* both the solutions attain the same molar concentration. As a result of osmosis the volume of (A) increases and increased quantity of water in the compartment A exerts a pressure on the separating membrane. This pressure exerted by excess of water, incorporated as a result of osmosis on the plasma membrane is called as the osmotic pressure.

The osmotic pressure of a solution is directly proportional to the concentration of the solute, *i.e.,* more the concentrated a solution is, higher the osmotic pressure exerted by it. For example, 1 gm of salt dissolved in 100 ml will have twice the potential osmotic pressure as compared to solution of 1 gm salt dissolved in 200 ml. This also indicates that the osmotic pressure is inversely proportional to the volume. Further more, it increases with the temperature, 1/273° for each degree rise in temperature. Solutions containing equal number of molecules exert equal osmotic pressure irrespective of molecular exert equal osmotic pressure irrespective of molecular nature as ions, undissociated molecules, aggregations of molecules etc. Thus, the osmotic pressure depends on the number of dissolved particles. In case of electrolytes, as dissociation increases strength (number) of ions, osmotic pressure is directly proportional to the degree of dissociation.

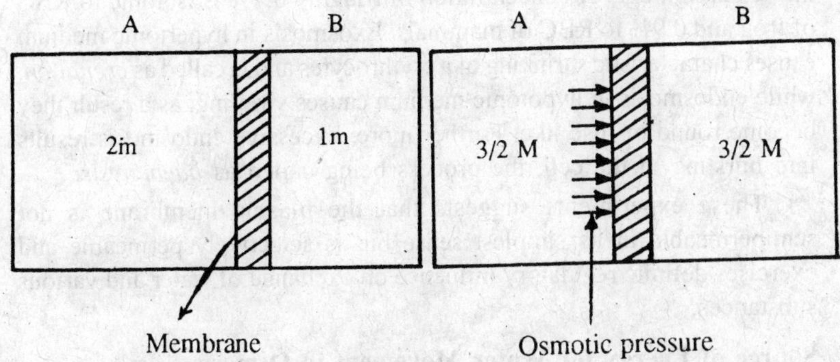

Fig. 6.7 : Concept of osmotic pressure.

A condition in which a pressure greater than the osmotic pressure causes migration of water from high concentration (A) to low concentration (B), is called *ultrafiltration.* In other wards, it can be considered as a diffusion under pressure. Thus, ultrafiltration, represents a condition opposite to the osmosis. Osmosis is the migration of water from the lower concentration to the higher concentration and is a mixing process, where as in ultrafiltration water migrates from higher concentration to lower concentration and is a separation process. Secondly, ultrafiltration is an active process and involves expenditure of energy while osmosis is rather passive process and does not involve expenditure of energy on the part of membrane. Ultrafiltration goes on in the Bowman's capsule of a nephron and plays an important role in the process of osmotic and ionic regulation of the body fluids.

Almost all biological membranes are permeable to the water and exhibit phenomenon of osmosis. The sea urchin egg in normal sea water retains its normal size because of isotonic (iso-osmotic) state of its protoplasmic contents with the medium. However, if it is transferred to the sea water diluted with distilled water, it swells and swelling increases with increasing dilution. As diluted sea water is hypotonic to the egg, a concentration gradient is established and water enters it by *endosmosis*. Increase in the dilution of the medium beyond a particular limit causes excessive endosmosis and subsequent bursting of the egg membrane (cytolysis). On the other hand, when the egg is placed into concentrated sea water, it shrinks. As the medium is hypertonic exosmosis is unavoidable and loss of water causes shrinking of the egg.

Experiments with R.B.C.s exactly give the same results as that of the sea urchin egg. A concentration of roughly 0.7% is isotonic to RBC of frog and 0.9% to RBC of mammals. Exosmosis in hypertonic medium causes characteristic shrinking of a erythrocytes and is called as *crenation*, while endosmosis in hypotonic medium causes swelling, as a result they become round or disc like. Further more, excessive endosmosis results into bursting of the cell, the process being called as *haemolysis*.

These experiments suggests that the plasma membrane is not semipermeable in its simplest sense but is selectively permeable and exercises definite regulatory influence on exchange of water and various substances.

Source of Energy for Water Movement in Osmosis

Transport through the plasma membrane involves an expenditure of energy. Molecules possessing sufficient kinetic energy to surmount the hurdles enter the cell membrane by diffusion, a process which does not involve actual expenditure of energy. However, when a substance moves against same gradient the process becomes *endergonic*. In osmosis, as water moves against concentration gradient, it is an active energy consuming process that is brought about at the expenditure of energy supplied from the metabolic pathways.

Active Transport or Concentrative Transport

Active transport is essentially an energy consuming process and involves transport of various substances against existing electro-chemical concentration gradient as compared to diffusion which is a passive and does not involve an expenditure of energy. It is also called as *concentrative transport* as substances move against existing concentration gradient *i.e.*, from lower concentration to higher concentration through the cell-membrane. Active transport is the main process by which major cellular transport goes on in the body,

The process involves carrier mediated mechanism. The carrier, associated with the membrane system, is essentially a protein component-which is highly selective and specific for a particular substance to be transported. For example, Velinomycin, a non polar fat soluble antibiotic, acts as a typical carrier, which is a polypeptide of 12 amino acids. When this is combined with phospholipid bilayer it enhances membrane permeability for potassium ions but not for sodium ions (specificity for potassium). This change in the membrane permeability is measured by change in the electric resistance across a phospholipid bilayer. The resistance in absence of carrier is several orders of magnitude then the resistance across a typical biological membrane: 10 million ohms cm^2 compared to 10 to 10,000 ohms cm^2. At this stage phospholipid bilayer is impermeable to small hydrophilic ions. But if the small amount of carrier (10^{-7} gram/millilitre of salt solution) is added to the system (phospholipid bilayer separating potassium solution), the resistance falls to a considerable extent and permeability of phospholipid bilayer rises equal to a biological membrane.

These observations clearly indicate that specific protein carrier systems are associated with the plasma membrane regulating an exchange of various substances. Such a carrier system for glucose transport by both intestinal and renal tubule epithelia is well established. This clearly indicates that membrane transport is the limiting factor in the movement of glucose and other substances from the tubule to the peritubular fluid or situations similar to this.

Basic Mechanism of Active Transport

The mechanism of active transport is believed to be similar for most substances and to depend on transport by carriers. A carrier substance meets two most important criteria:

(a) It must enhance permeability of the plasma membrane and

(b) It must be highly selective and specific for the substance to be transported. Valinomycin meets both the ideal conditions *i.e.*, it can dissolve bilayer portion of nonpolar fatty acid tail and secondly, it can diffuse between the two surfaces of the membrane and binds the potassium ions in such a way that its ionic charge is enshielded from the non polar region of the membrane. Finally, it is specific for potassium rather than sodium or other monovalent ions.

Transport with the carrier system involves mainly following steps:

(a) recognition of a substance to be transported as in the above case potassium ions,

(b) diffusion through the membrane barrier along with the substance, and

(c) release of substance on the other side of the membrane.

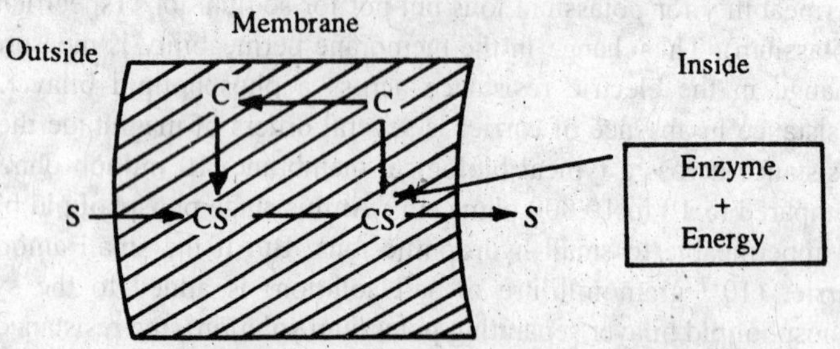

Fig. 6.8 : Mechanism of carrier-mediated transport.

Fig. 6.8 illustrates the basic mechanism, showing a substance 's' entering the outside surface of the membrane where it combines with carrier [(s) + (c) = (sc)]. At the inside surface of the membrane, 's' separates from the carrier and is released to the inside of the cell 'c' then moves back to the outside to pick up more 's'.

Though the mechanism by which energy is utilized to cause active transport is not entirely known, we do know some features of this process :

First, the energy is delivered to the inside surface of the membrane from high energy substances, principally ATP , inside of cytoplasm of the cell.

Second, active transport obeys the usual laws for chemical combination of one substance (the substance to be transported) with another substance (the carrier).

Third, a specific "carrier" molecule (or combination of molecules) is required to transport each type of substance or each class of similar substances.

Forth, a specific enzyme (or enzymes) is required to promote active transport.

From this information and as illustrated in Fig. 6.8 the carrier molecule has a natural affinity for the substance to be transported so that at the outer surface of the membrane the carrier and the substance readily combine. Then the combination of the two *diffuses* through the membrane to the inner surface. Here an enzyme catalyzed reaction occurs, utilizing energy from ATP to split the substance away from the carrier. In other words, enzyme-catalyzed reaction makes the affinity of the carrier for the transported substance very low and thereby displaces it from the combination. But the released substance, being insoluble in the membrane, cannot diffuse backward through the lipid matrix of the membrane. Therefore, it is released to the inside of the membrane while the carrier diffuses back to the outside surface to transport still another molecule of substance in the inward direction.

Examples of Active Transport

Accumulation of potassium in cells : Marked accumulation of potassium in many plant and animal cells can be explained by the process of active transport, for example, fresh water plant, *Nitella*, has 1065 times more potassium than the surrounding water. Similar high concentration of potassium is noticed in nerve and muscle cells. Active transport is an energy consuming process, it can be explained by a simple experiment; if a squid giant axon cell is placed under anaerobic condition, potassium leaks out as supply of energy required to retan is with held. Again, if oxygen is bubbled through the system, cells take up potassium.

Similarly, in case of human erythrocytes, if temperature is lowered down near to freezing point, potassium leaks out of it, while raising temperature reverses the process and potassium is again taken up.

From the above discussion, it is clear that cells maintain their internal environment, constant (homeostasis) with the help of characteristic devices employed by the selectively permeable plasma membrane and even slightest departure from the constancy of the internal environment leads towards collapsing of the cellular system and ultimately the death of an organism.

GENERAL TERMS

Osmotic pressure : Osmosis of water molecules can be opposed by applying a pressure across the selectively permeable membrane in the direction opposite that of osmosis. The amount of pressure required to oppose the osmosis exactly is called the osmotic pressure.

Osmoles : The ability of solutes to cause osmosis and osmotic pressure is measured in terms of "osmoles", the osmole is a measure of the total number of particles. *One gram mole of nondijfusible and nonionizable substance is equal to 1 osmole*. On the other hand, if a substance ionizes into two ions (sodium chloride into sodium and chloride ions, for instance), 0.5 gram mole of the substance equals 1 osmole. The obvious reason for using the osmole is that osmotic pressure is determined by the number of particles instead of the mass of the solute.

In general, the osmole is too large a unit for satisfactory use in expressing osmotic activity of solutes in the body. Therefore, the term milliosmole, which equals 1/1000 osmole, is commonly used.

Osmolality and osmolarity : The osmolal concentration of a solution is called its *osmolality* when the concentration is expressed in osmoles per kilo gram of water, when it is expressed as osmoles per litre of solution, it is called *osmolarity*. The term "osmolality" is generally preferred because the osmotic pressure of a solution is considerably more closely related to its osmolality than to its osmolarity in very concentrated solutions. However, in the very dilute solutions of the normal human body, the differences are so slight that the terms are frequently used interchangeably. Furthermore, it is so much easier to express the body fluid quantities in litres than in kilograms of water that almost all calculations are based on osmolarities rather than on osmolalities.

Osmoticity and tonicity : Two solutions that exert the same osmotic pressure are said to be *isomotic* to each other. If one solution exerts less osmotic pressure than the other, it is hypo-osmotic with respect to the other solution ; if it exerts more osmotic pressure, it is *hyperosmotic*. *Osmoticity* (or osmolarity) is defined on the basis of an ideal osmometer-one in which the osmotic membrane allows water to pass but completely prevents the solute from passing. Thus all solutions with the same number of dissolved particles per unit volume have the same osmoticity and are thus, defined as isosmotic. In contrast, *tonicity* is defined in terms of the response of cells or tissues (behaviour) immersed in a solution. If cells actually behaved as ideal osmometers, tonicity and osmoticity would be equivalent, but this is not generally true. For example, sea-urchin eggs maintain a constant volume in a solution of NaCl that is isosmotic relative to sea water, but swell if immersed in a solution of $CaCl_2$ that is isosmotic relative to sea water. The NaCl solution is therefore isotonic relative to the sea urchin egg, whereas the $CaCl_2$ solution is hypotonic relative to the sea urchin egg. The tonicity of a solution depends on the permeability of the cell membranes and tissues in question, as well as on the concentration of the solution. The more readily the solute passes through the cell membrane the lower the tonicity of a solution of given concentration or osmolarity. Thus, the terms isotonic, *hypertonic*, and *hypotonic* are meaningful only in reference to actual experimental determinations on living cells or tissues.

OSMOREGULATION

Osmoregulation is a problem faced by all living organisms, even those living in an isosmotic media. Term osmoregulation was coined by Hober (1902) referred to the collective activities of the variety of mechanisms used by organisms to control the water movement and water volumes. This implies the maintenance of an internal osmotic concentration which is different from the surrounding medium. Along with this it is also to be kept in mind that the distribution of ions also vary in the external and internal environment of an organism and also between the various compartments within the organisms. These ionic differences which are essential for proper functioning of tissues and cells are controlled by various mechanisms which fall under the study of *ionic regulation*. Because the water and ionic regulations are inseparable activities in organisms, as such the term *osmoregulation* is now considered to include both activities.

Study of osmoregulation has a wide field. Various overall mechanisms regulating the internal water and solute levels, the excretory organs, cellular activities basic to these processes and the molecular basis for these mechanisms are all included. It is also closely related to the homeostatic (some sort of internal) functions like pH and temperature regulation in which body water and ionic concentrations are involved.

If the water content of the body is to be maintained at a constant level, the amount of water entering the body must equal to the water which leaves the body. Water enters the animal body in a number of ways-by drinking, along with food, by oxidative reactions in body resulting in metabolic water or by osmosis from the surrounding medium. Water may leave the body through several ways-via urine, respiration, sweat, through the skin by osmosis and by exocytosis.

In general osmoregulatory studies includes, studies of the overall mechanism used to regulate internal water and solute contents; organs used for excretion, cellular activities which are basic to these regulatory mechanisms and the molecular basis for these mechanisms.

Osmotic Environment and Animals

So far as relation between body fluid concentration and the environmental concentration, and degree of internal environment are concerned, there exists a great, degree of variation in different groups of animals.

Animals that maintain their body fluid concentration more or less similar to that of the environment by time to time fluctuations in relation to changes in the latter, are called as *poikilosmotic* animals (Fig. 6.9a). A poikilosmotic animal thus shows osmotic dependence with respect to the environment. The osmotic pressure of body fluids, for example, in the marine annelid, *Arenicola*, almost matches that of the seawater in which it is dipped. Animals exhibiting this peculiarity in homeostasis are also called as conforms. In short, a poikilosmotic animal is an osmoconformer and responds to environmental osmotic change by drifting with it.

On the other hand, animals that maintain their body fluid concentrations more or less constant, irrespective of fluctuations in the environmental concentrations are called as homoiosmotic animals (Fig. 6.9 a). These forms engage metabolic work to oppose environmental changes, thereby maintaining their body fluid osmotic pressure and ionic concentration more or less constant.

The term homoiosmotic essentially suggests an osmotic independence of the animal with respect to the environment. Osmoregulation in this case, takes place at the level of outer exchange membranes of the body.

(a) contrast between a poikilo and homoiosmotic type of regulation;
(b) euryhaline poikilosmotic type of regulation;
(c) Stenohaline poikilosmotic type of regulation;
(d) euryhaline homoiosmotic type of regulation;
(e) Stenohaline homoiosmotic type of regulation; and
(f) hyperosmotic regulation.

Animals that live in aquatic media of a wide range of concentrations are called *euryhaline species*. This class includes *anadromous* (fishes that migrate from sea to freshwater rivers *e.g.*, salmon) and catadromous fishes (fishes that migrate from freshwater rivers to sea, *e.g.*, eel) and the wool handed crab, *Eriocheir* exhibiting catadromous migrations. Some euryhaline forms are capable of maintaining a rather constant internal pressure at the face of changing outside osmotic pressure (homoiosmotic) (Fig. 6.9b), while others body fluids follow more or less the outside osmotic pressure (Poikilosmotic) (Fig. 6.9 c) and they withstand large changes of concentration in their body fluids.

Animals that survive only within a narrow range of salinities and are restricted to environments of rather constant salt contents are called as *Stenohaline*. They do not employ osmoregulatory mechanism and if there is any change in the concentration of external and/or internal environment they cannot withstand the change. Many of the euryhaline species are more or less homoiosmotic (Fig. 6.9d) and inhabit more or less constant environment that is either hyper or hypotonic to their body fluids. A few stenohaline forms are poikilosmotic and tolerate a small range of salinity change (Fig. 6.9e).

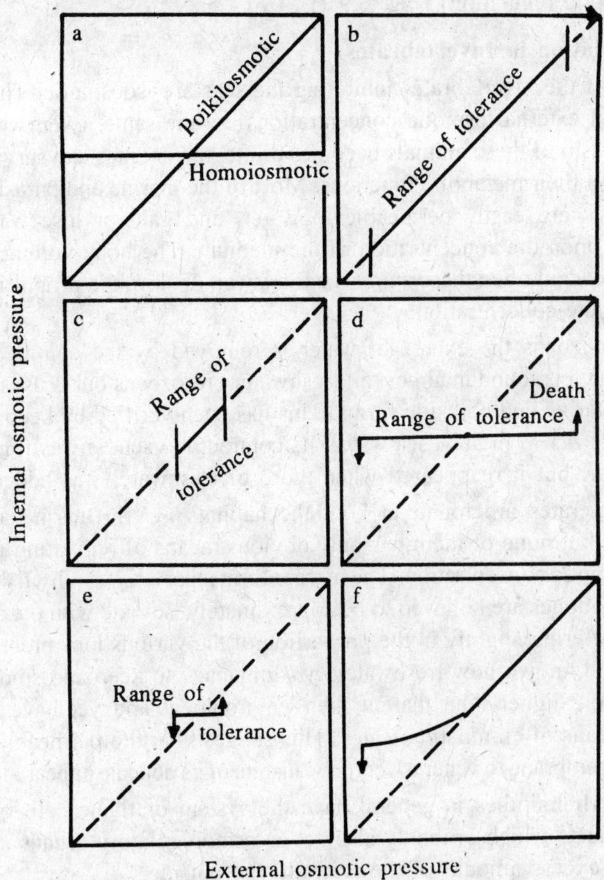

Fig. 6.9 : Diagrams to explain the terms, "piokilosmotic", "homoiosmotic", "stenohaline", and "euryhaline" relating external and internal osmotic pressures of aquatic animals:

There are few animals where a poikilosmotic animals becomes homoiosmotic, *i.e.,* poikilosmoticity is changed into homoiosmoticity and *vice versa* during osmoregulation over a wide range of concentration. Thus, initially the animal regulate its internal osmotic concentration (homoiosmotic regulation) only as long as the external medium is hypotonic. As soon as it becomes isotonic and further hypertonic, the internal osmotic concentration simply follows that of the external medium (poikilosmotic regulation) (Fig. 6.9 f).

Osmoregulation in Invertebrates

Most of the invertebrates inhibiting the seas are isoosmotic. Their internal and external osmotic concentrations are the same. Even when the protoplasm of these animals becomes dilute, the animals can survive and carry on their metabolic functions. Most of the marine and parasitic invertebrates are easily permeable to water, and gain or lose water depending upon the concentration of the medium. The body volume is not regulated and often these animals either swell or shirnk in proportion to their solute-concentration.

In protozoans the excess of water is removed by the contractile vacuole which is found in almost all freshwater protozoans but is usually absent in marine and parasitic forms. This has been verified by keeping *Amoeba verrucosa* in 50% sea water. Its contractile vacuole was found to disappear, but it reappeared when more of freshwater was added.

Coelenterates are found in both the habitats *i.e.,* in marine and freshwater, but none of them has only obvious means of regulating it's internal osmotic concentration. The marine forms like *obelia*, jelly fishes and sea-anemones are believed to be approximately isotonic with the sea although differing slightly in the proportion of the various ions present. It is not well known how freshwater *hydra* manage to keep an osmotic concentration higher than that of their environment and yet have no obvious means of eliminating water. This suggest that the permeability of the cell membrane to water is very low, inspite of its delicate appearance.

In platyhelminthes in general have the system of flame cells and excretory ducts which probably also act as osmoregulatory organs and pass some excess amount of the water to the outside.

The annelid worms, which include the marine polychaetes and freshwater and terrestrial oligochaetes, show little power of osmoregulation. Earthworms inhabits in high humid surroundings and it avoids desicating conditions and can be looked upon normally as being in a similar osmotic relation to its environment as is a freshwater animal.

It excretes through the nephridia a urine of lower osmotic concentration than its coelomic fluid from which the urine is principally derived. It thereby get rid itself of the excess water which enters the tissues through the gut and the skin.

Arthropoda includes animals which are adapted to many different types of habitats from the purely marine to esturine and from freshwater to an aerial environment. In general, marine forms such as the spider crab, *Maia*, has an internal osmotic concentration which is the same as that of the outside and any dilution of the medium in which it lives is closely followed by the dilution of its body fluids to the same level. The osmotic potential of the body fluids of freshwater form such as *Astacus* is greater than that of the water outside, so that there is continuous yet inward passage of water through the permeable regions of the body such as gills. The excess water is eliminated by the *green* or *antennary glands* which have been shown to produce urine with a very low salt content.

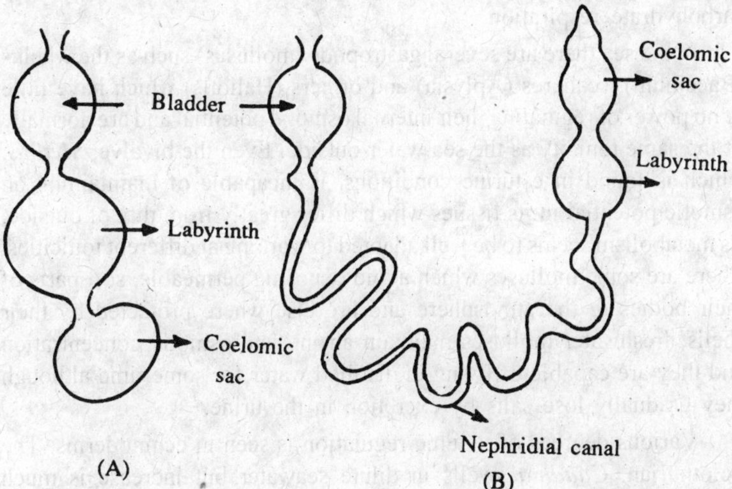

Fig. 6.10 : Antennary organ of (A) *Carcinus* and (B) *Astacus*.

The brackish-water animal from the sea like *carcinus* use all the methods of regulation. In hypo-osmotic media the production of urine by carcinus increases and some water is also secreted into the gut to be passed to the outside. The urine produced is hypo-osmotic to the blood but hyperosmotic to the medium and therefore the elimination of water by this method as entails some salt loss. The antennary organ is now though to be primarily as organ of ionic regulation. It produces a fluid, high in magnesium and low in sulphate and potassium by comparison with the medium. Salts loss can be compensated by the active uptake of salts from the medium by the gills.

There are many terrestrial animals found among Arthropoda ranging from crustaceans like tropical robber crabs which can live for short periods on the land, and wood-lice which are fully terrestrial but confined to humid places but eat nothing but very dry food as well. The chief features of these animals which enable them to reduce their water loss to extremely small amounts is the protection of much of body surface by a chitinous cuticle to which an almost impervious wax is added in the insects.

The insects excrete chiefly uric acid as their nitrogenous waste material and this is only slightly soluble and hence scarcely toxic. It is given out in the solid form and not as a solution, and so requires hardly any water for its carriage. Insects such as *flour beetles* and *wood beetles* depend for much of their water on that which is liberated from carbohydrate respiration.

In the sea there are several gastropods (molluscs) such as the whelks (Baccinum), seahares (Aplysia) and ormers (Haliotis) which have little or no power of regulating their internal osmotic potential and are normally of the same tonicity as the sea water outside. Even the bivalve, *Mytilus*, which is found in esturine conditions, is incapable of maintaining an osmotic potential in its tissues which differ greatly from that of outside. Its metabolism seems to be well adapted to working at different tonicities. There are some molluscs which avoid exposing permeable, soft parts of their bodies to the atmosphere and are else where protected by their shells, freshwater molluscs maintain an internal osmotic concentration and they are capable of living in distilled water for some time although they gradually lose salts by excretion in the urine.

Various degrees of volume regulation is seen in echinoderms. The holothurian, *Caudina* swells in dilute seawater but increase is much smaller. Echinoderms, such as echinoids, asteroids and ophiuroids due to their hard exoskeleton, cannot swell considerably.

Osmoregulation in Vertebrates

In vertebrates the process of osmoregulation is better understood as compared to invertebrates. Internal salt concentration is controlled chiefly by kidneys but permeability of the outer surfaces of the body play equally a important role in the maintenance of a steady internal state.

The osmotic pressure of the body fluids of animals are customarily measured by the depression of the freezing point they cause. This is expressed by the symbol Δ, the internal medium being represented by Δ_1 and the external medium as Δ_0.

Fishes

Fishes constitute a prominent group inhabiting aquatic environment. They are found both in fresh and marine waters. In addition, some fishes show migratory habits *e.g.,* anadromous and catadromous fishes. Thus, the nature of osmoregulatory problem is quite different in different environments and various groups of fishes inhabiting them have solved it by employing a variety of mechanisms.

(a) *Freshwater teleosts :* Freshwater teleosts are hypertonic (more concentrated) to their medium. The problem before such teleosts is to get rid of excess of water osmotically entered into the body and to compensate for the salts by diffusion.

Freshwater fishes drink little or no water and the excess of water is removed by the production of dilute urine (hypotonic). The production of hypotonic urine in large quantities adequately compensates for the excess of water uptake and maintains proper water balance.

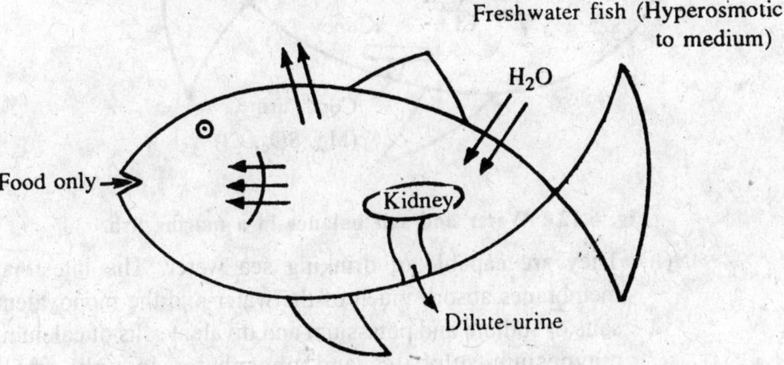

Fig. 6.11 : Water and salt balance in a freshwater fish.

The electrolyte balance is also achieved by the renal retention of salts. Kidney actively reabsorbs salts from the glomerular filtrate, thereby conserving salts otherwise lost in urine. In addition to renal retention of salts, some fishes obtain sufficient quantities of salts in their diets to-offset unavoidable salt loss. Still others are capable of active inward salt transport through the gill membranes. *Eel*, apparently depends entirely on salt uptake through food as the gills are incapable of actively transporting salts into the body. Thus, impermeable animals to a great extent depend on the salts in their food.

(b) *Marine teleosts* : They live in a hypertonic environment. Exosmostic water loss and salt gain (inward flow of salt) by diffusion through the permeable surfaces of the body create the potential hazards for life in hyperosmotic environment. They overcome these problems basically by following mechanisms.

(i) Marine teleosts possess relatively impermeable body surface. It is due to the thickening of the dermis and the presence of impermeable scales. Mucus covering of the body also helps in reducing the inflow of water.

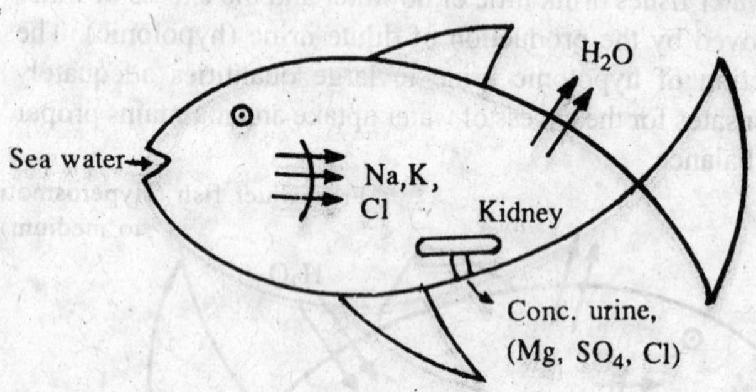

Fig. 6.12 : Water and salt balance in a marine fish.

(ii) They are capable of drinking sea water. The intestinal membranes absorb much of the water and the monovalent salts of sodium and potassium and divalent salts of calcium, magnesium sulphates and phosphates in only small quantities, most of them are passed with faeces. Moreover, divalent salts are also excreted by the kidney. The absorbed monovalent salts are eliminated by active transport through the gill membranes. Specific acidophilic cells, the chloride secreting cells at the base of the gills are considered to be responsible for the salt transfer.

(iii) As kidney is the main organ accounting for water loss through urine, it has undergone a marked structural and functional reduction, a change suitable for life in hyperosmotic environment. In renal physiology, the glomerular filtration is reduced considerably, even in some deep sea fishes (toad fish *Opsanus tau*), kidneys are without glomerular nephrons (aglomerular kidney). Thus, conserve water amount that must be lost as urine. Along with urine only some nitrogenous wastes are excreted.

(c) *Freshwater elasmobranchs* : The compensatory mechanisms of freshwater elasmobranchs are generally the same as those of freshwater teleosts *Carcharias gagenticus* and *pristis* have some urea in their blood. The tissues of the body are always in the uraemic condition. The urea is much less, about 0.6% and the salt content is also lowerer in comparison to marine fishes. They have to eliminate the large quantities of urine. Because both salts and urea in the blood make the internal concentration higher than of the freshwater, it has been noted that these fishes have become so adapted to this uraemic condition that in absence of urea, their heart fail to contract normally.

(d) *Marine elasmobranchs* : They use another mechanism to osmoregulate in their seawater environment. They make themselves iso-osmotic or even hyper-osmotic to the environment by conserving large amount of urea and trimethyl amine oxide (TMO) in their blood and tissues. The osmotic concentration of the blood is often sufficiently more than that of the sea water as such they can use mechanisms similar to those of freshwater fish for the excretion of water. There is a tendency from osmotic inflow and excess water is removed by the kidneys. However, inward diffusion of salt also occurs and this must be eliminated. Excess salts are eliminated not by gills but by specialized organs called the *rectal glands*. Thy can also eliminate excess monovalent ions. Kidneys eliminate divalent ions. The gut plays practically no role in water or solute balance in elasmobranchs. Some urea can be eliminated in the faeces.

(e) *Migratory fishes* : In migratory fishes, like *Anguilla*, both the adaptations to live in freshwater and seawater occur. These fishes which live in freshwater lakes migrate to the sea through rivers and in the sea. They may travel upto thousand of miles.

The young larval forms of these fishes called 'elvers', again migrate to the freshwater lakes. The eels have to regulate their concentration of blood, both in freshwater and in seas. In marine waters the blood concentration is maintained just like in marine fishes, by drinking seawater and secreting the extra salts through the chloride cells and making the urine isotonic with the blood. In freshwater ($\Delta^{-0.08°C}$) the internal concentration is $\Delta^{-0.63}$ which is less than in sea. This concentration is maintained as in freshwater fishes. Water in large amounts is removed in urine and the salts are reabsorbed. In the gills of these fishes, certain cells can extract the minute amount of salts from freshwater. These animals thus, have combination of freshwater and marine fishes features. Thus mechanism is controlled by the endocrine system.

Amphibia

The amphibians live largely in freshwater and have a body fluid which is hypertonic to the surrounding medium, so water enters osmotically at a slow rate due to the low permeability of skin. The water which enters is excreted as dilute urine. Salt is lost in the urine but is again absorbed from the pond water. The loss of salts is also minimized by active absorption in the kidney tubules and urinary bladder. Passive water reabsorption also occurs which increases the concentration of urine of some waste products that are not absorbed. The tubules of the kidney may also secrete some specific salts such as urea. Urine production is under the control of the neurohypophysis, which may altogether stop urine production when the animals stay on land.

Reptiles and Birds

Reptile and birds are closely related and have the same problems of osmoregulation. The reptilian skin is covered by scales and loss of water is thus minimized. The water content of tissues of *desert reptiles* is as high as the mammals. This is maintained by the conservation of water. The renal corpuscles of most reptiles are less poorly vascularized than in aquatic forms. The volume of urine excreted is small in terrestrial forms which may be even semi-solid. The cloaca may reabsorb water. In land reptiles loss of water is more by way of lungs and desert reptiles get most of their water from food. Lizards and snake often drink water to compensate its loss. Marine reptiles have special glands in the head (*nasal salt gland or orbital glands*) with openings in lachrymal of nasal ducts, these glands secrete salts and thus the excess salts of the body are removed, the marine iguana, *Amblyrhunchus cristatus* has acute salt problem because it feeds on high salt weed, but it can excrete a solution from its nasal glands that contain as much as 850 mm Na^+ per litre. Freshwater turtles go on land only for egg laying. Freshwater turtle, *Trinyx spinifer* possesses an active Na^+ uptake mechanism in its pharyngeal membranes. Some species of turtles (freshwater) also use the *cloacal bursa* or *accessory bladder* for Na^+ intake.

Unlike the reptiles, birds have a largely glomerulus and capsule and rely on the uptake from the long tubule to return and salts to the blood stream. A new additional part is present in the birds, which is called as the loop of Henle which is an integral part of salt and water uptake in these animals. Water is also reabsorbed from the cloaca of birds, through which the urine passes, and like the reptiles they make the use of uric acid, producing a semi-solid and hypertonic urine. In the large eggs of both reptiles and bird the nitrogenous waste products are stored up as the insoluble, non-toxic *allantoic acid.*

Marine birds have an internal osmotic pressure which is less than that of their environment so that their problems are much same as those of marine teleosts. Whether they drink sea water and feed on animals whose body fluids are isotonic with seawater, marine birds have an excessive intake of salts. The surplus salt in the most marine birds (*pelican, albatrosses and gannets*) is eliminated from the secretary glands present on head called the *nasal salt gland*. The domestic duck also possesses salt glands and can secrete solutions containing upto 540 $mMCl^-/l$.

Mammals

Mammals live in varied environmental conditions. Regulation of water content permits them to live in moist or dry air, in fresh or saltwater and over a wide range of temperature. They all have an almost impervious skin and are further protected by a hairy coat. On the other hand they have skin glands which can secrete fluid on to the surface and thereby play an important part in temperature regulation. They are all dependent on supplies of moist food or drinking water and they all excrete a hypertonic urine in which the chief nitrogenous waste product is urea. This has some advantages, it is soluble and nontoxic, so it is easy to excrete waste nitrogen with little water. The exact water content of the blood and tissue is maintained with considerable accuracy in most mammals by the action of the kidneys. Water loss during the respiratory exchange is reduced as far as possible by the construction of the lungs.

Terrestrial mammals usually obtain water by drinking but there are more desert animals which entirely depend on their food for water. They gain some water from metabolic reaction as well. In gerbils, *Gerbillus gerbillus* and sand rat, *Psammonamys obesus*, possess highly efficient kidneys that can reabsorb more of the water from urine.

Special Case of Camel

In mammals, camel is the best adapted animal to the dry conditions. It does not store water. In this, problem of osmoregulation is intimately related to temperature regulation. In summer, the camel varies its thermoregulation to a greater extent than in winter and may exhibit a morning temperature of 34°C and an afternoon of 41°C, a range of 7°C. Since an adult camel weights 450 kg, a considerable amount of heat must be absorbed for the gain of 7°C in body temperature and since the temperature is allowed to drop at night, the heat gained during day is dissipated. Thus, within limits, the camel warms up during the day and then dissipates the heat so gained during the night. Sweating is restricted and begins only when the maximum temperature of 40°C is approached, to ensure that this temperature is not exceeded. Additionally, in this animal the water withdrawn from the tissues and the blood volume and concentration remains practically constant.

The tolerance of tissue water depletion in this animal is some three times greater than that of most other mammals and unlike these it can eat normally until dessication becomes very severe. By means of these adaptations the camel can survive at least 17 days in summer on dry food without drinking and without using its fat to produce metabolic water. Camel can also conserve water because of the presence of micro-organisms in the gut, which convert urea back to protein, thus, making the water loss needed for urea excretion by the kidneys much less than it would normally be.

In man, the daily loss of water by kidneys, faeces, evaporation, sweat and lungs amounts to one to nine litres, depending on temperature, exercise, and other factors. This loss is compensated by water drunk, water in food and metabolic water. Urine production in man with the help of kidneys dependent on the temperature and body water load (working of kidney is dealt within the chapter excretion). In man, 1,100 litres of plasma circulated per day in the glomeruli yields 180 litres of filtrate, out of which 178.5 litres are absorbed leaving 1.5 litres per day of urine.

Hormones and Hydromineral Regulation in Vertebrates

The important hormones regulating water and salt balance in vertebrates are *Prolactin,* the neurohypophysial octapeptides, and the adrenocortical steroids. Hormones of the neurohypophysis and the *corpuscles* of *stannius* are also involved in some of the aquatic forms, while levels of calcium and phosphorus depend on the ultimobranchial bodies and parathyroid glands. The catecholamines and angiotensin have less direct effects but also form an integral part of this regulatory system. This group of substances operates, either individually or jointly on all the target organs like skin, gill, gut, kidney, urinary bladder, cloaca and salt glands concerned with water/ion balance.

Prolactin

It is now known that this hormone affects water/or electrolyte balance in all classes of vertebrates and may act on any of the osmoregulatory cells like gills, intestine, urinary bladder or salt glands. In teleosts it control all the target organs concerned with water, ion balance, (skin, gills, kidney and gut). In some amphibians, it acts on skin, and bladder, in birds it affects the nasal salt glands; in mammals it acts on kidney tubules, mammary glands, amniotic membranes and intestine.

The migratory physiology of the stickleback *Gasterosteus aculeatus* provides a good example of the role of this hormone in an animal's environmental reactions. Marine races of this small fish migrate into freshwater during the spring, prior to spawning. At this time, there are changes in osmoregulatory capacities, which involve the ability of the animal to excrete water and trap, or retain ions. During the autumn and winter, while the animals live in the sea, a sudden transfer to freshwater of low ion content (especially low calcium) is lethal; death is associated with the loss of salt and on inability to produce a copious urine of low ion content. Prolactin injections prior to the experimental immersion of "winter" animals in freshwater increases their survival time and prevent the excessive loss of salt. Thus, it appears that the marine stickleback is stenohaline during the winter but becomes euryhaline in the spring, further, it is indicated that prolactin secretion promotes the physiological change.

Neurohypophysial Hormones

Antidiuretic hormones (ADH) : This hormone play a major role in the adaptation of the vertebrates to habitates of varying salinity. This hormone cause two adaptations for water balance by two different ways:

1. Adaptations that are vascular and alter renal blood flow either by changing the systemic blood pressure or by specifically altering the glomerular blood flow; and
2. Adaptations that increase the water permeability of skin, urinary bladder or renal tubules.

In terrestrial vertebrates ADH is an antidiuretic. In amphibians antidiuretic action is glomerular as far as the circulation is concerned but in addition, ADH increases water permeability of skin, bladder and tubules. In adult mammals, the only physiological site of ADH action is on the tubules; glomerular and external organs are not involved, although ADH has a marked effect on the water permeability of the foetal bladder and some lesser effect on foetal skin and amnion. In reptiles and birds, the antidiuretic effects are both glomerular and tubular.

Adrenocortical Steroids

The adrenal cortex, or its homologue in the lower vertebrates, is the dominant chemical regulator of electrolytes in the vertebrates. In mammals, aldosterone is recognised as the most potent of the adrenal steroids concerned with electrolyte balance. Its major action is to increase the tubular reabsorption of sodium and to promote the renal excretion of potassium; in addition, aldosterone is physiologically important in reducing the loss of sodium and increasing the output of potassium through sweat glands, salivary glands and intestine.

In *non-mammalian* vertebrates, the extrarenal organs often play a dominant role in maintenance of water and salt balance, for example, the gills and intestine of fishes, the urinary bladder and skin of amphibians, the salt-glands in some elasmobranches, reptiles and birds and the coprodeum and lower intestine of reptiles and birds. Adrenocortical hormones alter the traffic of salt through the epithelial cells of these organs but the direction of movement if not the same for all of them; moreover, the mammalian distinction between "glucocorticoids" and "mineralocorticoids" is not faithfully maintained in the other groups of vertebrates. In general the action of the corticosteroids is adaptive, with salt output or retention altered in accordance with .environmental demands.

Renin-angiotensin System

Recently it is believed that renin-angiotensin system plays important role in regulating mineralocorticoids in mammals. There are two cellular components of this system : The *Juxtaglomerular cells (J G cells)* and the *Macula densa;* together they form the *Jaxtaglomerular apparatus or complex.* JG cells present in the form of modified band of smooth muscle cells in the median layer of the afferent glomerular arteriole at its junction with glomerulus which is a source of enzyme renin. Macula densa occur as a plaque near distal convoluted tubule. Enzyme renin acts on circulating plasma protein (synthesized in the liver) to convert it into a decapeptide called *angiotensin I.* This is followed by a second plasma reaction in which a converting enzyme splits off two amino acids to form the octapeptide *angiotensin II.* Angiotensin-II is a powerful constrictor of arterioles one of most potent vasopressor substances known. This initiates the release of aldosterone from the adrenal cortex. The sequence of biochemical steps leading to its release is as follows:

$$\underset{\text{(renin substrate)}}{\text{Angiotensinogen}} \xrightarrow{\text{renin}} \underset{\text{(decapeptide)}}{\text{Angiotensin I}} \xrightarrow[\text{enzyme}]{\text{converting}} \underset{\text{(octapeptide)}}{\text{Angiotensin II}} \xrightarrow{\text{initiates}} \text{adrenal cortex}$$

Previously, the renin-angiotensin system was thought to be primarily responsible for adjustments of the renal blood flow by regulating the systemic circulation. It was believed that the pressure-sensing JG cells in the walls of the afferent arterioles safeguarded the renal tissues from a sluggish circulation which would reduce urine formation. This action is now considered secondary to the regulation of water and electrolyte balance through the adrenocortical steroids. The enzyme renin has been found in kidneys of holocephalians, bony fishes and tetrapods.

Other Hormones

The hormonal regulation of water and electrolytes is an integrated process dependent on the co-operative action of several chemicals. The formation of hypertonic urine by the mammalian kidney depends on the control of membrane permeability by ADH and the regulation of sodium transport by aldosterone. In addition to these, several metabolic hormones are known to increase sodium transport by amphibian skin, for example, adrenaline, thyroid hormones and insulin have also been tested with positive results. In teleost fishes two unique endocrine structures - the urophysis and the corpuscles of Stannius-which may also play a part in hydromineral regulation.

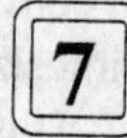

EXCRETION

During metabolic reaction a variety of by-products are formed, some are useless and injurious and must be removed from body. Sometimes a single substance may be act as excretory product and at other time, as an indispensable metabolite. Carbon dioxide although a metabolic by product, is also an important component in the synthetic and regulatory machinery of animals and plants, Urea act as a waste product, as well as perform useful function in some mammals. In the ruminant it is secreted in the saliva, passes back into the stomach and is a source of nitrogen for the microflora of the rumen. Thus, in one animal or another, almost all of these metabolic products which are commonly considered excretory, have found a use. Conversely, some compounds, not usually classed as waste, must be removed just an regularly as CO_2 or ammonia. Apart from their use, these wastes (CO_2, water, faeces, urea, ammonia, uric acid) causes some harmful effects and even fatal if accumulated in excess. There is no concise definition of excretion based solely on the chemical nature of the material removed. In general way excretion can be defined as "the process of removing wastes and excess substances from the internal environment".

The term excretion, is often taken synonymous with nitrogenous excretion-the waste products of protein and nucleoprotein metabolism. CO_2 elimination is often designated as *carbonaceous* excretion. The faeces are not regarded as excretory product because, they are mainly the undigested remains of the food. For the present, the term excretion will be confined to the ridding of the body materials which are chiefly the end product of nitrogen metabolism. In mammals most of the waste nitrogen comes from the elimination of amino acids taken in excess of the body requirements. For removal of nitrogenous waste a specialized system has come into existence in the form of the urinary system.

Nitrogenous wastes : The major nitrogenous wastes formed as a protein metabolism are derived predominantly from these three classes of metabolites : Pyrimidines, purines and amino acids. They include ammonia, urea, uric acid etc.

Ammonia : Ammonia (NH_3) is the primary nitrogenous waste product commonly produced by the catabolism of all types of nitrogenous metabolites. Following are the main reactions that evolve ammonia during protein metabolism (1) Transamination (2) Deamination-oxidative and non-oxidative, and (3) Hydrolysis of urea.

The ammonia is incorporated into metabolites through three fundamental reactions :

(1) Synthesis of amides from glutamic and aspartic acids with ammonia at the expense of ATP.

(2) Synthesis of arginine through the urea cycle, and

(3) synthesis of uric acid.

Free ammonia is usually toxic and rarely accumulates in living cells or their surrounding media. Only traces (0.1 to 0.2 mg per 100 ml) are found in human blood. Ammonia is freely soluble in water and thermodynamically it is most economical to remove by passive diffusion. Majority of aquatic invertebrates and vertebrates eliminate ammonia by this way. The animals that eliminate ammonia as the major excretory product of amino acid metabolism are called as *ammonotelic*.

The ammonotelism is always associated with availability of water and in case of animals those that face problem of water conservation and are associated with osmotically dry habitats (arachnides, insects, some gastropods, oligochaetes, and terrestrial vertebrates), elimination of ammonia becomes thermodynamically expensive. In such animals ammonia is converted into less toxic forms such as *urea* (Ureotelic animals) or uric acid (uricotelic animals), and same can be eliminated without considerable loss of water. Thus, adaptation of ureo-and urecotelism is associated with the osmoregulatory problems of the body.

Urea

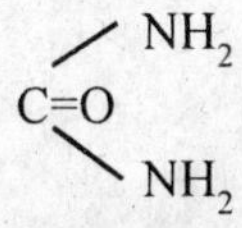

It is more soluble than ammonia as such water is used up for its elimination, but the amount required is much less than ammonia. It is less toxic than ammonia. Thus, marine elasmobranchs retain urea in their blood to avoid problem of osmotic dehydration.

In general, body tissues contain some amount of urea, however, any increase in it creates adverse effects. Thus, human blood normally contains 18 to 38 mg of urea per 100 ml plasma; some value above that 40 mg/100 ml brings about *uremia.* Those animals which excrete urea are known as *ureotelic.*

Chemically, urea consists of two molecules of ammonia united to one of carbondioxide.

$$CO_2 + 2NH_3 \rightarrow C(=O)(NH_2)_2 + H_2O$$

Urea

The excess amino acids are broken down in the body to supply part of energy, used by the body. This process involves splitting of amino group from amino acid. This amino group form ammonia, which is highly toxic, so it is immediately converted to less poisonous compound, the urea. Cells have a special way of combining the ammonia molecules which involves three organic molecules *i.e.,* ornithine, citrulline and arginine.

The steps of ornithine cycle can be summarised as follows:

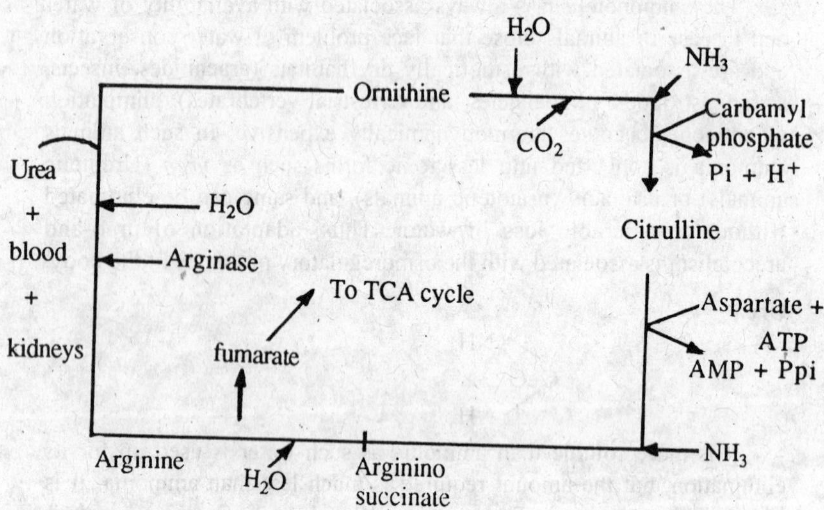

Fig. 7.1 : Urea biosynthesis by the Kreb's ornithine cycle.

First, one of the molecules of ammonia and a molecule of CO_2 combine with ornithine, forming a compound called *citrulline*. This *citrulline* combines with another molecule of ammonia, forming what is called *arginine*. Arginine then combines with water and splits into urea plus ornithine *i.e.*, a product with which the cycle started. Thus, a biochemical cycle, continues. Each turn of the cycle takes, up two molecules of ammonia and forms one molecule of urea. No molecule of ornithine is destroyed—they are used over and over again.

Modern tracer and microchemical techniques have now added two additional links:

1. *The carbamyl phosphate link*, through which one unit each of CO_2 and NH_3 are added between ornithine and citrulline, and
2. *The Arginino succinic acid link*, which adds the second amino group to the cycle.

1. *Carbamyl phosphate link*, Carbamyl phosphate, the compound which primarily fixes the components, of urea. The necessary energy for this reaction is provided by an associated phosphate bond. Carbamyl phosphate is present in all living organisms and it is synthesized in two steps and the process consumes two molecules of ATP. The reaction is catalysed by the enzyme, *carbamyl phosphate synthetase* and contain cofactors like *magnesium*. The overall reaction goes on as follows:

$$NH_3 + CO_2 + H_2O + 2ATP \xrightarrow[\text{phosphate synthetase}]{\text{Carbamyl}} \underset{\text{Carbamyl phosphate}}{H_2C\text{—}\overset{\overset{\displaystyle O}{\|}}{C}\sim P} + 2ADP + Pi$$

2. *Argino-succinic acid link :* In this link also, aspartic acid is the central key point. Aspartic acid, produced by amination of oxaloacetic acid, couples to citrulline to form argino-succinic acid which then splits up to form arginine for the ornithine cycle and releases fumaric acid which subsequently enters TCA cycle. Thus, through oxaloacetic acid, argino-succinic acid link is connected with TCA cycle. Overall reaction consumes an ATP molecule during the formation of argino-succinic acid. During the synthesis of a molecule of urea thus 3 ATPs are consumed which is subsequently the metabolic cost of detoxifying ammonia.

3. *Uric acid and uric acid cycle:*

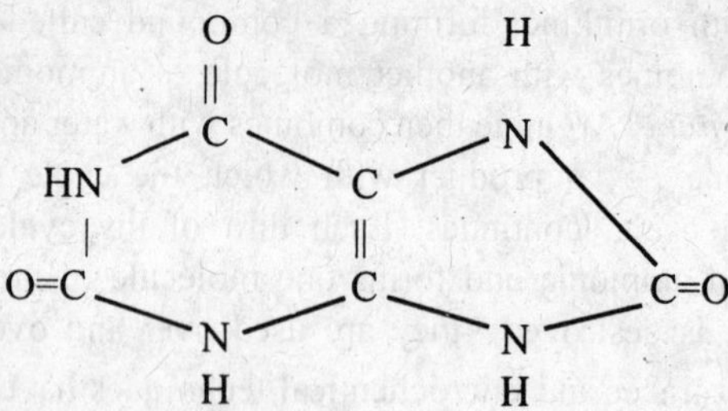

This is the third type of nitrogenous waste formed during the detoxification of ammonia. It is highly insoluble and easily precipitated from a supersaturated colloidal solution. It is only the nitrogenous waste which is eliminated in solid form, it permits nitrogen excretion without the loss of water. All successful groups of animals inhabiting arid lands (pulmonate snails, insects, reptiles, birds etc.) are *uricotelic.*

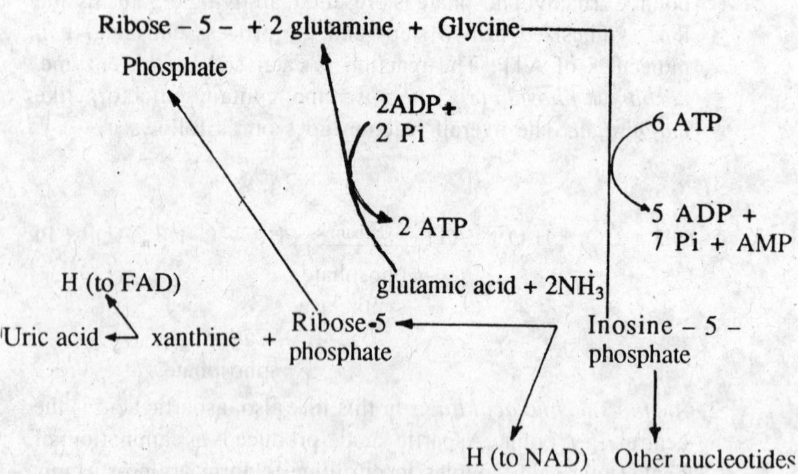

Fig. 7.2 : The outline of the uric acid cycle.

Uric acid is a member of the purines. Its formation is more complex than urea. It involves a series of reactions. The essential features in its formation are the incorporation of the amino acid, glutamic acid and glycine and the hexose sugar ribose into a nucleotide, inosine-5-phosphate, from which the ribose is eventually removed to leave, after the further dehydrogenation of uric acid.

Other Excretory Products

Apart from various excretory products discussed, there are many other miscellaneous products of nitrogen metabolism which are restricted to specific groups of animals.

1. *Amino acid :* The excess of amino acid the end product of protein digestion is excreted as such by certain animals such as *Unio*, *Limnaea, Asterias, Paracentrotus* (echinoderms).
2. *Trimethylamine oxide (TMO) :* It is the excretory product mainly of marine teleost fishes, which are confronted by serious osmotic problems of retaining sufficient water. It is soluble nontoxic substance whose mode of synthesis is not fully known.
3. *Hippuric acid :* It is formed when benzoic acid enters into the diet of a mammal. The benzoic acid combine with glycine forming hippuric acid (benzoyl-glycine).
4. *Ornithinic acid :* This acid is formed in birds, when benzoic acid present in the food combines with arnithine, ornithinic acid is formed.
5. *Creatinine :* It is formed in the body from creatine. The normal level of creatinine in the blood is normally 1 mg/100 ml. The excess amount is excreted out.
6. *Creatine :* Sometimes creatine may also be excreted unchanged along with urine, when it is excess. The normal level of creatine is 2 to 8 milligrams/100 ml of blood.
7. *Purine and pyrimidine :* A relatively small amount of nitrogen waste is derived from the breakdown of nucleic acid. The nucleic acid mainly breaks into purines and pyrimidines. Some animals excrete them as such but the flat worms, annelids and many other animals possess enzymes that convert purine into *xanthine*, from which uric acid is formed.
8. *Allantoin :* In those animals where uricase enzyme is found, the uric acid is further degraded by this enzyme into allantoin which may be excreted in many-forms.

Table 7.1: Major nitrogenous end products of different groups of animals.

Mode of nitrogen excretion	Major nitrogenous end product	Representatives
Ammonotelism (aquatic)	NH_4^+	Fresh water and marine invertebrates. Fresh water and marine teleosts, larval and permanently aquatic amphibians.
Ammonotelism	NH_3	Terrestrial isopods
Mixed ammonotelism -ureotelism	NH_4^+-urea	Earthworms, metamorphosing amphibians
Ureotelism	Urea	Land planaria; adult amphibians; mammals.
Mixed ureotelism–uricotelism.	urea-uric acid	Chelonid (tortoise) and rhyncho-cephalid (sphenodon) reptiles.
Uricotelism	uric acid	Terrestrial gastropods, terrestrial insects; squamata reptiles (lizards, snakes), birds.
Mixed ammonotelism-uricotelism	NH_4^+-uric acid	Crocodilid reptiles.
Guanotelism	Guanine	Scorpions; spiders.

URINE

The amount of urine eliminated per 24 hours varies tremendously depending upon the water intake state of mental and physical activity, environmental temperature and food intake. The volume of urine is decreased in several pathological disorders, such as dehydration, arterial hypotension, edema and kidney disease. The stage is called *oligouria.* On the otherhand the increased urine is called *polyuria* or *diuresis*. It may be due to nervousness, fear, alcoholic beverages and cold climate. *Anuria* or *suppression* is the stage where kidney fails to secrete urine.

1. *Colour :* The colour of normal urine is transparent and pale yellow. The colour is due to the presence of pigment called *urochrome.* The intensity of the colour increases in the concentrated urine and lightens in the dilute urine sample.
2. *Reaction :* Normal freshly voided urine is usually clear and acidic in reaction with a pH value as low as 4.5 and as high 8.2. The mean pH of the normal mixed 24 hour urine is about 6.0.

The urine becomes alkaline on standing because of conversion of urea to ammonia and loss of CO_2 in air. It may also be alkaline after excessive vomiting, at least at the early stage and after meals due to H^+ secretion in the stomach (alkaline tide). When the protein intake is high, the urine is acid. Because, excess phosphate and sulphate are produced in the catabolism of protein.

3. *Specific gravity* : In normal urine specific gravity varies between 1.01 to 1.05 and may be subject to wide fluctuation. As a result of excessive water intake, specific gravity may fall to 1.003 and on the other hand may rise to 1.040 or higher because of haemoconcentration due to excessive perspiration. The specific gravity of urine is directly proportional to the solute content and varies inversely with the volume.
4. *Turbidity* : Usually freshly void urine is transparent but alkaline urine on standing may become cloudy due to precipitation of calcium phosphate. In pathological condition the urine may be turbid due to presence of mucoid, nucleoprotein, epithelial cells, pus cells, etc.
5. *Odour* : The odour of normal urine is faintly aromatic and is due to presence of number of volatile organic substances. In diabetes, urine gives a sweetish odour but in extreme condition of the diatebes when excessive ketosis occurs, urine has got the characteristic odour of acetone. Normal urine on standing gives an ammonical odour because of the conversion of urea to ammonia.
6. *Osmotic pressure* : Osmotic pressure of the urine is much above that of blood plasma. The depression of freezing point Δ of plasma is only 0.56°C, whereas that of the urine varies between 0.87°C and 2.71°C.

COMPOSITION OF URINE

Normal constituents of urine : Urine consists of total organic and inorganic constituents which are as follows :

(A) Organic constituents

1. *Urea* : It constitutes about half of the total urinary solid and is the principal end product of protein metabolism. In human beings, it represents about 80-90% of the total urinary nitrogen. About 25-30 g of urea are excreted per 24 hours. Generally, the quantity of urea excreted is proportional to the total protein

metabolism including food protein and tissue protein undergoing catabolism.

2. *Ammonia :* It is the second and most important nitrogenous constituent. Ordinarily there is very little ammonia in the freshly voided urine. It is about 2.5 to 4.5 % of the total urinary nitrogen and in average 0.7 g is excreted per day.
   In severe nephritis, urinary ammonia is greatly decreased because capacity of the kidney to form ammonia is impaired. But in cystitis, urinary ammonia is greatly increased due to excessive hydrolysis of urea by the bacteria in the bladder.
3. *Uric acid :* It is the end product of the purine metabolism in the body. About 0.7 g uric acid is excreted through the urine per 24 hours. It is derived both from the dietary nucleoprotein and from the breakdown of cellular nucleoprotein.
4. *Creatinine and creatine :* Creatinine is the product of the breakdown of creatine. The amount of creatinine excreted through the urine by an adult individual is about 1.2 to 1.7 g per 24 hours. Excretion of creatinine per 24 hours is practically constant in the subject with creatinine-free diet.
   Creatine is present in the urine of children and in much smaller amounts in a normal adult men. It is observed, that normal males excrete about 6% of the total creatinine output of creatine (60-150 mg/day). In females, this amount is higher than that of in males.
5. *Oxalate :* Normal urine contains about 10-30 mg of oxalate per 24 hours. Though some quantity of oxalic acid comes from the metabolism of glycine and ascorbic acid, major portion of oxalic acid comes from the diet such as asparagus, spinach. Excretion of oxalic acid is increased in diabetes, in certain liver diseases. In normal urine, sometimes oxaluric acid is present in traces. This acid is a combination of oxalic acid and urea. Upon hydrolysis oxaluric acid breaks up into oxalic acid and urea.
6. *Amino acids :* In adults about 150-200 mg of amino acids are excreted through the urine in 24 hours. All the naturally occurring amino acids are excreted through the urine in small amounts although its renal threshold is quite high.
7. *Hippuric acid :* It is chemically benzoyl glycine. It is detoxication products of benzoic acid with glycine. The quantity of hippuric acid excreted through the urine is about 0.7g (ranges about 0.1 to 1.0g).

8. *Allantoin* : It is derived from partial oxidation of uric acid and present almost in all mammals. In human beings, it is present in very small amount.
9. *Vitamins, hormones and enzymes* : are also excreted in normal urine. In adults 15-50 mg of ascorbic acid are excreted per 24 hours. Meabolic degradation, products of adrenocortical hormones are excreted through the normal urine of both males and females.

(B) Inorganic Constituents

1. *Chloride* : Next to urea, it is the chief solid constituent of urine. Generally, 6-9 g per 24 hours as chloride and 10-15 g as sodium chloride are excreted through the urine. Chlorides are mainly excreted as sodium chloride.
2. *Phosphate* : The amount of phosphate excreted through the urine varies widely and it depends largely upon the diet. It is normally excreted 0.8-1.3 g of p per day. Urine phosphates are combination of Na^+ and K^+ phosphates as well as calcium and magnesium phosphates.

   Urinary phosphates comes largely from the breakdown of phospholipids, nucleoprotein, nucleotides and phosphoprotein of the diet and tissues. *Phosphaturia* is a condition where urine contains a crystalline precipitate of magnesium ammonium phosphate. This occurs due to decreased acidity of the urine. Kidney and bladder stones are the cause of precipitation of the insoluble inorganic phosphates. .
3. *Sulphates* : Urinary sulphates are derived mainly from the metabolic degradation of sulphur-containing amino acids-methionine, cystine and cysteine. The quantity of excretion of sulphate depends upon the protein consumption and the breakdown of tissue protein.
4. *Minerals* : The four cations –Na^+, K^+, Ca^{++} and Mg^{++} are present in the urine. The quantity of sodium is excreted through the urine normally ranges from 4-5 g per 24 hours. Urinary potassium is about 2.5 to 3.0 g per day and rises when the intake is increased or in presence of excessive tissue catabolism. Potassium and sodium ratio is about 3:5. In Addison's disease (hypofunctioning of adrenal cortex) sodium excretion is increased and potassium excretion is decreased.

Calcium and magnesium are practically excreted through the faeces and very little amount is excreted through the urine. Daily excretion of calcium is about 0.1 to 0.3 g and of magnesium is about 0.1 to 0.2 g. The excretion of these two ions are dependent upon the nature of diet.

Iodine, arsenic and lead are also excreted.

Table 7.2 : Normal and abnormal constituents of urine.

Normal constituents of urine		**Abnormal constituents of urine**
(A) Organic constituents		
1. Nitrogen (total) ...	25-35 g	1. Protein
2. Urea	25-30 g	(a) Albumin
3. Creatine	60-150 g (approx)	(b) Globulin
4. Creatinine	1.4 g	(c) Bence Jones proteins
	(1.2-1.7 g)	2. Sugar
5. Ammonia	0.7 g	(a) Glucose
	(0.3-1.0 g)	(b) Fructose
6. Uric acid	0.7 g	(c) Galactose
	(0.5-0.8 g)	(d) Lactose
7. Hippuric acid	0.1-1.0 g	(e) Pentose
8. Oxalic acid	10-30 mg	3. Ketone bodies
9. Amino acids	150-200 mg	4. Indican
(Amino acid nitrogen)		5. Blood
10. Allantoin	Small quan.	6. Pigments
11. Vitamins, hormones		(a) Bile pigments
and enzymes	Small quan.	(b) Urochromogen
(B) Inorganic constituents	[per 24 hours)	(c) porphyrin
1. Chloride	6-9 g	(d) Melanin
Chloride as NaCl..	10-15 g	7. Casts
2. Phosphate as P	0.8-1.3g	8. Calculi or stone
3. Sulphate (total sulphur)	0.8-1.4 g	9. Pus
	(average 1.0 g)	10. Hormones
4. Potassium	2.5-3.0 g	
5. Sodium	4-5 g	
6. Calcium	0.1-0.3 g	
7. Magnesium	0.1-0.2 g	
8. Iodine	50-250 μg	
9. Arsenic	50 μg	
10. Lead	50 μg	

Abnormal Constituents of Urine

1. *Protein :* Normally very little protein is excreted through the urine and is not more than 20-80 mg per 24 hours. But in abnormal condition as much as 20 g of protein are excreted through the urine.

Proteinuria (Albuminuria) is the condition where albumin and globulin are frequently present in abnormally high concentration in the urine. Besides these, nucleoprotein, fibrin, myoglobin, haemoglobin, proteoses, peptones and Bence Jones proteins are present in the urine.

Nephritis is the condition which represents a diffuse inflammation of the glomeruli and is always associated with urinary albumin, casts, haemoglobin, etc. In glomerulonephritis, glomeruli are characterised by inflammation along with secondary changes in the tubule.

Nephrosis or generative nephritis is always characterised by degenerative changes in the tubules and also in the glomeruli both. Nephrosis is always associated with albuminuria, haematuria (blood in the urine), oedema, hypertension and anuria.

Nephrosclerosis is the condition where there are pathological changes in the glomeruli as well as marked arteriosclerosis of the arteries and veins of the kidney.

Bence Jones protein : It is considered as a low-molecular weight-globulin and may occur in the urine of patients with multiple myeloma, leukaemia (rarely), Hodgkin's disease and also in lymphosarcoma.

2. *Glucose :* In normal urine very negligible amount of glucose is present in the urine and it is clinically insignificant. About 140 mg per 24 hours, are excreted through the urine. Abnormal excretion of glucose through the urine is called *glycosuria.* In diabetes mellitus, excessive glucose is excreted through the urine. About 20 % or more glucose is excreted through the urine. This is associated with the increased blood sugar levels exceeding the threshold level.

(C) OTHER SUGARS

(i) *Fructose–fructosuria* is a condition when excess fructose is excreted through the urine. It is observed in severe cases of diabetes mellitus in which fructose in excreted along with glucose.

(ii) *Galactose-Galactosuria* is a condition in which galactose is excreted through the urine of nursing infants.

(iii) *Lactose :* It is frequently present in urine (lactosuria) of lactating mother as because the lactose may frequently come from the mammary gland in the general circulation. Since lactose as such is not utilised by the tissue, it is excreted.

(iv) Pentose-Pentosuria is the condition in which transient excretion of pentose is observed through the urine. Congenital pentosuria is a benign genetic defect which is characterised by inability to metabolise L-xylulose.

4. *Ketone bodies :* In normal individual 3-15 mg of ketone bodies are excreted through the urine per 24 hours. In diabetes, starvation, pregnancy and ether anaesthesia, excessive ketone bodies are excreted. The ketone bodies come from the excessive oxidation of fatty acids.

5. *Indican :* It is indoxyl potassium sulphate and is formed from indole. Indole is formed in the large intestine due to putrefaction of protein food. Indole is absorbed in the blood and being toxic to the body, is detoxified in the liver with the formation of indican, the less toxic and excretable substances. In normal urine very little amount of indican is formed but in abnormal condition when excessive putrefaction of proteins occurs, excess indican is excreted through the urine.

6. *Blood :* In cases of acture inflammation of the kidney blood may be present in the urine (haematuria) which may be the result of a lesion in the kidney or urinary tract (*e.g.,* after trauma in the urinary tract). In tuberculosis, cancer and renal stone, haematuria is frequently observed.

7. *Pigments :* A number of pigments are found in the urine. These are urochromogen, bilirubin, porphyrine and melanine. Urochrome gives a normal colour of the urine. This urochrome comes from haemoglobin through series of reactions. In tuberculosis, urochromogen is excreted through the urine instead of urochrome.

Bilirubin is excreted through the urine in obstructive jaundice when bile is reabsorbed from the biliary tract into the blood stream. Bile pigment makes the urine a greenish-yellow or golden-brown colour. In chronic malaria, wasting diseases, melanin is excreted through me urine.

8. *Calculi and casts* : Mineral salts may precipitate and form calculi or stones. These stones may be formed in any part of the kidney tubules. These calculi or stones may be present in the urine.

   In some abnormal conditions, kidney tubules become lined with substances that harden or form a cast inside the tube. These casts are excreted through the urine.

9. *Pus* : Pus cells often are formed in the urine in suppurative condition of the urinary system.

10. *Hormones* : Urinary excretions of different adrenal steroid hormones and gonadal hormones are altered considerably in different physiological and pathological conditions. Urinary neutral 17-ketosteroids are the reflection of the androgenic function of the subject. In adrenocortical carcinoma, hyperplasia of the cortex and testicular tumours, excretion of urinary 17-ketosteroids are tremendously increased. Excretion of 17-ketosteroids is decreased greatly in Addison's disease, pituitary dwarfism, simmond's disease, etc. Pituitary gonadotrophins and placental gonadotrophins are also excreted through the urine in different physiopathological conditions of the organ.

FORMATION OF URINE

The functional unit of the vertebrate kidney is a tubule, the *Nephron* (Fig. 7.3). At its proximal end, the nephron begins with a filter, the renal corpuscle; this tiny structure consists of a double walled cup *Bowman's* capsule enclosing a knot of blood capillaries called *glomerulus*. Bowman's capsule continued in different tubules like proximal, distal, Henle's loop, collecting tubule etc. These nephrons or uriniferous tubules of kidney form urine from the blood circulating in the glomerulus. Since the only source for the urine formation is blood plasma and since the urine is so different in composition from plasma. From the Table 7.3, it is apparent that some major changes in the composition takes place during the formation of urine.

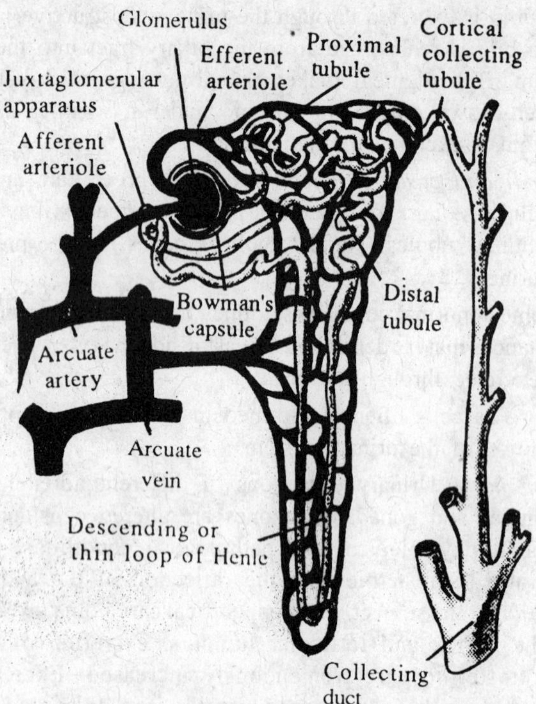

Fig. 7.3 : Structure of uriniferous tubule.

Table 7.3 : Showing relative concentration of some of the components of urine and blood plasma.

Component	Concentration	
	Urine	Plasma
Water	97%	91.5%
Protein	0% (normally)	8.0%
Glucose	0% (normally)	0.1%
NaCl and other salts	0.6%	0.85%
Urea	2.0%	0.03%
Creatine	0.1%	0.001%
Uric acid	0.05%	0.004%

Formation of urine by the kidneys is considered to be due to three types of activities or mechanisms :

1. Glomerular filtration;
2. Selective reabsorption and
3. Tubular secretion.

1. *Glomerular filtration or ultrafiltration :* The initial stage of urine formation is the filtration of plasma and the accumulation of the ultra filtrate in the lumen of Bowman's capsule. Ultrafiltration takes place in the malphigian body which acts as a biological filter. Its histological structure shows that a very thin membrane, about 2μ thick separate blood in the afferent arterioles from the cavity of the capsule and also it is with micropores of about 800 to 1000 A° diameter and thus functions like a sieve. Secondly the glomeruli are enormous in number and their capillaries offer a very large surface (1.5 square metres in mammalian kidney) for the process of filtration.

Third significant feature is the peculiar renal circulation : (a) Renal artery is a short wide branch of the aorta that branches immediately after entering the kidney, as a result, blood enters at a relatively high pressure, (b) the efferent glomerular arteriole is narrower than afferent; as a result the glomerular blood pressure remains sufficiently high to bring about active filtration. Means filtration process occurs when the blood pressure in the glomeruli is greater than the sum of the osmotic pressure of the plasma proteins and the pressure in Bowman's capsule. This is known as *effective filtration pressure.* The hydrostatic pressure of blood at the afferent glomerular anteriole is about 75 mm Hg, in contrast to 25 mm Hg in other capillaries throughout the body. In the efferent arterioles the pressure goes down to 18 mm Hg. The colloidal osmotic of plasma proteins averages only about 30 mm Hg. The hydrostatic pressure in Bowman's capsule (intra-capsular hydrostatic pressure) is about 20 mm Hg (interstitial pressure, 10 mm Hg and intratubular fluid pressure, 10 mm Hg) of these three factors, blood pressure is the motive force for filtration. The other two oppose the process of filtration. So, the net or *effective filtration pressure* is about 25 mm Hg and this pressure is sufficient to overcome other resisting forces and brings about *ultrafiltration.*

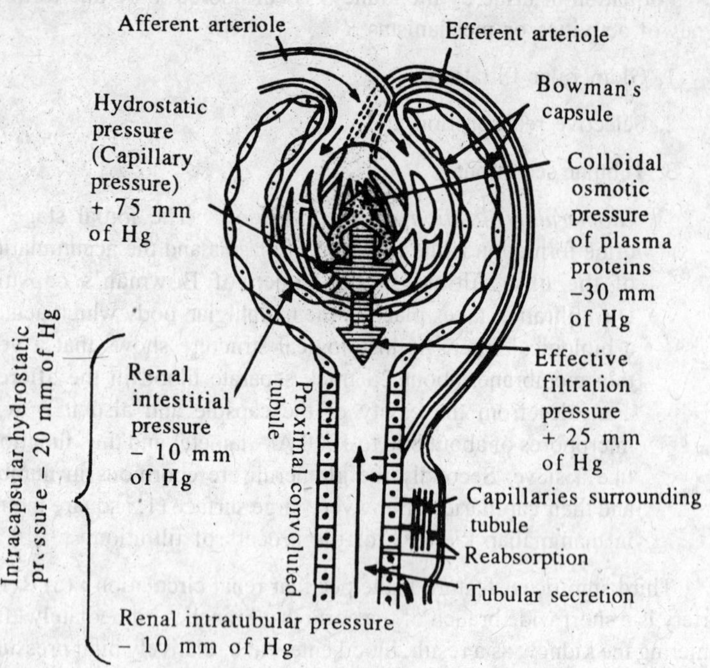

Fig. 7.4 : Diagram showing the factors controlling the net or effective filtration pressure (15 mm Hg) within the glomerulus.

Regulation of Glomerular Filtration Rate (GFR)

The glomerular filtration rate is about 125 ml per minute which is actually the volume of the plasma filtered per minute. GFR can be calculated as :

$$GFR = \frac{UV}{P}$$

where, U = mg of the filtered substance per ml urine.

V = ml of urine per unite, and;

P = mg of filtered substance per ml of plasma.

The filtration rate is directly proportional to the filtration pressure. Therefore, any factor that changes the filtration pressure also changes the filtration rate.

Afferent arteriole constriction decreases the rate of blood flow into the glomerulus and thereby decreases the glomerular pressure and the filtration rate.

Constriction of the efferent arteriole increases glomerular filtration. In addition to this, to maintain sufficient pressure nervous and hormonal control is also evolved.

As a result of .ultrafiltration except blood corpuscles, high molecular weight plasma proteins and certain dyes, rest of all other substances are filtered off at the malphigian body. Experimentally it has been proved that substances with molecular weights lesser than 60,000 to 70,000 are filtered off. Thus, gelatin (molecular weight 35,000) and egg albumin (34,500) are filtered, whereas serum albumin (67,500) and serumglobobin (103,000) are not removed.

At the end of this process, glomerular filtrate contains low molecular weight proteins, near about 95% water, glucose, salts, urea etc. In short, glomerular filtrate is identical to plasma but without its high molecular weight proteins.

2. *Selective reabsorption :* Reabsorption is carried out in the tubular part of the nephron which is richly supplied with blood vessels branching out from the efferent glomerular artery.

The glomerular, filtrate is much dilute as compared to the urine that is eliminated out. During this state, concentration of the filtrate is brought about by the process of selective absorption. It involves the reabsorption of a number of substances like glucose, amino acids, salts, water etc. Which are filtered off unavoidably at the glomerulus during ultrafiltration. At the same time non-essential substances like excess of water and electrolytes and waste products like urea, uric acid etc. are allowed to pass out from subsequent elimination.

The term *renal threshold* denotes the plasma concentration above which a given substance appears in the urine. For example in man renal threshold for glucose varies between 125 to 160 mg/100 ml plasma. The substances which are reabsorbed completely are known as *high threshold substances* (water, glucose etc.). The substances reabsorbed only slightly are called low *threshold substances* (urea, and those which are not reabsorbed at all are the athreshold or *nonthreshold substances*, like uric acid).

Plasma clearance is another term which accounts for the elimination of various substances from the plasma. The term is used to express the ability of the kidneys to clean or "clear" the plasma of various substances. This, if the plasma passing through the kidneys contains 0.1 gram of a substance in each decilitre, and 0.1 gram of this substance also passes into the urine each minute, then 1 decilitre of the plasma is cleaned or cleared of the substance per minute. Plasma clearance for any substance can be calculated by the formula:

$$\text{Plasma Clearance (ml/min)} = \frac{\text{Quantity of urine (ml/min)} \times \text{Conc. of urine}}{\text{Conc. in plasma}}$$

When we say plasma clearance of glucose is 0, it means no glucose appears in the urine. The plasma clearances of the usual constituents of urine are shown in the last column of Table 7.4.

The proximal convoluted tubule is ideally structured for the massive reabsorption of salts and water. Reabsorption of the substances fall under following categories.

Reabsorption of Substances of Nutritional Value

Five different substances in the glomerular filtrate of particular importance to bodily nutrition are glucose, proteins, amino acids, acetoacetate ions and vitamins. Normally all of these (except proteins) are completely or almost completely reabsorbed by active processes in the proximal tubule. Protein filtered (about 30 gm each day) into the glomerular filtrate, attaches itself to the membrane of the proximal tubule, and this portion of the membrane then invaginates to the interior of the cell. This process takes place in the brush border of the proximal tubule and is called as *pinocytosis*. The protein is digested and converted into amino acids which are then absorbed through the wall of *pinocytic vesicles*.

Reabsorption of Metabolic end Products

The metabolic end products like urea, creatine, urates etc. show poor reabsorption. Urea is reabsorbed in small quantities. About 40% of the urea filtered, are reabsorbed. The urate ions are absorbed much more than urea, About 86% of the total are reabsorbed. Other end products, such as sulphates, phosphates, and nitrates are transported in much the same way as urate ions. Creatine is not reabsorbed in the tubules at all.

Reabsorption of ions : The rates of flow of different ions decrease markedly as the tabular fluid progresses from glomerular filtrate to urine. Positive ions are generally transported through the tubular epithelium by active transport processes, whereas negative ions are usually transported passively as a result of electrical differences developed across the membrane when the positive ions are transported.

Table 7.4 : Relative concentrations of substances in the glomerular and in the urine.

	Glomerular Filtrate (125 ml/min.)		Urine (1 ml/min.)		Conc. Urc./Conc. Plasma
	Quantity/min.	Concentration	Quantity/min.	Concentration	(Plasma clearance per min.)
Na^+	17.7 mEq	142 mEq/L	0.128 mEq	128 mEq/L	0.9
K^+	0.63	5	0.06	60	12
Ca^{++}	0.5	4	0.0048	48	1.2
Mg^{++}	0.38	3	0.015	15	5.0
Cl^-	12.9	103	0.134	134	1.3
HCO_3^-	3.5	28	0.014	14	0.5
$H_3PO_4^-$ } HPO_4^-	0.25	2	0.05	50	25
SO_4^-	0.09	0.7	0.033	33	47
Glucose	125 mg	100 mg/dl	0 mg	0 mg.dl	0.0
Urea	33	26	18.2	1820	70
Uric acid	3.8	3	0.42	42	14
Creatinine	1.4	1.1	1.96	196	140
Inulin	–	–	–	–	125
Diodrast	–	–	–	–	560
PAH	–	–	–	–	585

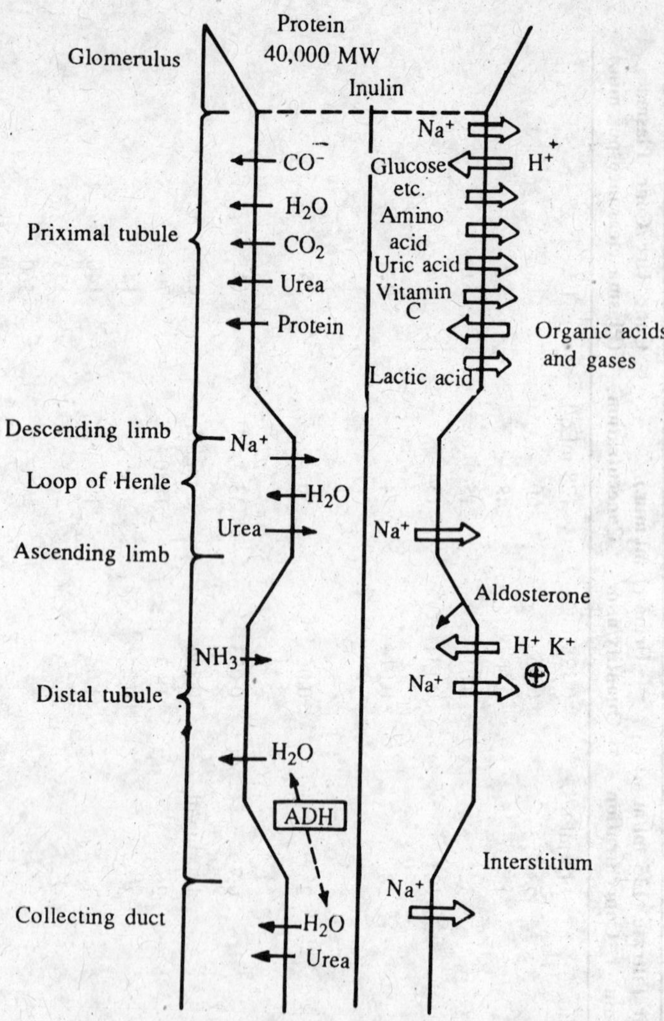

Fig. 7.5 : Diagram showing tubular reabsorption and secretion Transport mechanism indicated by ⇒ ; diffused by → ; and exchange pumping by ⊕.

As for example, in the proximal tubule 75% of the Na^+ is removed from the lumen by active transport, and a nearly proportional amount of water and certain other solutes such as Cl^-, follow passively.

Reabsorption of Water

Out of 2400 ml of water intake, approximately 1400 ml is lost in urine, 100 ml is in the sweat, 200ml in the faeces and remaining 700 ml is lost by evaporation through the lungs or by diffusion through skin.

About 80% of the water is reabsorbed in the proximal tubule passively. This portion of the reabsorbed water occurs as a function of the law of osmosis. So it is referred to as *obligatory reabsorption.* This water reabsorption is controlled by sodium transport and by water carrier molecules. When sodium and other substances are transported from the tubular lumen across the tubular membrane into the peritubular fluid, it causes increase in the solute concentration in the peritubular fluid medium. The proportion of water in the tubular lumen becomes higher in relation to tubular sodium. Thus, an osmotic gradient is established between the tubular fluid and the peritubular fluid and water starts diffusing into the peritubular fluid.

Passage of most of the remaining water in the filtrate can be regulated by ADH. When the blood water concentration is low, the posterior pituitary releases ADH, a hormone that increases the permeability of the plasma membranes of the distal tubule and collecting duet cells. As the membranes become more permeable, more carrier molecules can pass in and out of the cell, carrying water molecules with them. This *facultative reabsorption* is responsible for about 18% of the water in the filtrate.

3. *Tubular secretion :* Tubular secretion adds material to the filtrate from the blood. So those products of metabolism which are not at all required by the body, rather they are injurious to health, are secreted out by tubular epithelium in the tubular filtrate. The secreted substances include potassium, hydrogen, ammonia, creatine, uric acid, and the drugs penicillin and para-amino hippuric acid.

Tubular secretion has two principal effects. It rids the body from certain materials and it controls the blood pH. The more important aspect of tubular secretion is the shift of K^+ and H^+ ions from epithelial cells to renal filtrate in exchange of Na^+ ions present in renal filtrate.

A certain amount of CO_2 normally diffuses from the peritubular blood into the cells of the distal tubules and collecting ducts. Inside the epithelial cells, the CO_2 combines with water to form carbonic acid (H_2CO_3) which then dissociates into H^+ ions and bicarbonate ($H_2CO_3^-$) ions. A low blood pH stimulates the cells to secrete the hydrogen ions into the urine, for each H^+ ion secreted into the tubular filtrate, one sodium ion is absorbed by the tubular cell. Bicarbonate ions obtained from carbonic acid dissociation, and the sodium ions absorbed from the renal lumen diffuse into the blood stream in the form of sodium bicarbonate. The H^+ ions, secreted into the tubular filtrate combine with HCO_3^-, HPO_4^- and NH_3 to form H_2CO_3, H_2PO_4 and NH_4, respectively. Such reactions therefore fix up the H^+ ions in the tubular fluid and prevent their reabsorption.

The counter-current mechanism for excreting a concentrated urine :

This mechanism is exceedingly important to concentrate the urine as much as possible so that excess solutes can be eliminated with as little loss of water from the body as possible–for instance, when one is exposed to desert conditions with an inadequate supply of water. Fortunately, the kidneys have developed a special mechanism for concentrating the urine called the *counter-current* mechanisms.

The counter-current mechanism depends on a peculier anatomical arrangement of the *loops of Henle and vase recta* (peritubular capillaries). In the human being, the loops of Henle of the third to one fifth of the nephrons dip deep into the medulla (descending loop) and then return to the cortex (ascending loop). This group of nephrons with the long loops of Henle is called the *Juxtamedullary* nephrons. Paralleling the long loops of Henle are loops of peritubular capillaries called *vasarecta*; these also loop down into the medulla from the cortex and then back out to the cortex. These arrangements of different parts of the Juxtamedullary nephron and the vasarecta are diagrammed in Fig. 7.6. The term counter-current refers to the fact that the movement of fluid., in descending limb and then from the tip of the loop to the ascending limb, is in the opposite direction. A small difference in the osmotic pressure between the descending and ascending limbs is always maintained by the differential permeability for water and salts at various levels of loop of Henle. Further, due to counter-current flow, the effect of osmotic difference at a given level is amplified as fluid courses from the bottom of the loop to the top of it. Hence the system is called as *counter-current multiplier* system. Hypothetically it works as follows:

1. The descending limb of loop of Henle is freely permeable to water and ions like Na^+ and Cl^- but the ascending limb of the loop is absolutely impermeable for water. It has a mechanism that actively transports Cl^- from the filtrate into the interstitial fluid of the medulla. The peculiarity of the loop is very important in relation to concentration of urine.

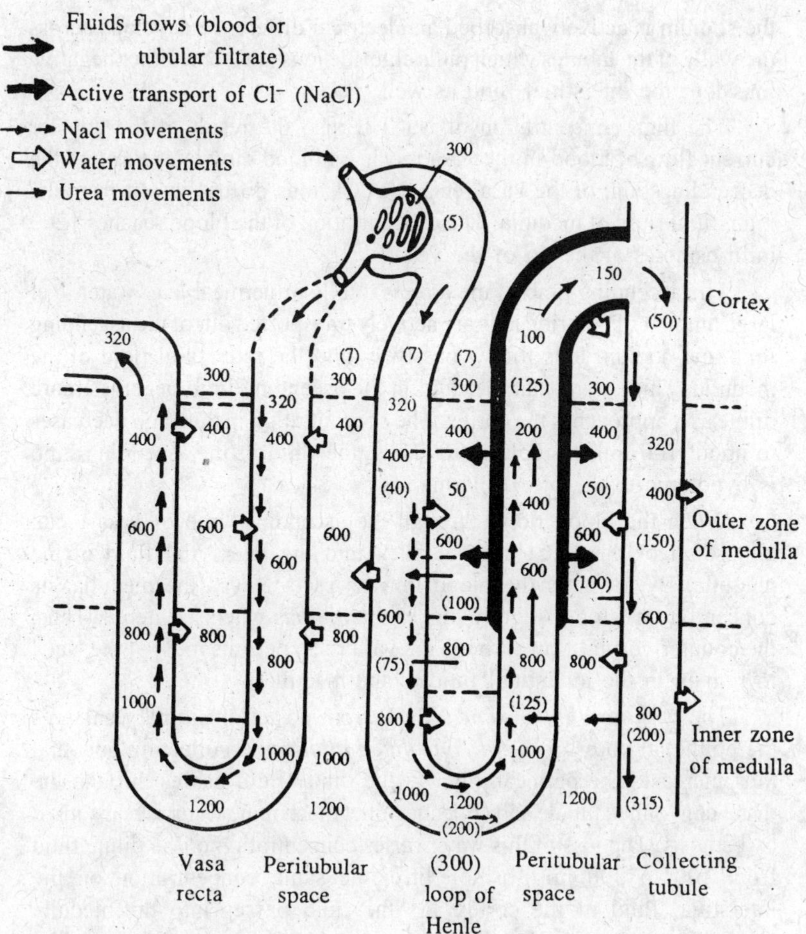

Fig. 7.6 : Diagram of the counter current multiplier mechanisms of the mammalian kidney.

The normal osmality of the glomerular filtrate as it enters the proximal tubules is about 300 milli-osmoles/litre. The osmality of the interstitial fluid increases gradually. It is 300 milli osmoles/litre in the cortex and 1200 milli-osmoles/litre in the pelvic tip of the medulla. This increase is due to the active transport of sodium out of the loop into the medullary interstitial fluid. The very dark arrows through the wall of the ascending limb of the loop of Henle, illustrate the active absorption of sodium. As the sodium is actively absorbed an electrical difference develops across the walls of the tubules which pulls chloride ions and some other negative ions into the interstitial fluid as well.

The high concentration of NaCl is also the result of the counter current flow of blood in the vasa recta. As blood circulates through the descending limb of the vasa recta, Na^{+} Cl^{-} ions diffuse into it from the interstitial fluid of medulla. The concentration of the blood reaches 1200 milli-osmoles at the tip of the vessel.

The ascending limb of the loop is totally impermeable to water. Yet large amount of chloride ions are actively transported out of the ascending limb and sodium ions follow passively into the interstitial fluid of the medulla. This means that the fluid in the ascending limb becomes more dilute as it approaches the cortex. The concentration in this limb decreases to about 100 milli-osmoles/litre. Thus, the fluid in the ascending limb is hypotonic to the blood plasma.

When the blood flows through the ascending limb of vasa recta, almost all of the NaCl diffuses back into the interstitial fluid of the medulla. By the time the blood in vasa recta leaves the medulla, its concentration is only slightly higher than it was when it entered. Thus, the counter-current flow through the vasa recta permits most of the NaCl to remain in the interstitial fluid of the medulla.

The *antidiuretic hormone* (ADH) from posterior pituitary enlarges the epithelial pores of *distal convoluted tubule* and collecting duct and thus increases the permeability. As the dilute fluid passes through the distal convoluted tubule and collecting duct most of the water is reabsorbed by osmosis. The loss of this water raises concentration of the dilute fluid from 100 to 300 milli-osmole/litre, the same concentration on the interstitial fluid of the cortex. As the fluid passes into the medulla through the collecting duct, it is exposed to the hyperosmotic interstitial fluid of the medulla. As a result, large amounts of water are absorbed by osmosis into the interstitial fluid of the medulla from the collecting duct.

The highly concentrated interstitial fluid of the medulla causes the rapid osmosis of water when the epithelial pores are opened by ADH. Thus, in the collecting duct the concentration of the fluid approaches 1200 milli/osmoles/litre which is equal to the concentration of the interstitial fluid of the medulla. The fluid that enters the papillary ducts, calycs, renal pelvis and ureter, flows into the urinary bladder is a very concentrated urine.

Blood Supply of Renal Organ

The kidney has a rich blood supply with a specialized relationship of circulatory vessels to the nephron. At the hilus of the kidney, the renal

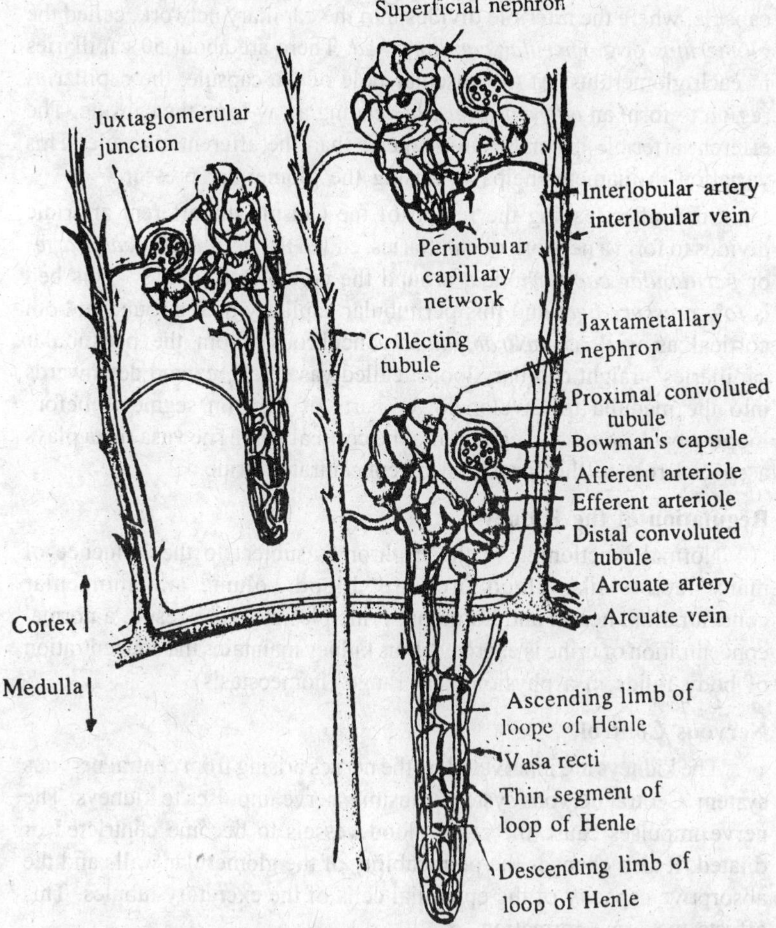

Fig. 7.7 : Diagram showing three nephrons of the mammalian kidney with their blood supply. On the right, compare the cortical with the juxtaglomerular nephron, the long loop of Henle in the latter penetrates deep into the medulla and is associated with a parallel capillary loop, the vasa recta. Arrows indicate direction of blood flow. Although the juxtaglomerular units comprise only 15 per cent of all nephrons, they serve the important function of concentrating thé urine.

artery divides into four or five large branches then runs to the boundary between cortex and medulla. Here the branches turn and divide again forming *arciform arteries*. These give rise to smaller *interlobular* arteries, which pass to the cortex of the kidney and divide into still smaller *afferent arterioles*. One afferent arteriole is distributed to each glomerular capsule, where the arteriole divides into the capillary network, called the *glomerulus* or *glomerular capillary bed.* There are about 50 capillaries in each glomerulus. At the vascular pole of the capsule, the capillaries region to form an *efferent arteriole*, leading away from the capsule. The efferent arteriole is smaller in diameter than the afferent arteriole. This variation in diameter helps in raising the glomerular pressure.

Soon after leaving the region of the capsule the efferent arteriole divides to form a network of capillaries, called the *peritubular capillaries* or *peritubular capillary bed*, around the convoluted tubules. This bed is *low pressure bed*, and this peritubular capillary bed is found in both cortical as well as *Juxtramedullary* nephrons. From the peritubular capillaries/straight capillary loops, called vasa recta, extend downwards into the medulla to envelop lower parts of the thin segments before looping back upward to empty into the cortical vein. The vasa recta plays a special role in the formation of concentrated urine.

Regulation of the Kidney

Normal functioning of the nephron is subject to the influence of many factors like blood pressure, blood volume and molecular concentration, neural and hormonal principles etc. As a result, a normal concentration of urine is excreted, thus kidney maintains the concentration of body fluids in a physiological range (homeostasis).

Nervous Control

The kidneys are innervated by the nerves arising from central nervous system. Central nervous system transmits nerve impulses to kidneys. The nerve impulses cause the renal blood vessels to become contricted or dilated. It also changes the permeability of the glomerular walls and the absorptive capacity of the epithelial cells of the excretory tubules. This affects the urine formation.

Hormonal Control

Hormonal system plays major roles in the urine formation. The hormones taking part in the regulatory mechanisms are as follows :

1. *Aldosteron or mineralo-corticoid :* This hormone is secreted from adrenal cortex (zona glomerulosa) and its secretion inturn

under the control of *Adrenocorticotropic hormone* (ACTH) of the pituitary, osmotic concentration of blood plasma and *renin angiotensin mechanism*. Renin-angiotensin mechanism activates when podocyte cells of the nephron secrete an enzyme *renin* that catalyzes the plasma protein *angiotensin* into *angiotensin* I which is then converted into angiotensin II in the presence of converting enzyme. Angiotensin II increases the production of aldosterone and also causes vasoconstriction of the systemic arterioles.

Aldosterone increases the sodium reabsorption of the tubules along with chlorides, but it also brings about excessive potassium elimination. In the absence of aldosterone secretion, the kidneys lose tremendous quantities of sodium and chloride in the urine, consequently, large amounts of water lost, thereby reducing extra-cellular fluid volume and blood volume below normal. This condition is called *Addison's disease*. If the loss continues for more than 4 to 5 days, the effect can actually cause death because of development of *circulatory* shock.

2. *Antidiuretic hormone (ADH) :* It is secreted from posterior lobe or neurohypophysis of pituitary gland, It regulates the amount of water excreted in urine. It increases the reabsorption of water in the distal tubule and collecting duct. Normal concentration of ADH results in normal reabsorption of water and thereby normal output of water in urine. Under secretion of ADH results *diuresis* or *diabetes insipidus*, or *polyuria*, whereas over secretion of the hormone results more reabsorption of water and less output of water. It causes *edema* or *oedema* (swollen state of tissue). It is interesting to note that the secretion of the ADH varies with the intake of water. If less water is taken more ADH is produced to reduce the volume of urine and when more water is taken less ADH is secreted so that only a small amount of water is reabsorbed and the excess is allowed to go in urine.
3. *Parathormone (PTH) :* It is secreted by parathyroid glands. It increases renal tubular calcium reabsorption, thus decreasing urinary calcium excretion. It also reduces the renal tubular reabsorption of phosphate, thus, raising its urinary excretion and lowering extracellular phosphate concentration.
4. *Thyroxine :* It is secreted by thyroid gland. The principal effect of thyroxine seems to be on general metabolic activities of the

animal. But additionally it also controls mineral metabolism, meaning it influences electrolyte and water metabolism. Hyperthyroidism mobilises Ca and P from bones making them porous. But small amounts of thyroxine increase Ca retetion in growing animals as a secondary effect. In hypothyroidism retention of sodium, chloride and water has been noted, administration of the hormone under such condition causes loss of sodium and water.

Autoregulation in Kidney

Apart from secondary functional regulation through nervous and hormonal factors, kidney is capable of autoregulation. This type of regulation is independent of extrinsic nervous and hormonal factors and may involve a myogenic response of smooth muscles in the arterioles to the changes in presence of the blood within. Alternately, autoregulation may be dependent on a neural and or hormonal.

The precision with which glomerular filtration rate must be autoregulated demands that there be an effective means for controlling this filtration rate. Fortunately, each nephron is provided with not one but *two* special feedback mechanisms which add together to provide the degree of glomerular filtration autoregulation that is required.

These two mechanisms are :

1. an afferent arteriolar vasodilator feedback mechanism, and
2. an efferent arteriolar vasoconstrictor feedback mechanism.

In each of these mechanisms, the degree to which the fluid entering the distal tubule has been processed is detected, and appropriate signals are fed back to the afferent and efferent arterioles to increase or decrease the glomerular filtration rate as required. The combination of these two feedback mechanisms is called *tubuloglomerular feedback.* And the feedback process probably occurs either entirely or almost entirely at the *juxtaglomerular complex,* which has the following characteristics.

The juxtaglomerular complex : Fig. 7.8 illustrates the juxtaglomerular complex showing that the initial portion of the distal tubule, immediately after the upper end of the thick segment of the ascending limb of the loop of the Henle passes in the angle between the afferent and efferent arterioles, actually *abutting* (connecting) each of these two arterioles. Furthermore, those epithelial cells of the distal tubule that come in contact with the arterioles are more dense than the other tubular cells and are collectively called the *macula densa.* The macula densa cells appear to secrete some substance toward the arterioles because the Golgi apparatus, an intracellular secretory organelle, is directed toward the arterioles and not toward the lumen of the tubule, in contrast to all the other tubular epithelial cells. Note also in Figure that the smooth muscle cells of both the afferent and efferent arterioles are swollen and contain dark granules where they come in contact with the macula densa. These cells are called *Juxtaglomerular cells*, and the granules are composed mainly of inactive renin. The whole complex of macula densa and juxtaglomerular cells is called the *juxtaglomerular complex*.

Thus, the anatomical structure of the juxtaglomerular apparatus suggests strongly that the fluid in the distal tubule in some way plays an important role in helping to control nephron function by providing feedback signals to both the afferent and efferent arterioles.

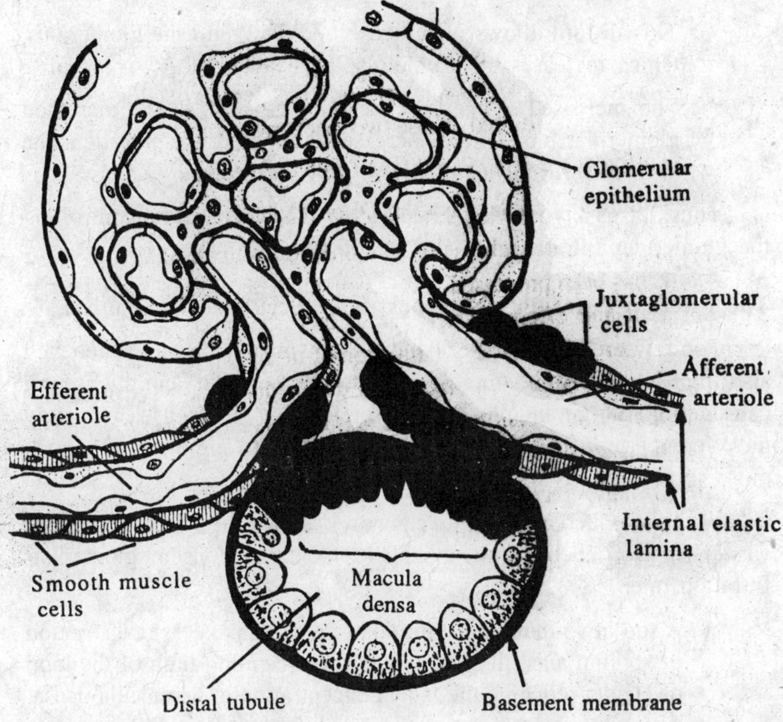

Fig. 7.8 : Structure of the Juxtaglomerular apparatus, illustrating its possible feedback role in the control of nephron function.

The Afferent Arteriolar Vasodillator Feedback Mechanism

A low rate of glomerular filtration causes over reabsorption of sodium and chloride ions in the ascending limb of the loop of Henle and therefore decreases the ionic concentration at the macula densa. This decrease in ions in turn initiates a signal from the macula densa to dilate the afferent arteriole. Putting these two facts together, the following is the postulated mechanism by which the afferent arteriolar vasodilator feedback mechanism, controls glomerular filtration rate:

1. Too little flow of glomerular filtrate into the tubules causes decreased sodium and chloride ion concentration at the macula densa.
2. The decreased ionic concentration causes afferent arteriolar dilatation.
3. This in turn allows increased blood flow into the glomerulus, which increases the glomerular pressure.
4. The increased glomerular pressure, as well as the increased glomerular blood flow, increases the glomerular filtration rate back toward the required level.

Thus, this is a typical negative feedback mechanisms for controlling the glomerular filtration rate at a steady rate.

The Efferent Arteriolar Vasoconstrictor Feedback Mechanism

Too few sodium and chloride ions at the macula densa are believed also to cause the juxtaglomerular cells to release renin, and this in turn causes formation of angiotensin. The angiotensin then constricts mainly the efferent arteriole because it is highly sensitive to angiotensin II, much more so than is the afferent arteriole.

With these facts in mind, we can now describe the efferent arteriolar vasoconstrictor mechanism that helps to maintain a constant glomerular filtration rate:

1. A too low glomerular filtration rate causes excess reabsorption of sodium and chloride ions in the ascending limb of the loop of Henle, reducing the ionic concentration at he macula densa.
2. The low concentration of ions then causes the JG cells to release renin from their granules.
3. The renin causes formation of angiotensin II.

4. The angiotensin. II constricts the efferent arterioles, which causes the pressure in the glomerulus to rise.
5. The increased pressure then causes the glomerular filtration rate to return back toward normal.

Thus, this is still another negative feedback mechanism that helps to maintain very constant glomerular filtration rate; it does so by constricting the efferent arterioles at the same time at the afferent vasodilator mechanism described above dilates the afferent arterioles. When both these mechanisms function together, the glomerular filtration rate increases only a few per cent even though the arterial pressure changes between the limits of 75 and 160mm Hg.

8

MUSCLES

Movement is a characteristic and fundamental attribute of all forms of life. In higher animals, muscles are specialized structures which help to move the whole or the part of their bodies (heart beat, peristalsis etc.). They also maintain a particular posture of the animal besides producing heat during muscular activity. They mainly consists of elongated cells, organized in a variety of ways and bound together by connective tissue. The cells have the power of contraction when they are activated either by means of a stimulus, transmitted down the nerve that innervates them or in some otherway.

Classification of Muscles

There are three types of muscles in the body which differ histologically, anatomically, functionally and neurogenically. (1) striated muscle, (2) smooth muscle and (3) cardiac muscle. Approximately 40% of the body is striated and almost another 10% is smooth and cardiac muscles.

1. *Striated or voluntary muscle :* These are also called *stripped* or skeletal and composed of a large number of elongated cylindrical cells or muscle fibres. Several such muscle fibres are bound together by areolar connective tissue into *muscle bundles* or *fasciculi.*

The spaces between the fibres within a fasciculus are filled by delicate connective tissue, the endomysium. Each fasciculus is surrounded by a stronger connecting tissue sheath, the *perimysium.* The perimysium extends between the fasiculi and is continuous with the tough fibrous sheath, the epimysium, which envelops the whole muscle.

Muscle Fibres

Muscle fibres are elongated cells ranging between 10 and 100μ in diameter. The length of the fibres varies with the size and shape of a muscle, most fibres extending the entire length of the muscle, while a few end in connective tissue intersections within the body of the muscle.

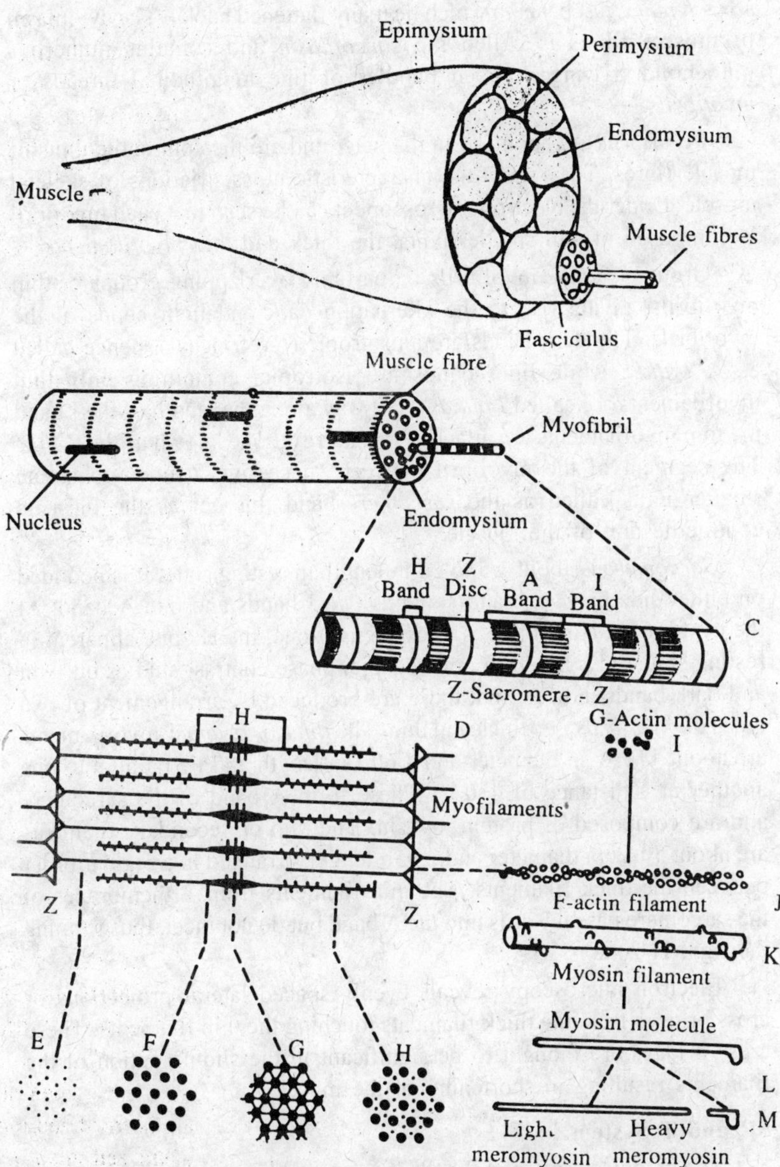

Fig. 8.1 : Organisation of skeletal muscle, from the gross to the molecular level.

Each fibres is surrounded by a cell membrane known as the *sarcolemma,* just beneath which lie many flattened nuclei. The cytoplasm of muscle fibres is called the *sarcoplasm* and contains numerous mitochondria lying between bundles of fine longitudinal threads or *myofibrils*.

Myofibrils are about 1μ in diameter and are the contractile units of muscle fibres. They show the characteristic cross striations of skeletal muscle. Under the electron microscope it can be seen that each myofibril is composed of still smaller units, the thick and thin *myofilaments*.

Groups of *thick* myofibrils lie partially overlapping groups of thin myofibrils, giving rise to the alternating dark and light bands of the myofibrils. The dark bands are anisotropic (birefringent), hence called as A *bands*, while light bands are isotropic, containing only thin myofilaments are called *I bands*. Half way along the length of the I band the thin myofilaments are attached to a narrow zone known as the Z *line*. The segment of the myofibril between successive Z lines constitute smaller units called as the *sarcomeres* and this act as the ultimate contractile unit of the muscle.

Sarcomere is about 1.5 to 2μ in length in resting state. It is bounded on either side by Z line and contains two I bands and one A band. At the centre of A band there is a less dense zone, the H zone apparent in resting state only. Electron microscopic, phase contrast studies on light and dark bands indicate that these are produced by arrangement of two types of *myofibrils i.e.,* thick and thin. The *thick or primary* myofilaments are about 110A° in diameter and 1.60μ in length and lie parallel to one another at a distance of 450A°. These form A band of the sarcomere and are composed of protein myosin. The thin or secondary filaments are about 50A° in diameter and 2.05μ length, arranged in a regular order between the thick filaments. The thin filaments from Z membranes of the sarcomere pass inwards into the A band but do not meet, thus forming the light H zone.

Electron microscopy reveals evenly spaced lateral projections or cross bridges from the thick filaments touching the thin filaments. These cross bridges are thought to be significant in the sliding action of the filaments resulting in shortening of the muscle.

SR and T System

The cytoplasm of animal cells is pervaded by a complex system of membranes which form tubules, vacuoles and other variously shaped compartments. The *endoplasmic reticulum* (ER) forms the major component of this vacuolar system ; within muscle cells it is termed the *sarcoplasmic reticulum* (SR).

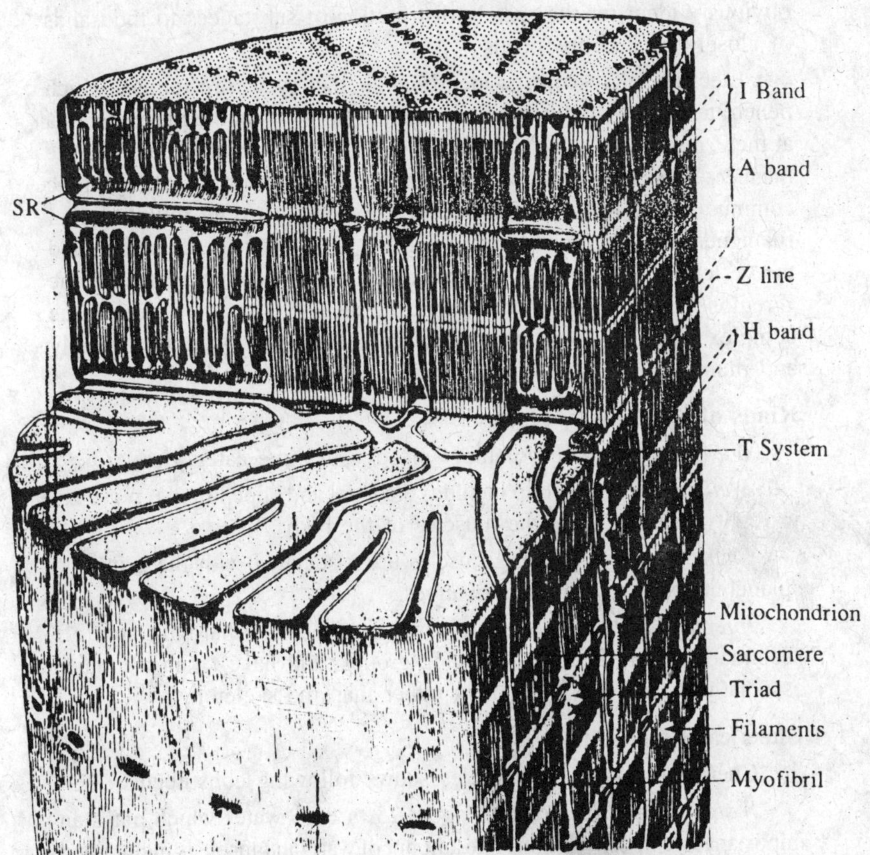

Fig. 8.2 : Three dimensional diagram of vertebrate striated muscle to show sarcoplasmic reticulum and muscle filaments in longitudinal sections with the transverse T system of tubules in cross sections and their interconnections (triads) at the Z regions.

The organization and distribution of sarcoplasmic reticulum varies considerably in different muscles and in various animals. Its salient features are shown in the three-dimensional diagram shown in Fig. 8.2. Many tubules, often standing like columns parallel to the myofilaments, are connected by transverse channels in the Z and H regions of the fibre.

This system of tubules and cisternae forms a loose network which ensheathes the greater part of the surfaces of the myofibrils. The tubules are dilated and particularly extensive in the Z region. Such a system is obviously ideal for the speady distribution of substances to thousands of closely packed myofibrils.

Electron microscopists, identified another system of tubules which penetrate the muscle fibres transversely from pores in the plasmalemma at the Z region and which interconnect with one another in an elaborate manner. This transverse or T system, shown to provider a telegraphic communication from the surface of the fibre to excite multitudes of filaments in a synchronous way. Fig. 8.2 show, that the T-tubules and the vesicles or sacs of the sarcoplasmic reticulum come together in the Z region to form a TRIAD. In short, the SR and T systems provide the complex machinery required for speedy communication, energy supply and plumbing for thousands of closely packed fibrils.

Kinds of Voluntary Muscles

Wilder classify the voluntary muscles in three categories :

Metameric : The group includes the axial and appendicular muscles, in reality takes in most the muscles of the body.

Branchiometric : These muscles are associated with the primitive splanchnocranium and its derivatives.

Integumenteric : This group consists of muscles that have split off secondarily from the two preceding groups, and have taken up major associations with the integument rather than the skeleton,

Chemical Composition

Chemical analysis of muscles shows following constituents :

Water : A muscle contains about 75 to 80% water which plays an important role in contraction. The amount of water in muscle is maintained by osmotic forces. It prevents the muscle dehydration.

Proteins : The proteins constitute about 80% of the dry weight of muscle. The muscle proteins, *actin* and *myosin*, associated with the contractile mechanism comprising about 60% of this and the remaining two-fifth of muscle protein is shared equally by protein enzymes and by stroma proteins.

Myosin : Myosin has a characteristic shape-like a golf club, with a short compact head and long shaft. The length of the molecule is 1500A° and its diameter is 20-40 A°. When the myosin molecule is treated with the proteolytic enzyme trypsin, it separates into two parts.

The *light meromyosin* (LMM) and *heavy meromyosin* (HMM). The LMM constitutes the major part of the tail region, it is a simple linear strand 20 A° in diameter and 1000 A° long. It forms only the backbone of the thick filament and possess only structural function. The HMM (300 A°) molecules have a large globular head (40A° diameter). This contains all the enzymatic and actin binding activity of the parent molecule.

Actin : It is a globulin and being structurally attached to the Z-membrane and is difficult to extract from the muscle. It has molecular weight about 60,000. The actin filament resembles two strings of beads twisted into a double helix. Each 'bead' is a molecule of G-actin (globular actin) having 55 A° diameter. It shows high affinity for calcium ions. In the presence of salts (KCl) and ATP, it is converted into fibrous actin which is denoted as *f-actin* (fibrous actin). The f-actin molecules are in the form of a two stranded rope. The f-actin double helix has a pitch of about 710A°, so that its two strands cross over each other once every 355 A° f-actin represents the polymerised form of G-actin. Actin filaments are about 1 μm long and 80 A° thick, and they are joined at one end to the material that constitute the Z-lines.

Tropomyosin

This protein constitutes about 3 to 8% of the total protein content of the muscle filament. It has a molecular weight of the order of 70,000. It is about 400 A° long and has 20A° diameter. It lacks ATPase activity. There are two known forms of tropomyosin. *Tropomyosin* A and tropomyosin B. Tropomyosin A which is also known as *paramyosin* can be salted out in dilute ammonium sulphate solution, while tropomyosin B is water soluble. When tropomyosin is mixed with actomyosin, it can inhibits *calcium activated ATPase*. It does not inhibit the *magnesium activated ATPase*. It is the constituent of Z-line and extends into thin filaments.

Troponin : It is attached to each tropomyosin, is a complex of globular protein molecules collectively called troponin. The troponin complexes are spaced out along the actin filament of intervals of about 400 A°. This protein inhibits the interaction of myosin and actin. Ca^{++} brings about a structural change in troponin and thus abolishes the previous repression of interaction, of myosin and actin. Actomyosin complex can then be formed resulting in contraction of the sarcomere.

Actinin : This is protein having a molecular weight of about 160,000. It is present in Z-line. It can strongly react with actin and can form cross linking with f-actin filaments.

Nervous Control of Muscles (Fig. 8.3)]

The contraction of the muscles is under the control of the nervous system. *Motor fibres* are those nerves that initiate the contraction of muscles, while *inhibitory fibres* prevent the contraction. Some of the nerve fibres regulate the continuously contracting muscles as the heart muscles. These are referred to as regulatory fibres. The supply of all these fibres to a muscle is called its innovation. *Myoneural junction* or *neuromuscular junction* is the point where a synapse of an efferent nerve makes contact with the muscle fibre. The sensory nerve supply to the muscle is known as the *afferent* supply, while the motor supply is the *efferent* supply.

A single motor nerve may supply several fibres of muscle or fibres of different muscles. A *polyneural junction* is one in which muscle fibres receive innervation from two or more efferent axons. When a muscle fibre is innervated by several branches of one or more axons, the condition is called as *multiterminal innervation*.

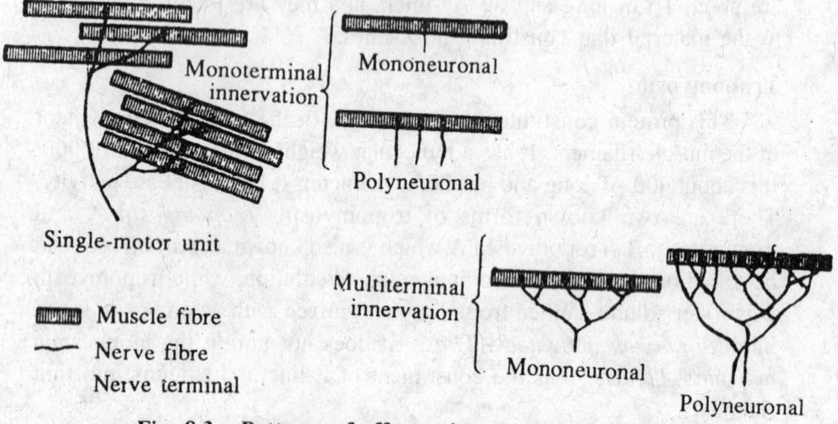

Fig. 8.3 : Patterns of efferent innervation of muscle.

Motor Unit

In an organism, excitation of skeletal muscle is under the control of nervous system. In man hundreds, or even thousands of nerve fibres innervate each muscle, each fibre dividing further into many branches. Thus all the muscle fibres are controlled by a single neuron constituting *motor unit*. The number of muscle fibres forming a motor unit varies from 2 to 6 as in eye muscles to several hundreds in the limb muscles of the mammals. The motor units are usually smaller where the movements are delicate. Though all the muscle fibres are controlled by single *motor unit*, however, there is no protoplasmic continuity between the neuron and muscle fibre. There remains a potential space between the two cell membranes called *myoneural junction*. The portion of the muscle membrane directly under the end of the axon is called a *motor end plate*. Motor end plate invaginates into the muscle fibre but lies entirely outside the muscle fibre membrane. At the tip of the many nerve branches in the end plate are sole feet. The invagination of the muscle fibre membrane is called the *synoptic gutter*, and the space between the sole foot and the fibre membrane is, called the synoptic *cleft* or *subneural cleft*. The synaptic cleft is filled with a gelatinous "ground" substance through which diffuses extracellular fluid.

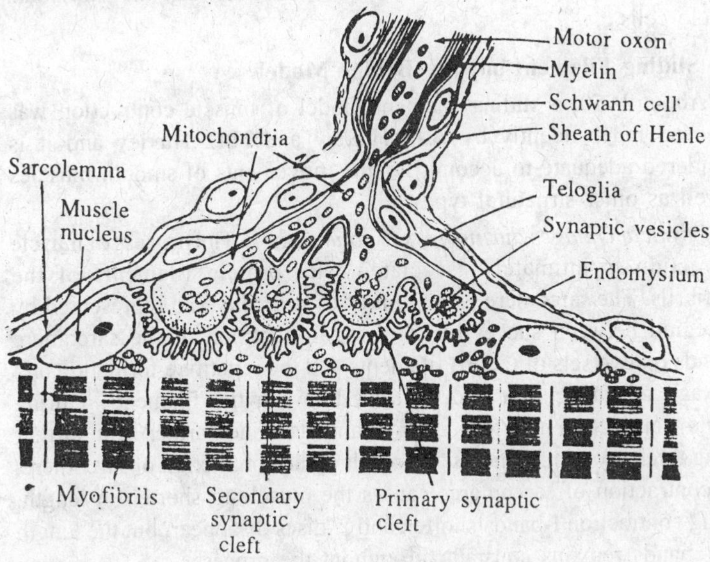

Fig. 8.4 : Diagram of the structure of the motor end plate of mammalian skeletal muscle.

Stored in the nerve terminals of the motor end plate are many small vesicles containing the neurotransmitter *acetylcholine*, which is synthesized by the cytoplasm of the nerve terminals.

When a nerve impulse reaches a motor end plate, calcium ions diffuse from the extracellular fluid into the nerve terminals causing the vesicles to rupture and release acetylcholine into the synaptic cleft. The acetylcholine, which acts at specific receptor sites in the muscle membrane, causes depolarization of the underlying sarcolemma and initiates contraction of the muscle fibres. Almost immediately after depolarization of the muscle fibre the acetylcholine is destroyed by the enzyme *cholinesterase*, which is present in the synaptic cleft.

Contraction of Muscle Fibres

For more than a century, muscle physiologists have wrestled with two major problems. One is the mystery of the actual movement or change in length of the muscle and second problem concern the mechanism which excites and energizes thousands of myofilaments to work simultaneously. The first analysis has now firmly focused on sliding molecules of fibrous-protein while the second analysis has revealed a unique telegraphic communication within and between the individual muscle cells.

The Sliding Filament-moving Bridge Model

About 1950, a sliding filament model of muscle contraction was proposed independently by A.F. Huxley and H.E. Huxley and it is considered adequate to account for the movements of smooth muscles as well as other structural types.

Physical changes during muscle contraction : The process of muscle contraction is intimately associated with protein filaments of the myofibrils. The sarcomere is the unit of contractility and represented by the region between successive Z-discs. Contraction of the sarcomere depends on two sets of (actin) filaments and the repetitive formation and breakage of *linkages* or *crossbridges* between the filaments. During muscle contraction the thin actin filaments slide farther and farther among thick myosin filaments and result in the contraction of sarcomere. The contraction of sarcomeres causes the muscle to shorten in length. During contraction I-bands shorten and Z-discs disappear, but the length of A- bands remains constant throughout the process.

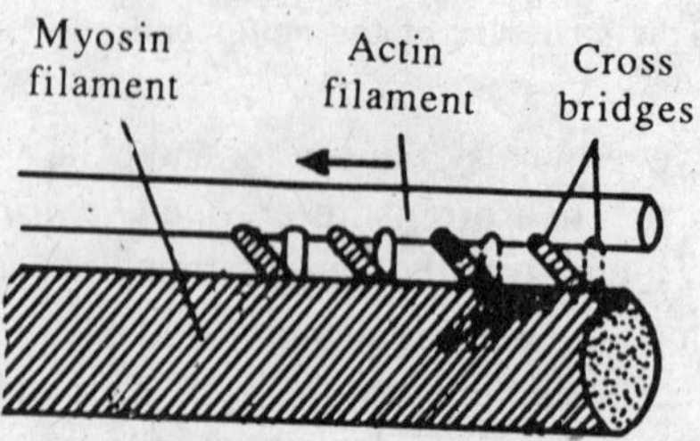

Fig. 8.5 : Position of cross bridges between myosin and actin filaments during sliding.

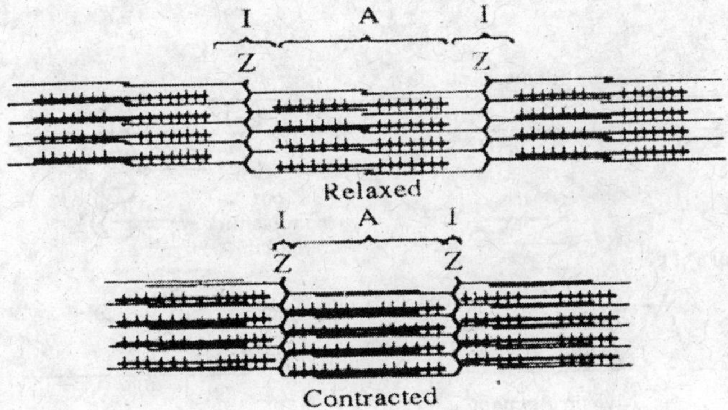

Fig. 8.6 : The relaxed and contracted states of a myofibril, showing sliding of the actin filaments into the channels between the myosin filaments.

Chemical Changes During Muscle Contraction

A resting muscle fibre is electrically polarised at its membrane surface. Its inner surface is –vely charged. The motor nerve stimulates the muscle cells to contract. The arrival of the nerve impulse by the way of motor nerve axon produces acetylcholine. It initiates a wave of depolarization altering the permeability of the membrane to sodium ions. This depolarization or action potential reaches the sarcomeres through sarcolemma insertions of T-system and triggers the release of stored Ca^{++} ions by the sarcoplasmic tubules of the triad. The T-system and sarcoplasmic reticulum thus serve to synchronise the activity of myofibrils.

The released Ca^{++} ions brings about two instant actions. The first is the "release of break" which prevents the sliding of myofilaments and second is to start chemical plant which generates the phosphate bond energy. In a nonreactive muscle, troponin prevents the interaction between actin and myosin. However, the Ca^{++} ions now released, change the structure of troponin and thus abolish the repression of actin-myosin interaction. Actin and myosin filaments are not contractile by themselves but actomyosin complex is contractile in presence of ATP. The complex involves the following reactions.

(i) Myosin + ATP $\rightarrow$ Myosin – ATP complex

(ii) Actin + Myosin – ATP $\xrightarrow{K^+}$ Actomyosin – ATP

(iii) Actomyosin – ATP $\xrightarrow[Ca^{++}]{\text{ATPase}}$ Actomyosin + ADP
(contracts)

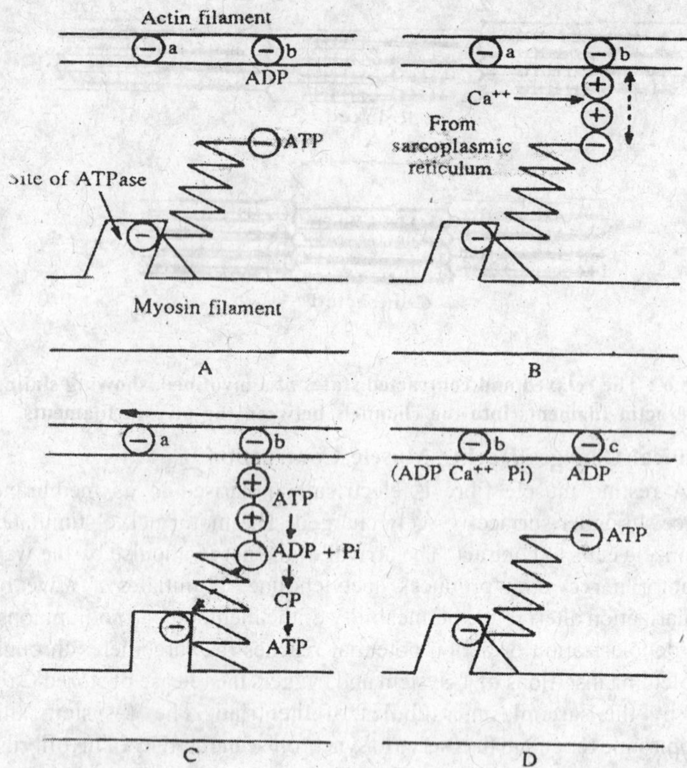

Fig. 8.7 : Electro-chemical events in muscle contraction.

ATP plays a very important role in muscle contraction. In the resting state ATP which contains energy rich phosphate bonds is attached to myosin. ATP has two actions. Its breakdown and release of energy catalyses the combination of actin and myosin resulting in contraction. In the absence of further nerve impulses ATP once more combines with myosin; actin-myosin link is broken and the muscle is allowed to relax.

ADP + Actomyosin $\rightarrow$ ADP + Actin + Myosin

From the above discussion we can conclude that muscle contraction is the repetitive, formation and breakage of linkages between actin and myosin by the crossbridges of thick filaments of A band. As the connections are formed and broken the two sets of filaments are induced to slide past one another resulting in the shortening of the sarcomere. The bridges are formed when ATP is broken down whereas they rupture in the presence of ATP. The free calcium ions couple the excitation of the plasma membrane with both the contractile system and the metabolic system; and is described as *excitation contraction coupling*.

The Source of Energy for Muscle Contraction

We have already seen that muscle contraction depends upon energy supplied by ATP. Myosin in addition to its structural role has an ATPase activity which catalyses the breakdown of ATP to ADP. This breakdown provides the energy required for the movement of the cross-bridges. Fortunately, after the ATP is broken into ADP, the ADP is rephosphorylated to form new ATP within a fraction of second. There are several ways or sources of the energy for this rephosphorylation.

The first source of energy that is used to reconstitute the ATP is the substance *phosphocreatine*, which carries a high energy phosphate bond similar to those of ATP. The high energy phosphate bond of the phosphocreatine has a slightly higher amount of free energy than that of the ATP bond. Therefore, it is instantly cleaved and the released energy causes bonding of a new phosphate ion to ADP to reconstitute the ATP.

$$\text{ADP} + \text{phosphocreatine} \xrightleftharpoons[\text{kinase}]{\text{creatine}} \text{Creatine} + \text{ATP}$$

The next source of energy used to reconstitute both phosphocreatine and the ATP is energy released from foodstuffs-from carbohydrates, fats and proteins. A small amount of this energy is released during the initial breakdown of glucose and glycogen in the cells, which is the process of glycolysis. However, about 95% of the energy is released during final oxidation of the food stuffs, which occurs almost entirely in the mitochondria. Both these processes utilize the energy released from the foodstuffs to form new ATP. The importance of glycolysis is that, energy can be released to form new ATP about 2.5 times as rapidly by this mechanism as by the oxidative mechanism. However, the glycolytic mechanism also rapidly builds up glycolytic end-products in the muscle cells so that glycolysis can usually sustain maximum muscle contraction for only about one minute. On the other hand, oxidative release of energy is exceedingly efficient and can also use other food substrates such as fats and proteins in addition to glucose and glycogen. Allowing continued muscle activity for many hours, though at a level of energy release only about one fourth that which can be achieved during the first few seconds of exercise.

Smooth Muscle

These are also called *unstriated* or *involuntary muscles* and are devoid of any cross striations. They are widely distributed in the visceral organ systems; so usually referred to as visceral muscles. These cells form sheets or bands but may occur as isolated units among the connective tissue fibres.

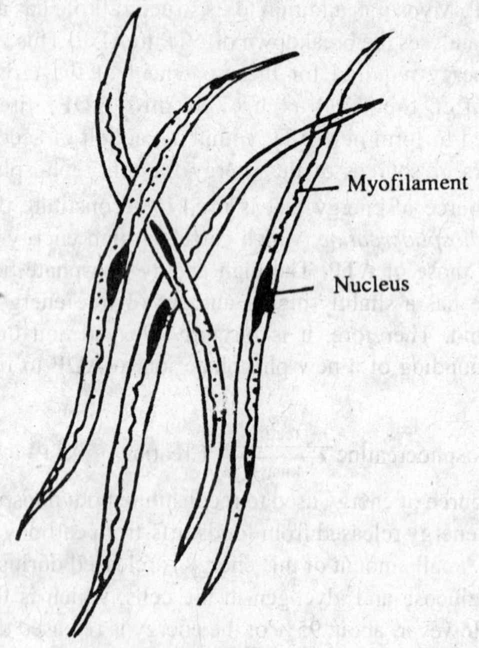

Fig, 8.8 : Smooth muscle fibres.

The cells are roughly parallel to each other but are irregularly and densely packed together. The shape varies according to the organ containing the muscle *e.g.,* very long and slender in the walls of the intestine, short and thick in arteries, twisted and folded in large arteries. The diameter varies from 3 to 8 μ and the length from 5 to 200μ.

The shape of the nucleus is oval, elongated or flattened and it conforms the outline of the cell. The *cytoplasm* contains the organelles mitochondria, a Golgi complex, centrioles, endoplasmic reticulum and ribosomes. It also contains glycogen and fat droplets. In addition, it has longitudinally arranged *myofibrils* which are specialised structures for contraction. They represent aggregates of the myofilaments which can be seen in electron microscope and they may probably contain actin and myosin contractile proteins. The *plasma membrane* of the smooth muscle cells shows outer and inner layers. The outer layers of the membranes of adjacent cells form specialised zones of contact known as nexuses or close *junctions* or 'gap' junctions. The nexus serves as an intimate union of cells and probably useful in transmission of impulses for contraction from one cell to another.

Each smooth muscle fibre (cell) is surrounded by a layer of glycoprotein. The contraction of smooth muscle is apparately dependent upon the sliding of myofilaments but details of the contractile mechanism are not well understood. The smooth muscle cells show nerve endings and they are not richly supplied with blood vessels.

Smooth muscles are found in the wall of the alimentary canal, gall bladder, hepatic ducts, ureter, bladder, blood vessels, spleen, oviducts, uterus and vagina etc. Since smooth muscle contraction is involuntary and slow, therefore it can work for longer period without fatigue.

Cardiac Muscle

The most characteristic feature of the cardiac muscle is that it possesses inharent rhythmicity. It is also known as *myocardium*. It shows some common characters between smooth and striated muscles. It is found only in the heart and is involuntary in its action. The cardiac muscle fibres are about 80μ long and 15μ thick. They are joined end to end and show frequent branchings. Where the cell branches join, a bridge is said to have formed. The fibres are separated by strands of loose connective tissue or *endomysium* through which enters numerous blood and lymph capillaries and nerve fibres.

The sarcolemma of cardiac muscle cells is similar to but more delicate as compare to striated muscles. Each muscle cells contains 1-2 large, oral nuclei, which like those of smooth muscles are placed centrally. The sarcoplasm is abundant and with numerous mitochondria. The myofibrils show cross-striations.

The angulated dark areas crossing the cardiac muscle fibres are called *intercalated* discs, they are actually cell membranes that separate individual cardiac muscle cells from each other. That is, cardiac muscle fibres are made up of many cardiac muscle cells connected in series with each other. It is supposed that intracellular current (ions) is transferred from one cardiac muscle cells to another at the *intercalated discs*.

Therefore, cardiac muscle is a *syncytium*, in which the cardiac muscle cells are so tightly bound that when one of these cells becomes excited, the action potential spreads to all of them, spreading from cell to cell and spreading throughout the latticework interconnections.

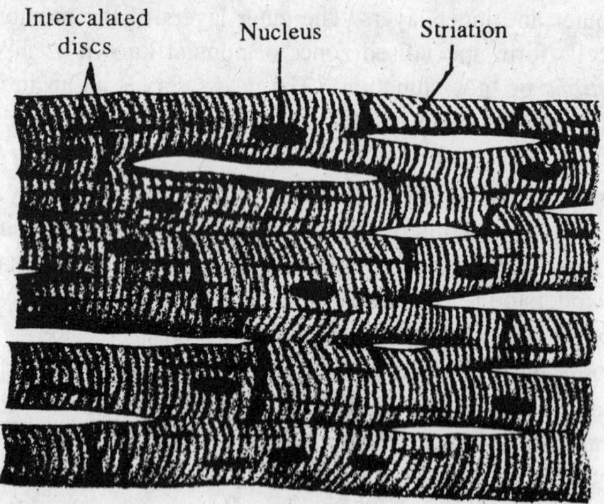

Fig. 8.9 : The "syncytial" interconnecting nature of cardiac muscle.

Under the endocardium which lines the internal surface of the heart, there is a network of modified cardiac fibres called *Purkinje fibres*, which form a special impulse-conducting system.

Properties of Muscle

All the types of muscles exhibit some common properties which are as follows:

1. *Irritability* : It is the ability of muscle tissue to receive and respond to stimuli. A stimulus is a change in the internal or external environment strong enough to initiate a nerve impulse.
2. *Contractibility* : It is the ability to shorten and thicken or contract, when a sufficient stimulus is received. Contraction is faster in skeletal muscle, intermediate in cardiac and of slower degree in involuntary muscle.
3. *Conductivity* : Once a part of the muscle is stimulated by a stimulus of adequate strength, it is conducted within no time to all its other parts. This property is fast in skeletal muscle than other.

4. *Extensibility and elasticity* : Muscles have stretching ability *i.e.,* they extend, however on releasing the tension they return to its original shape or length due to their elastic properties.
5. *Tonicity* : It can be defined as involuntary resistance to passive stretch. All the muscles in the body at a given time are never found in a perfect relaxed state. They are in a state of mild contraction which causes them to resist being stretched. This is the tonicity of the muscles.
6. *Refractory period* : If two stimuli are applied one immediately after the other, the muscle will respond to the first stimulus but not to the second. This brief period during which the muscle does not respond to the second stimulus is called as the *refractory period*, or *period* of lost irritability. Its duration varies with the muscle involved. Skeletal muscle has a short refractory period. Involuntary muscle has medium refractory period and cardiac muscle has a long refractory period.
7. *The all or none law of muscle contraction* : Skeletal muscle, fibres contract in response to nervous stimuli, and the weakest stimulus that can initiate contraction is known as the threshold or *liminal stimulus*. When muscle fibres receive a stimulus strong enough to elicit a response the fibres contract with the maximum force possible or they do not contract at all. They are unable to respond with partial contraction. This is known as the all or none law. This however is not true of a muscle as a whole. In a whole muscle contraction is graded, *i.e.,* contraction may be weak or strong depending on the number of muscle fibres responding to a stimulus.

Stimulation of Muscle

A stimulus is a sudden change in the environment. Strong enough to excite the living body or its organs. If the stimulus is strong enough to evoke a response, it is called as *adequate stimulus*. The stimulus may be physical, mechanical, chemical or electrical in nature. The muscle responds to the stimulus despite its nature; by contracting.

The lowest strength of stimulus sufficient to elicit an action potential is called as *threshold stimulus*. This value differs in various tissues. Excitable tissues require lower threshold of stimulus than the less excitable tissues. If a stimulus is less than threshold value, it fails to create a response. Such a stimulus is called as *subthreshold stimulus.* A maximum response is produced by the *suprathreshold stimulus*. However, further increase in the threshold shall not add to the strength of the response. When any, say electrical stimulus is applied to the muscle or its nerve, muscle contraction results due to the shortening (contraction) of the fibres of the muscle. This muscle contraction can be recorded by Kymograph where a simple muscle curve is formed on smoked paper, mounted on the drum of a kymograph apparatus. A time tracing below it, gives the duration of its various phases.

Isotonic and Isometric Contractions

These types of contractions are related to the load applied to a muscle. The muscle is said to be in an *isotonic condition* when it

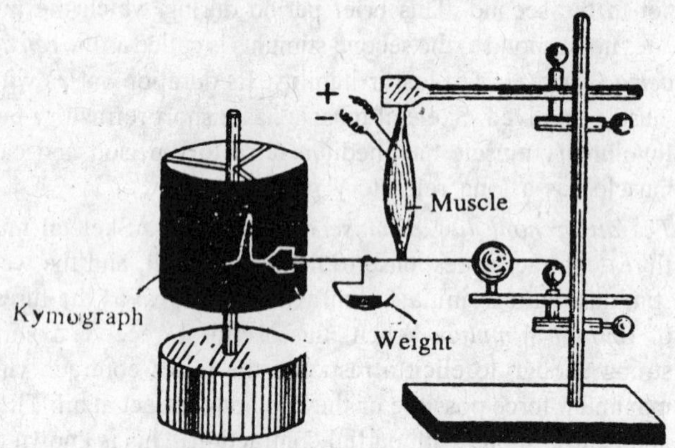

Fig. 8.10 : Isotonic contraction of muscle.

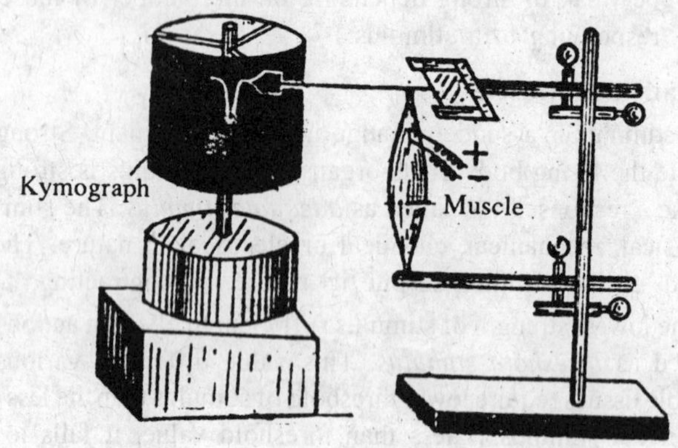

Fig. 8.11 : Isometric contraction of muscle.

contracts with a constant load that it can lift. During this phase, the muscle maintains an equal tonus or tension (iso; same; tonus, tension).

On the other hand, when a muscle contracts against a weight that it cannot lift, it is said to give an *isometric* (iso, same; metric, length) contraction, since it maintains uniform length. In other words, during isotonic contraction, there is a change in the shape of the muscle, while there is no such change of shape in isometric contraction.

Simple Contraction or Muscle Twitch

The response of a muscle to a single brief stimulus, such as an electric shock is known as twitch. A *twitch* can be divided into three phases (Fig. 8.12).

1. A latent period in which the length of the muscle remains constant.
2. A contraction period during which the muscle shortens, and
3. A relaxation period in which the length of the muscle and its tension reach the normal level.

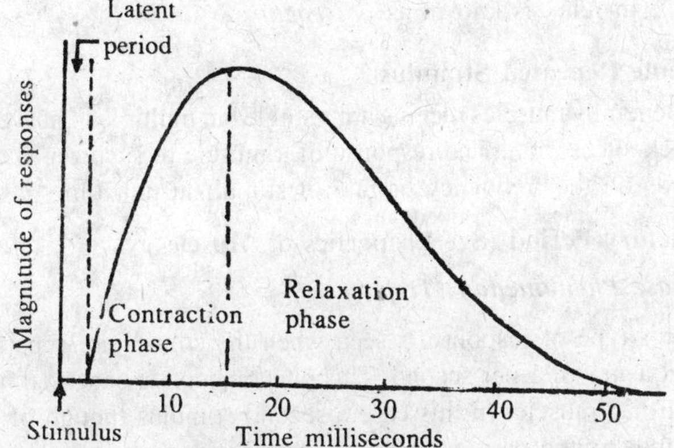

Fig. 8.12 : Single contraction of skeletal muscle showing different components.

1. *Latent period* : This period is nothing but the time between the stimulation and activation of the lever or the short lapse of time that occurs between the application of stimulus and the beginning of the response. The latent period of simple muscle curve is about 0.01 sec. The duration of the latent period varies with the species, type of muscle, temperature and internal conditions of muscle.

2. *Contraction period :* is the period during which a muscle reaches a peak of contraction. In isotonic contraction shortening of the muscle filament takes place. The dark bands of the fibrils become shorter and wider. The light bands also decrease in length in isotonic contraction and may slightly increase in length during isometric contraction. During the phase of shortening of the muscle fibres, external work is done. The work done by a muscle is dependent on the size of the muscle, the type of muscle, its nutritive condition, and upon external conditions such as temperature. This period is marked by the point of contraction to the crest of the muscle curve. It is about 0.04 sec.

3. *Relaxation period :* is the reversal of the contraction phase, it is the time that elapses between the crest of the curve until the muscle resumes its normal length. This phase consumes more time than the contraction process, it is about 0.16 sec. but it also dependant upon certain conditions in the muscle. Cold prolongs the relaxation process and also in fatigue. If there is rise in temperature, span of this period will fall. The failure of a muscle to relax is known as *contracture.*

Multiple Repeated Stimulus

Generally muscles receive not a single but multiple of nerve impulses in quick succession. The response of a muscle to such repeated stimuli depends on the frequency or rate of stimuli in unit time.

Refractory Period (See Properties of Muscles)

Staircase Phenomenon (Treppe)

This type of response is seen when the stimuli are separated with the frequency of 1 per second. This phenomenon is observed in skeletal and cardiac muscle. In this case a second stimulus though of the same magnitude as the previous one, elicits a better response. Thus each of the first few twitches is a little greater than the previous one. This is known as *staircase phenomenon* or *treppe*. The accumulation of metabolic products formed during earlier activity and slight increase in temperature of the muscle possibly creates more favourable conditions for excitation-contraction coupling work. The first contraction as if proves beneficial to the succeeding ones. Hence, this phenomenon is also described on beneficial effect.

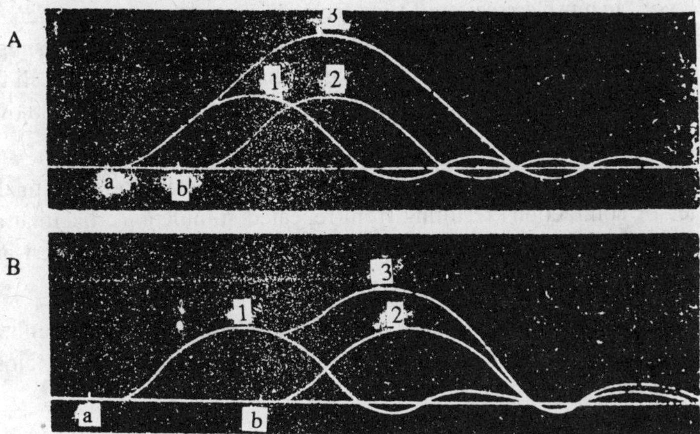

Fig. 8.13 : Staircase phenomenon. (a) point of first stimulus; (b) point of second stimulus; (1) Contraction due to first stimulus; (2) contraction to second stimulus; (3) Summated contraction, (A) Second stimulus during contraction phase; (B) Second stimulus during relaxation phase.

Summation : When the pre-synaptic portion of a nerve is stimulated more than two limes, it tends to have an additive effect on the post-synaptic portion. In the case of muscles, the effects may either be-mechanical or electrical; accordingly summation or addition takes place in the electric behaviour of the membrane of the muscle fibre and in the contractile elements. However, as the electric membrane responses

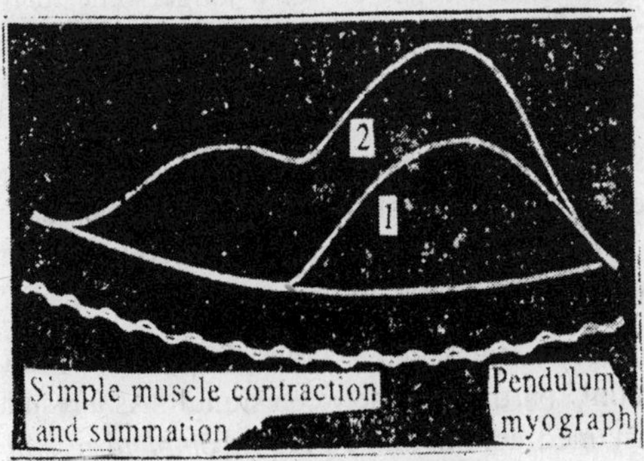

Fig. 8.14 : Showing summation.

are of short duration, it is essential that the stimulations should be at short intervals. In muscles a series of stimuli causes contraction, which gradually increase and the resulting final contraction is greater than a simple contraction, excited by a stimulus of greater intensity and excites all the fibres of a muscle. The additive effect of repeated contractions is known as summation.

Facilitation : In contrast to summation, facilitation, refers to the series of contractions resulting from repeated stimulations. Facilitation is not a single phenomenon and various theories have been put forward to explain this process.

(i) the stimulation of pre-synaptic portion releases more transmitter substance with each stimulation if the impulses are at close intervals,

(ii) with each stimulus more transmitter substance is added to the previous one as it is not completely inactivated,

(iii) the membrane is kept activated by the pre-synaptic stimulation until the next impulse arrives and may consist in the mobilization of certain chemical processes,

(iv) facilitation may consist in the rearrangement of contractile filaments and finally,

(v) it may also be affected by the activation of certain metabolic processes which supply energy. Facilitation takes place within a definite period of time and does not proceed indefinitely.

If the stimulation are repeated for a longer time than the optimal value, contractions gradually decrease and may altogether stop.

Tetanus

If the muscle fibre is stimulated before it relaxes for a second time, it can contract again. Therefore, a muscle can be maintained in a continuously contracted phase, if stimulated frequently within a given time. A continuous contraction of this type is known as "*tetanus*".

If a frog muscle is stimulated at a rate of 20 to 30 stimuli per second, the muscle can only partly relax between stimuli. As a result, the muscle maintains a sustained contraction called *incomplete tetanus*. Increased stimuli at a rate of 35 to 50 stimuli per second, result in *complete tetanus*, a sustained contraction that lacks even partial relaxation.

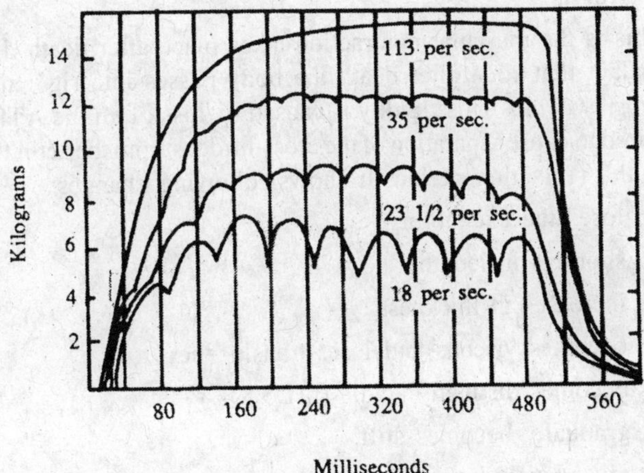

Fig. 8.15 : Complete and incomplete tetanus due to stimuli on the gastrocnemtus muscle.

Muscle Fatigue

When repeatedly stimulated, the muscle has lost its irritability becomes gradually less excitable and ultimately ceases to respond. This phenomenon is called *fatigue*. So it can be defined as the inability of muscle to do further work.

Though the exact reason for fatigue is not known, various explanations have been made:

1. the depletion of the metabolic sources of energy.
2. accumulation of the end products of chemical reactions, such as lactic acid, CO_2, ketone bodies etc.
3. loss of potassium ions from the post-synaptic cell and accumulation of the same in the extracellular space.
4. increase in the concentration of sodium ions in the post-synaptic cell.
5. decrease of local synthesis of acetylcholine like susbstances during prolonged exercise. Experiments have shown that removal of the waste products formed during contraction by repeatedly washing the muscle in a balanced salt solution, delays fatigue. Recovery of the fatigued muscle takes place if allowed to rest for a particular time.

Rigor Mortis

This is the muscular contraction takes place after death. It is well known fact that soon after death the body passes into rigor mortis or *stiffening of death*. This rigidity is caused by loss of all the ATP, which is required to cause separation of the cross-bridges from the actin filaments during the relaxation period. It shows following changes:

1. loses the excitability,
2. shortens in length,.
3. increases in thickness,
4. becomes viscous and loses translucency,
5. becomes distinctly acidic (pH 5.8),
6. gradually becomes stiff,
7. glycogen disappears, and
8. the muscles gives off carbonic acid.

On the average rigor mortis starts in the second hour and is completed in three hours after death. The muscles remain in rigor until the muscle proteins are destroyed, which usually results from autolysis caused by enzymes released from the lysosomes some 15 to 25 hours later. This phenomenon helps in finding out approximate time of death of a individual.

Attachments of Muscle and Movements

At the extremities of the muscles the connective tissue of the endomysium, perimysium and epimysium unite to form strong, fibrous, non-elastic cords called *tendons*. Tendons attach a muscle to the periosteum of a bone, and vary in length from a fraction of an inch to more than a foot. Sometimes they form a broad, flat expansion called an *aponeurosis*.

Most skeletal muscles are attached to bones, although a few, such as the muscles of facial expression, are attached to the soft tissues of the face, and others are attached to cartilage or ligaments.

Some tendons, for example those of the wrist and ankle, which pass under ligamentous bands or through bony tunnels, are enclosed in sheaths of synovial membrane called *tendon sheaths*. These facilitate smooth, frictionless movement of the tendons.

In situation where a muscle or tendon comes in contact, with or moves over a bony prominence, or where the skin moves directly over bone, the pressure is relieved by a small synovial sac, called a bursa. *Bursae* are usually located near joints, for example the olecranon bursa over the olecranon process of the ulna; the prepatellar bursa where the skin moves over the front of the patella.

Bursae may become inflamed, usually as a result of repeated minor injury (*e.g.,* prepatellar bursitis or 'housemaid's knee'.)

Actions of Muscles

The main mass of a muscle is termed the belly, and lies along the shaft of a bone, never over a joint. Muscles are firmly attached at each end to different bones and it is the tendons which cross a joint. When a muscle contracts, a pull is exerted on both bones but one is stabilized by isometric contractions of other muscles and the contraction pulls the other bone toward it. For example, the belly of the biceps muscle lies parallel to the shaft of the humerus in the upper arm. The two tendons at the upper end of the biceps are attached to the scapula, while the tendon at the lower end crosses the elbow joint and is attached to the radius. Contraction of the biceps muscle draws the lower arm toward the upper (Fig. 8.16).

The fixed point of muscle attachment is called the *origin*, while the movable point of attachment is called the *insertion*. In the example above the muscle attachments into the scapula form the origin of the biceps muscle and the attachment into the radius forms the insertion. Muscles which stabilize the bone giving origin to the muscle are known as *fixation muscles*.

Muscles which bend a limb at a joint are called *flexors*. Muscles which straighten a limb at a joint are called *extensors*. Muscles which move a limb away from the midline of the body are known as *abductors*, while those that move the limb toward the midline are called *adductors*. Some muscles cause *rotation* of a limb. In movements of the wrist joint, *supinators* turn the hand palm upward and *pronators* turn the palm downward. In movements of the ankle joint *dorsiflexors* turn the foot upward and *plantarflexors extend* the foot toward the ground. Muscles which raise a part of the body are called *levators* and those which lower a part are known as *depressors*.

Movements are complex and the performance of any given movement, *e.g.,* flexion of the elbow joint, requires the co-ordination of several muscles. Muscles which initiate and maintain a movement are called *prime movers* or *agonists*, while those which oppose a movement or reverse it are known as *antagonists*. Thus when the biceps muscle contracts to raise the lower arm towards the shoulder it is the prime mover. The triceps muscle, which can oppose this action and straighten the elbow, is the antagonist. However, actions which require a joint to be held rigid will cause simultaneous contraction of both prime movers and antagonists.

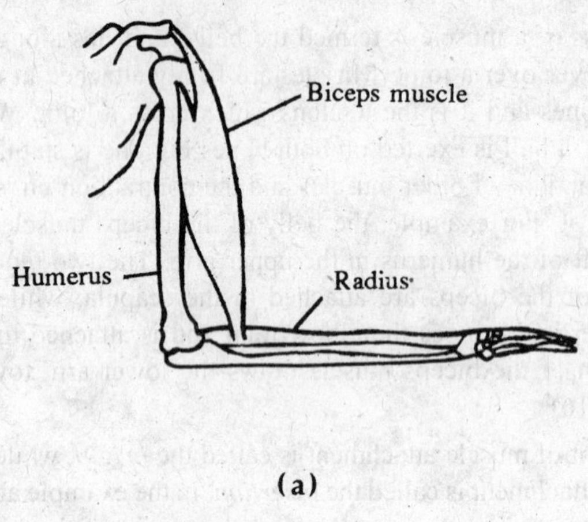

(a)

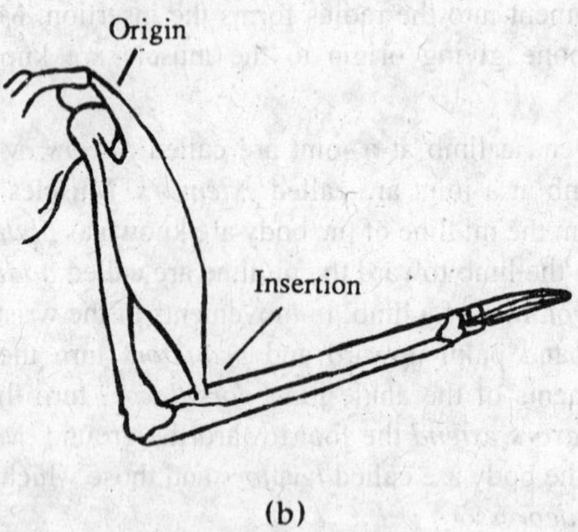

(b)

Fig. 8.16 (a), (b) : Muscles are attached to two bones across a joint, contraction of the muscle pulls is on the bone into which the muscles is inserted producing movement.

Synergists are muscles which assist a prime mover by stabilizing a joint crossed by the tendon of the prime mover, thus allowing it to produce a more effective movement.

Muscles may be named according to one or more of the following.

1. Function, *e.g.,* flexors, extensors, abductors, etc.
2. Attachments, *e.g.,* sterno-mastoid.
3. Shape, *e.g.,* deltoid (like Greek letter D or Δ).
4. Position or direction, *e.g.,* pectoralis major (large breast muscle), rectus abdominus (straight abdominal muscle), the oblique and straight muscles of the eye.
5. Formation *e.g.,* biceps = two heads; triceps = three heads; quadriceps = four heads.

NERVOUS SYSTEM

The nervous system is the most important organisation which controls and integrates the different bodily functions and likewise maintains a stability or constancy of the internal environment despite extreme changes in the external environment. The activities of the nervous system depends upon a complex interplay of numerous dynamic interactions or regulatory reactions. This system is absolutely necessary for the reception, storage and release of different informations for regulating or initiating a particular behaviour of the individual ranging from the cellular to the gross animal being. Simple organisms are simply structured and organised but a large animal with a complex structure requires this system to overcome the problems of recognition of stimuli, storage of information (memory), communication between the various parts of its body, and the execution of effective responses.

Nervous system includes brain, spinal cord, peripheral nerves and autonomic nerves innervating body organs. It constitutes about 2.4% of the body weight. Brain alone weights about 1400 gm, spinal cord 35 gm, spinal nerves about 150 gm and the cranial nerves about 12 gm. This system may be divided into 3 parts : the central nervous system (brain and spinal cord), the *peripheral nervous system* (cranial and spinal nerves) and *autonomic nervous system* (Parasympathetic and sympathetic nerves). The principal constituents of this system are the neuron and neurolgia.

Neuron : (Fig. 9.1). It is the structural and functional unit of the nervous system and is the largest cell in the body and there are about 10 billion neurons are present in human beings. It may be round, flask shaped, oval, triangular and star shaped. It is made up of 3 distinct parts (1) Cell body or cyton (2) Dendrites and (3) Axon.

(1) *Cell body or cyton or perikaryon* : This consists of a well-defined nucleus and nucleolus surrounded by a granular cytoplasm. Within the cytoplasm are several mitochondria, golgibodies and Nissil granules. Nissil granules consists of

nucleoprotein' and organically combined iron and may be concerned with continued synthesis of new cytoplasm. These bodies disappear during fatigue and injury to the nerve cell and reappear again after a rest. There is no *centrosome* in cytoplasm and due to lack of this full matured nerve cells never multiply and when damaged, are never replaced. Each neuron usually gives off a single cylindrical axon from a funnel-shaped area

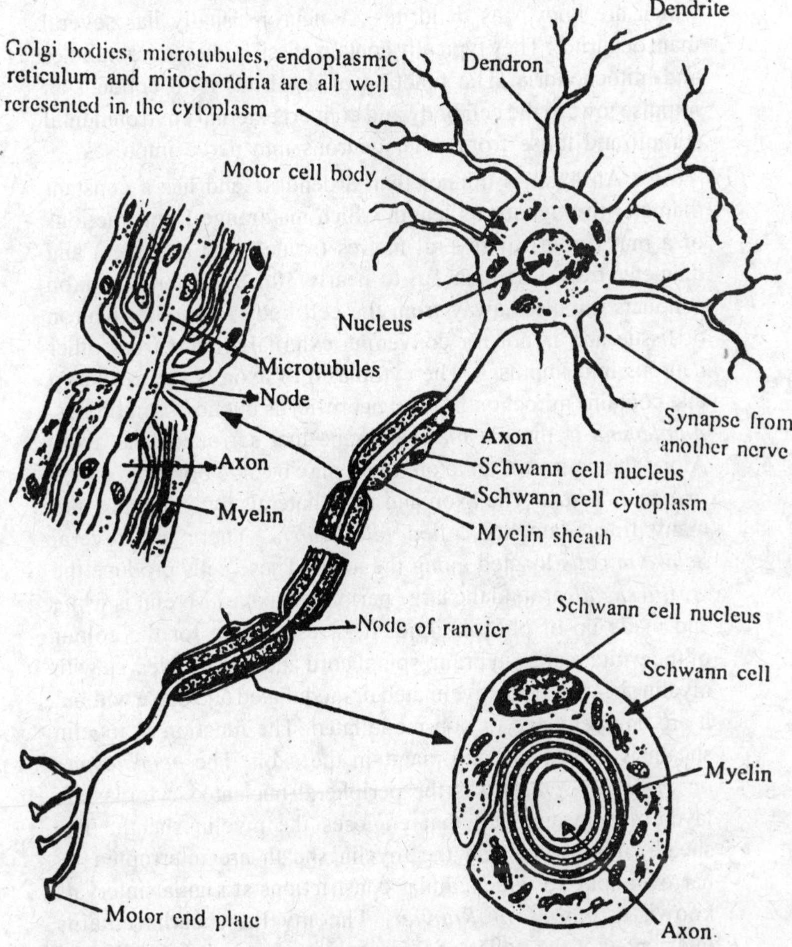

Fig. 9.1 : The structure of a motor neuron.

called axon hillock. This portion is found to be rich in *neuro-fibrillae.* Neurofibrils are five filaments passing through the cytoplasm from the dendrite to the axon. These are composed of microtubules and may perform a function of support.

A longitudinal section through a node (left) and a transverse section through the axon (right) are also shown.

(2) *Dendrites (G. dendron = tree) :* The cell membrane, of the cell body is projected in the form of certain filamentous structures which are known as dendrites. A neuron usually has several main dendrites. They typically contain Nissil bodies, microtubules and mitochondria. The function of dendrites is to conduct an impulse toward the cell body and convert external environmental stimuli and those from other neurons into nerve impulses.

(3) *Axon :* An axon is thinner than a dendrite and has a constant diameter throughout its length which may range from fractions of a mm (brain) to several metres (spinal cord and toes) and diameter from less than 1μ, to nearly 30μ. Functionally, axon conducts impulses away from the cell body to another neuron or tissue and is not for convening external stimuli from other neurons into impulses. The cytoplasm of axon is the *axoplasm* that contains mitochondria and neurofibrils but no Nissil bodies. *Amolemma* is the plasma membrane that surrounds the axon. Along the course of an axon, there may be side branches called *axon collaterals.* The axon and its collaterals by branching into many fine filaments called *telodendria.* There are several *Schwann cells* located along the axon. These cells produce the *myelin sheath* around the large peripheral axons. Myelin is white and made up of phospholipid. It is responsible for the colour of the white matter in brain, spinal cord and nerves. Nerves with myelin sheath are the myelinated or medullated and those without it are unmyelinated or non-medullated. The function of myelin sheath is to insulate and maintain the axon. The *neurolemma or sheath of schwann* is the peripheral nucleated cytoplasmic layer of schwann cell that encloses the myelin sheath. The sheath of schwann and the myelin sheath are interrupted by narrow about 1μ wide annular constrictions at regular intervals known as *nodes of Ranvier.* The myelin sheath remains interrupted at the nodes of Ranvier. If axon gives off collateral branches, these arise from a node of Ranvier. The length of the

internodal segments varies in different species and in different nerve fibres from about 200 to over 2000μ.

Neuroglia (C. glia = glue), or satellite cells constitutes the accessory tissue of the central nervous system. They include *astroglia, oligodendroglia,* ependyma, microglia, and the schwann cells. These cells have different forms and different functions like nutritive, supportive, limiting, phagocytic and insulative. The main difference between neurons and neuroglial is that these cells can multiply throughout the animal's life.

On the basis of their function, neurons are distinguished into:

(1) *Afferent or sensory or receptor neurons :* These are bipolar cells whose processes bring impulses generated at the receptors located in the skin, tendons, visceral organs, etc. to the central nervous system.

(2) *Efferent or motor/effector neurons :* These carry particular impulses from the central nervous system along their axons to effectors such as glands, muscles, stimulating them to appropriate actions.

(3) *Association or internuncial or connector or adjuster neurons :* These are present only in central nervous system. They perform the function of co-ordination, integration and connecting links between the sensory and motor neurons.

(4) *Neurosecretory neurons :* These are the special motor neurons and are specialised for the production of hormones when are transported along the axon to its distal tip. The axons terminate at blood capillary walls and the hormones are released into the blood stream through which they reach to their target organs.

On the basis of the chemical substances released by the neurons, these are categorised into.

(a) *Adrenergic neurons* are those, releasing substances of hormonal nature. Majority of post ganglionic sympathetic fibres releasc sympathin, a similar hormone to adrenaline (epinephrine), hence are often known as adrenergic neurons.

(b) *Cholinergic neurons* are those, which produce a substances called acetylcholine. Post ganglionic parasympathetic and sympathetic fibres of sweat glands and uterus belong to this category.

Functional properties of the neurons and nerve fibres :

(1) *Excitability* : The neurons can be stimulated by a stimulus of mechanical, electrical, chemical and thermal of adequate strength.

(2) *Conductivity* : The place of stimulation or excitation does not remain at the site of its origin. It is transmitted along the nerve fibres normally in one direction. This property of conduction is called the conductivity. The velocity of conduction depends upon the diameter of nerve fibres and temperature.

(3) *All or none law* : If the stimulus be adequate the neuron will always give a maximum response. If the strength or duration of the stimulus be further increased no alteration in the response will take place.

(4) *Refractory period* : When the neuron or the nerve fibre is once excited, it will not respond to a second stimulus for a brief period. This period is called *absolute refractory period.* The absolute refractory period means that the nerve is completely refractory to stimulation-in other words, is incapable of eliciting an action potential at any intensity of stimulation. During the absolute refractory period there is total inactivation of the sodium carrier mechanism and as the Na^+ ions cannot enter the fibre, there is no development of the action potential. Immediately following this, there is a brief relative refractory period. During which the excitability is subnormal but gradually rising. In large mammalian nerve fibres the durations are as follows : Absolute refractory period 2 to 3 milliseconds in frog but in mammals it is 0.5 millisecond. Relative refractory period 10 to 30 milliseconds in frog but in mammals 3 milliseconds.

(5) *Summation* : In a nerve fibre summation of two submaximal stimuli is possible. A current above the rheobase (magnitude of current just sufficient to excite nerve or muscle is called rheobase), but applied for a time less than that required on the basis of the strength-duration curve, fails to evoke a response in a neuron. However, if the same stimulus is repeatedly applied for a sufficient number of times, stimulation occurs by summation provided the sum of all the application of the stimulus is greater than the minimum demanded by the strength-duration curve. Summation, though adequated will not stimulate if the time elapsed between stimuli is increased beyond a certain limit, because the neurons recover from each stimulus.

(6) *Adaptation* : The nerve fibre quickly adapts itself. Due to this adaptation there is no excitation during the passage of a constant

current. Only when the strength of the current is suddenly altered or the current is made or broken excitation takes place. A gradual change will fail to excite.

(7) *Accommodation :* If a stimulus even with stronger strength is applied slowly to a nerve, then there may have no response only due to lack of attaining the threshold strength. This phenomenon is called accommodation *i.e.,* slowly applied stimulus is accommodated by the nerve no matter how strong the stimulus is applied.

(8) *Indefatigability :* In the nerve muscle preparation, if the nerve is stimulated repeatedly, then after a certain period the muscle fails to give any response. Now if that nerve is isolated from the muscle and placed on a fresh muscle, then application of stimulus will excite the muscle. This shows that nerve is not fatigued.

Information : Information means variety of different things, such as knowledge, facts, quantitative values, intensity of pain, light, temperature and any other aspect of the body or its immediate surroundings that has meaning. Pain from a pin prick, pressure on the bottom of the feet, degree of angulation of the joints and a stored memory in the brain are some of the examples of information.

Impulses : Informations cannot be transmitted in its original form but in the form of action potentials called nerve Impulses. Thus, a part of the body that is subjected to pain must first convert this information into nerve impulses; specific areas of the brain convert abstract thoughts also into nerve impulses that are then transmitted either elsewhere in the brain or into peripheral nerves to motor effectors throughout the body. The retina of eye converts vision into nerve impulses;, is one of the example where information is converted into nerve impulse.

Signals : In the transmission of information, it is frequently not desirable to speak in terms of the individual impulses but instead in the form of overall pattern of impulses; this pattern is called a signal. As an example, when pressure is applied to large area of skin, impulses are transmitted by large numbers of parallel nerve fibres, and the total pattern of impulses transmitted by all these fibres is a signal. Thus, we can speak of visual signals, auditory signals, some aesthetic signals, motor signals and so forth.

Though there are differences in size, position and structure, nerve cells can be functionally distinguished into 3 regions (Fig. 9.2).

(a) *Generator region* restricted to the dendrites, soma and collaterals
(b) *conductile region* is the axon and
(c) *transmissional region* comprises the nerve ending or nerve terminals.

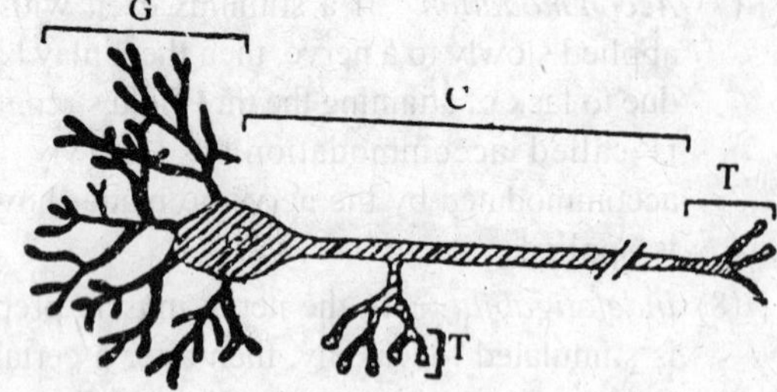

G = Generator region, C = Conductile region, T = Transmissional region.

Fig. 9.2 : Functional Organisation of Neuron.

Nerve impulse : A nerve impulse has been defined differently by several workers. *Prosser* has defined nerve impulse as "the sum total of physical and chemical reactions which take place in the propagation of the wave of physiological activity along the nerve fibre." According to *Githlin* "nerve impulse is a phenomenon which involves both physical and chemical action." A neuron represents transmissional unit of the nervous system and performs the function of an impulse transmission from receptor to effector and *vice-versa.* Neuron is capable of doing this because of many factors governing its physiological behaviour, among which the most important is *Donnan equilibrium.*

Donnan equilibrium : Maintenance of cell volume for normal activities depends not only on osmotic gradients, but also on chemical and electrical gradients. Thus, as a result of the electro-chemical gradient maintained by the cell, the ionic flux inside and outside of it is distributed in a peculiar manner. This ionic inequilibrium on the cell membrane is specified on Donnan's equilibrium and is maintained at the expenditure of energy.

A Donnan model of a hypothetical cell may be postulated as follows : interior of the cell has non-diffusible anions (chloride) which maintain a permanent internal negative charge with respect to the exterior of the plasma membrane which is positively charged because of the excess of cations (sodium). If this cell model is immersed in a solution of potassium chloride, both chemical and electrical gradients will drive potassium to the inside of the cell. The concentration gradient will drive the chloride to the inside while the electrical gradient will drive at the outside of the cell. At equilibrium, there will be a high concentration of potassium inside than outside, while a lower concentration of chloride inside than outside. By applying the law of Mass Action, Donnan has showed that at equilibrium,

$$(K^+)_{in} + (Cl^-)_{in} = (K^+)_{out} + (Cl^-)_{out}$$

where the product of the concentrations of diffusible ions is equal inside as well as outside.

Actually, due to unequal distribution of ions like sodium, potassium and chloride (constituting major ionic flux for membrane's environmental fluid) inside and outside of the cell, a resting potential is developed and the membrane becomes *charged* and *polarized*. Particularly the sodium ions are more outside and potassium and chloride ions inside. As a result, outer surface of the membrane becomes positively charged with respect to the inner surface when is negatively charged. Thus, a resting nerve cell (unstimulated) maintains a transmembrane potential due to Donnan equilibrium.

Speed of nerve impulse in the nerve fibres is different in the different animals. In the larger nerve fibres of mammals this impulses travel at a relatively slow speed as compared to medullated. Usually impulses that a nerve fibre can transmit is 500-1000 impulse per second.

Conduction of nerve Impulse In non-medullated nerve fibres (Fig. 9.3) : Nerve impulse travels along a nerve fibre by a series of steps. These steps are both chemical and electrical in nature. Each nerve impulse is of the same nature and is similar in all the nerves. Registering of different sensations in the brain is not dependent on the nature of the impulse but on the area in which it is received. The chemical reactions of the nerve impulse at any given segment of a fibre consume oxygen and require energy. In addition CO_2 is produced and a rise in temperature occurs. Electrical changes accompany these localised chemical changes.

The electrical activity that accompanies the nerve impulse along a fibre has been studied extensively Like all other cells, the nerve cells exist in a fluid environment (interstitial fluid) in which salts and ions are dissolved. The neurilemma is impermeable to most of these ions, permitting only potassium (K^+) ions to diffuse freely and keeping sodium (Na^+) and chloride (Cl^-) ions outside.

Resting potential : At rest there is a considerable difference between the ion concentration outside and inside the plasma membrane. In a resting neuron or fibre, there is a difference in electrical charges on either side of the membrane. This difference is called the potential difference.

This difference is mainly due to the unequal distribution of sodium and potassium ions on either side of the membrane. Potassium ion concentration inside the neuron is about 30 times greater than it is outside. Similarly, sodium ion .concentration is about 10 times greater outside than inside. Another significant factor is the presence of large non-diffusible negatively charged ions trapped in the cell, most of them are proteins. Neurons also contain a large number of negative ions on the inside that cannot diffuse outside or diffuse very poorly. Sodium ions are positive and develop a positive charge outside the membrane. Though potassium are also positive and are actively transported to the inside of the cell, these are insufficient to equalize the larger number of non-diffusible negative ions trapped in the cell. Thus, the inside of the membrane has a negative charge. This difference in charge on either side of the membrane of a resting neuron is the *resting potential or membrane potential*. At rest the value of resting potential is about –70 millivolts (mV). The membrane at this stage is said to be the *polarized membrane*.

Depolarization : When a stimulus of any kind, mechanical, electrical or chemical impenges upon the nerve fibre, a momentary local increase occurs in the permeability at the site of stimulus which permits more sodium ions to rush into the cell. This results in change in potential of inner membrane from-70 mV towards zero. At this stage membrane is said to be depolarized. The inward movement of sodium ion continues thus the membrane potential is reversed-the inside of the membrane becomes positive and the outside negative. This changed electric potential of neurilemma is known as *action potential*.

The initial change produces an ionic imbalance in the membrane on either side of the point of stimulus producing local electric current. These areas of negative depolarization, in turn initiate changes in the membrane adjacent to them. A wave of electric change runs along the length of fibre and, thus, represents the path of nerve impulse.

The propagation of nerve impulse can be compared to the pushing over of a *row of* dominoes. Energy (ATP) is required for the initial disturbance, but after that the displacement of domino works to displace the next and once the stimulus has set off a nerve, the impulse passes without any change down the length of the fibre. The membrane restores the original positive ion concentration by the outside movement of Na^+ ions from the inner side of the membrane (sodium pump), during this potential value is changed from zero to + 30 mV. This is known as *repolarization*. This process of change requires some time during which

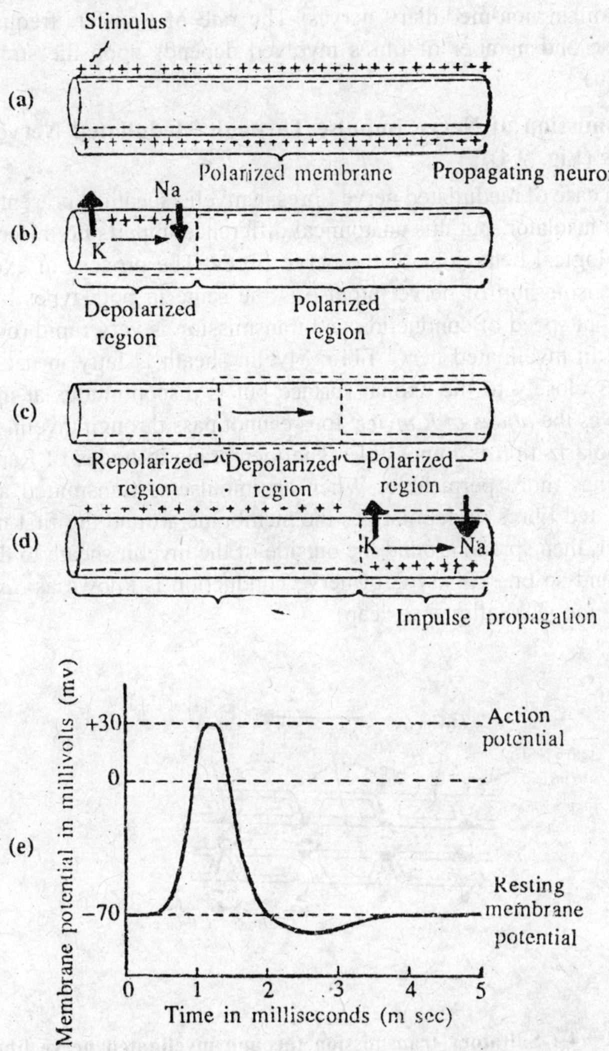

Fig. 9.3 : Initiation and transmission of a neuron impulse.

the nerve cannot be stimulated again. This is known as *refractory period.* Meanwhile, the membrane restores to the original resting state (*i.e.,* from + 30 mV to –70 mV), the dominoes set up the same changes again. The neuron is now prepared to receive another stimulus and transmits in the same manner. Such type of conduction and transmission of impulse is common in non-medullary nerves. The rate of transfer, frequency of impulse and number of fibres involved depends upon the strength of stimulus.

Transmission of Nerve Impulse Through Medullated Nerve Fibres (Fig. 9.4)

In case of medullated nerve fibres, a myelin sheath is present, which acts as insulator, but this anatomical difference imparts no difference in physiological behaviour of the nerve fibres. The process of excitation and transmission of nerve impulse is the same in both types of nerve fibres but speed of conduction and transmission is very rapid (over 100 m/sec) in myelinated nerve fibre. Myelin sheath is fatty in nature and adheres closely to the axonal surface but is discontinuous at intervals known as the *nodes of Ranvier*. Ions cannot pass through myelin sheath, so depolarization is impossible. The membrane at nodes of Ranvier is 500 times more permeable. When an impulse is transmitted along a myelinated fibres, it depolarizes the membrane around the first node of Ranvier, then spread around the outside of the myelin sheath to the next node, and so on. This type of nerve conduction is known as *Saltatory conduction* (L. Salire = to leap).

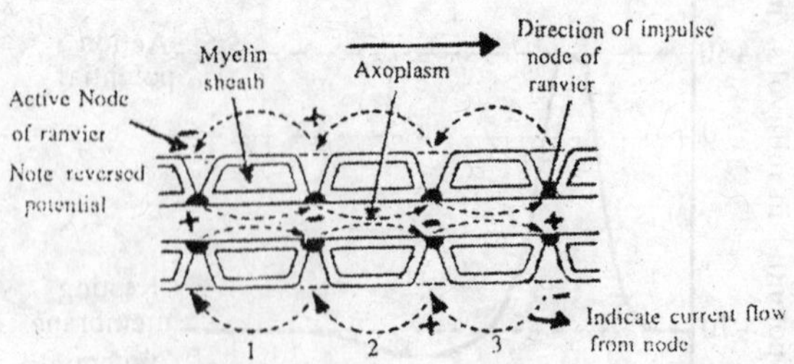

Fig. 9.4 : Saltatory transmission through myelinated nerve fibre.

Saltatory conduction is important for many reasons. First, by causing the depolarization process to jump long intervals along the axon, it greatly increases the speed of impulse conduction. Second, it results in substantial economy of energy expenditure because of the transmembranal movement of the ions during repolarization (an energy requiring process) occurs at the nodes of Ranvier and not throughout the axon and thirdly, avoids dissipation of impulse into adjacent fibres.

NERVE IMPULSE

Neurones specialize in IRRITABILITY and in CONDUCTION of IMPULSES. In RESTING (INACTIVE) NERVE FIBRE.

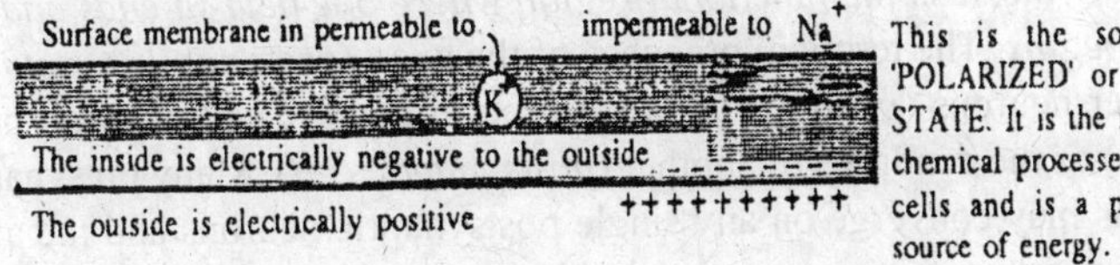

When *NERVE FIBRE is STIMULATED* (e.g. electrically or chemically) ELECTRO-CHEMICAL CHANGES occur at point of stimulation. The resting potential is abolished

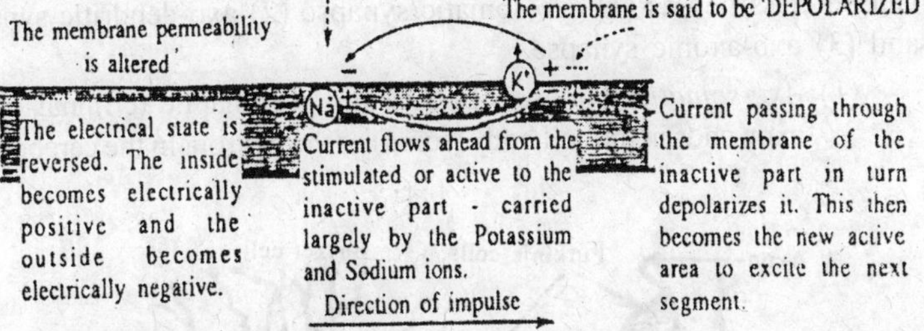

In *MYELINATED NERVE FIBRE*

The active region still 'triggers' the resting part ahead of it by causing an outward flow of current but this occurs only at the Nodes of Ranvier. i.e. The Nerve Impulse is propagated from Node to Node.

This increase speed of CONDUCTION along these large fibres.

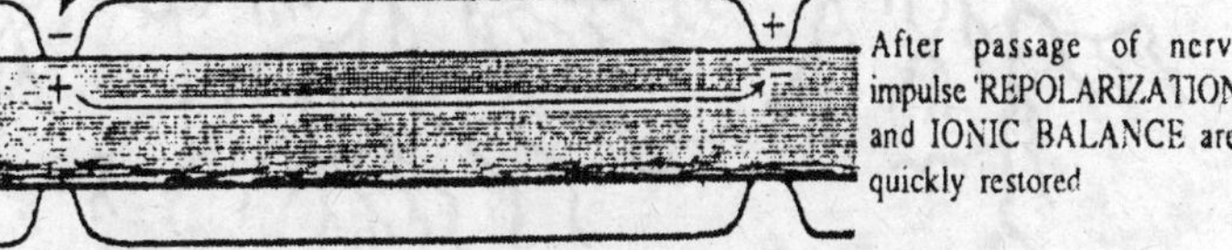

A nerve impulse is the same whether it is in a sensory nerve taking messages to be brain or in a motor nerve taking impulses from the brain to the muscles, etc.

Fig. 9.5 : Short summary of nerve impulse (Illustrative).

The Synapse : As we are now aware that information is transmitted in the central nervous system mainly in the form of nerve impulses through a succession of neuron, one after another. The axonic endings may either be associated with an effector organ such as a muscle fibre or gland cell, or, if the axon belongs to a sensory neuron or intermediate neuron, will make connections with other neurones. Regions where two neurons are functionally connected are known as Synapses, or, in other words, *Synapse is the junctional region where one neuron ends and the other begins.* The terminal branches of the axon (*presynaptic terminals*) of other neurons (*presynaptic cell*) come in contact with the cell body (Soma) or the dendrites of another (*postsynaptic cell*). Many presynaptic neurons may converge on any single postsynaptic neurons and the axon of any presynaptic neuron may divide into multiple branches and may diverge to end on multiple postsynaptic neurons.

Classification : According to the nature of connections, the synapses can be classified as (1) axo-somatic synapse (2) axo-dendritic synapse and (3) axo-axonic synapse.

(1) *Axo-somatic synapse* : In this, the presynaptic terminal of the axon ends in the cell body (soma) of the neuron. In the cerebellum,

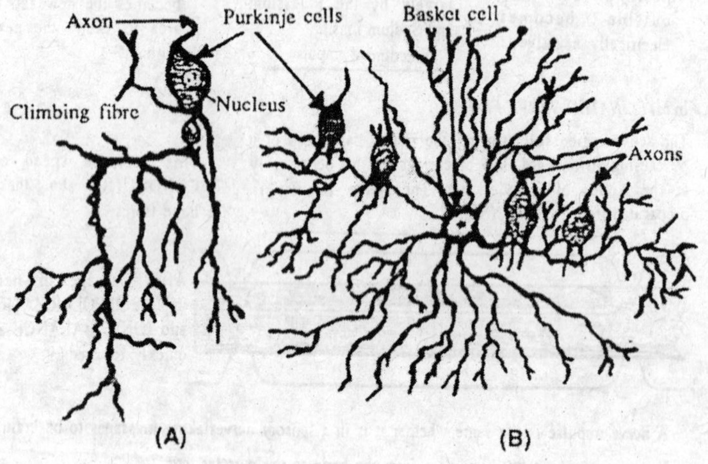

Fig. 9.6 : Diagrammatic representation of almost parallel axo-dendritic synapses upon the dendrites of a Purkinje cell of the cerebellum showing climbing fibres (left side) and axo-somatic synapses of the axon of a basket cell upon the Purkinje cells of the cerebellum (right side).

synaptic connections in between the basket cell and the Purkinje cells are of axo-somatic type. The axons of basket cell make synapses with the soma of the Purkinje cells. This type of synapse is also present in cerebral cortex where basket cell makes synapse with the soma of the pyramidal cells. (Fig. 9.6).

(2) *Axo-dendritic synapse* : Here, the presynaptic fibres of any axon end in the dendrites of the postsynaptic cell. This type of synapse is also present in cerebellum where climbing fibres from axo-dendritic connections with the dendrite of the Purkinje cells. (Fig. 9.6).

(3) *Axo-axonic synapse* : In this presynaptic fibres of any axon ends in the axon of the postsynaptic cells.

Ultrastructure of synapse : Minimum two neurons are needed for the formation of each synapse. The nerve cell which contributes the transmissional terminal is called the *presynaptic* neuron, while that which contributes the generator region is called the *postsynaptic* neuron. The presynaptic terminals are usually in the form of small bulbous swellings and are therefore known as *synaptic knobs*, axon *knobs, synaptosomes, bouton terminaux, end bulbs* or end feet. The synaptic knob contains a large number of two very important structures, the

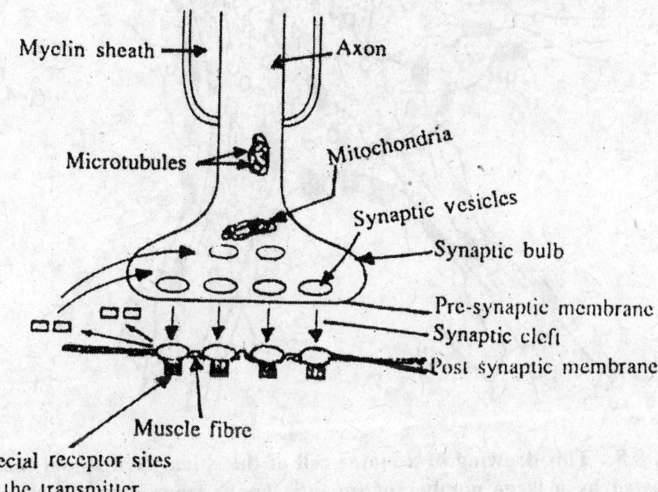

Fig. 9.7 : A neuromuscular junction.

synaptic vesicles and *mitochondria*. Many hundreds of the synaptic knobs lie on the surfaces of the soma and the dendrites (Fig. 9.8). A small intercellular space, the *synaptic cleft*, usually having a width of about 200 to 300 A° units (20-30 nm) separates the membrane of the presynaptic knob from the membrane of the postsynaptic cell. The synaptic vesicles contain a *transmitter substance* which, when released into the synaptic cleft, either it *excites* or *inhibits* the neurons excites if the neuronal membrane contains *excitatory receptors*, inhibits if it

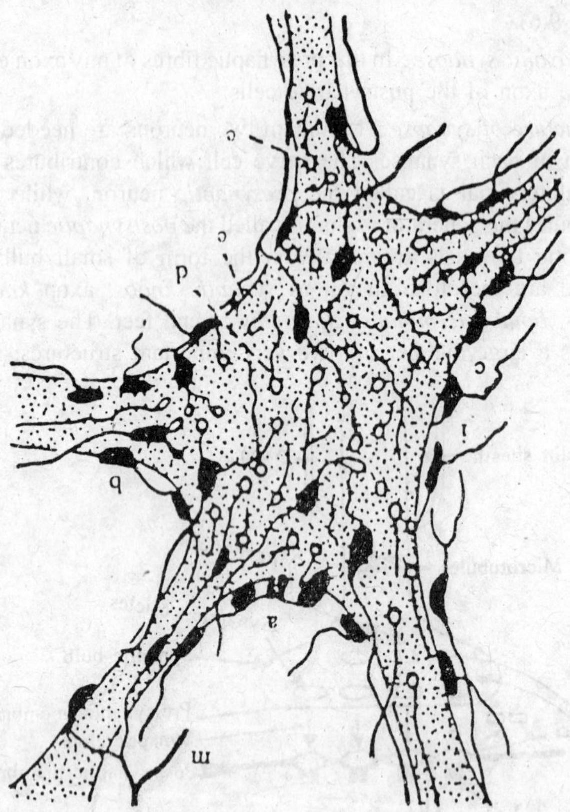

Fig. 9.8 : This drawing of a motor cell of the spinal cord shows that it is invested by a large number of synaptic knobs from many neurons. The synaptic density is about 20 per 100 m². The surface area of a motoneurone is on average 165000 m². This gives about 33000 synapses. a, b, strong bulbs; c, i, terminal buttons; d, e, fine bulbs, m, terminal nerve fibre.

contains *inhibitory receptors*. The mitochondria provide ATP, which is required to synthesize new transmitter substance. The transmitter must be synthesized extremely rapidly because the amount stored in vesicles is sufficient to last for only a few seconds to a few minutes of maximum activity. The membrane of the synaptic knob is known as *presynaptic membrane* and that of the soma, the *postsynaptic* (subsynaptic) membrane

Properties of Synapse

Synaptic response : At the synaptic junction, impulses are received and discharged. But there is no relationship between the receipt and discharge of impulses. Sometimes many impulses are received from different sources but the neuron discharges its own. So it may be said that the synapse not only acts as a relay station but it may also act as an integrator. The integrating mechanism of the synapse is found in the cerebral cortex.

Law of forward conduction : An impulse is allowed to pass through a synapse in one direction only, viz, from the axon of one neuron to the dendrite of the next. But some synapses can transmit impulses in both directions. They are bidirectional and usually electrical in nature, where presynaptic and postsynaptic membranes are in close apposition and often fused at several points.

Synaptic delay : The impulse while passing through a synapse takes a certain length of time. The time between the arrival of the impulse and causing initial depolarization is called *synaptic latency*. The depolarization gradually rises to a spike height. So the synaptic delay is the *sum of the synaptic latency and the time taken for depolarization leading to a spike height in the neuron.* Synaptic delay in chemical synapses is less than 0.5 millisecond whereas in electrical junctions they are extremely short as there is no release of chemicals.

Seat of fatigue : The physiological seat of fatigue is in the central nervous system, probably at the synapses. The mechanism underlying the synaptic fatigue is presumably due to exhaustion of transmitter material from the synaptic vesicles following repeated presynaptic stimulation at a faster rate.

Inhibition : Inhibition may be defined as *an active process which either prevents the onset of activity in a Structure or stops the activity already present.* It may be either postsynaptic or presynaptic and direct or indirect. Inhibitory impulse causes hyperpolarization of the cell membrane beneath the synapse. This is known as inhibitory postsynaptic potential (IPSP). This is due to increased permeability of the cell membrane to K^+ and Cl^- caused by the liberation of an inhibitory chemical transmitter. Na^+ permeability is decreased; and efflux of K^+ and influx of Cl^- from postsynaptic terminals hyperpolarize the postsynaptic membrane. The net effect is increased negativity in the cell with increased membrane potential (–90 mV). Thus the inhibitory postsynaptic potential is developed. The inhibitory postsynaptic potential (IPSP) opposes the excitatory postsynaptic potential (EPSP).

Mechanism of synaptic transmission : The transfer of information across a synaptic junction is called *synaptic transmission* and these transmissions are brought about either by chemical or by electrical or by both processes.

Nerve action potential (NAP) arriving at the axonal terminals, initiates a series of events, causing either a transmission of an excitatory or inhibitory in nature across the synapse or neuro-effector junctions.

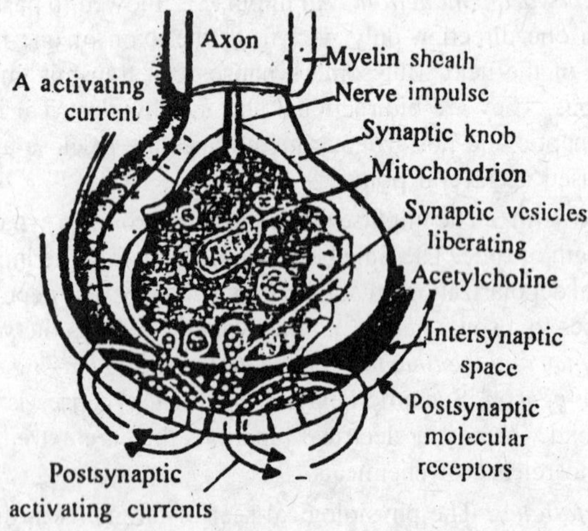

Fig. 9.9 : Schematic representation of synaptic excitation. The transmission of nerve impulse is linked to a specific electro-chemical process. Activating current first travels along neuronal process, afterwards radiates over the synapse and causes the liberation of acetylcholine contained in the synaptic vesicles. Acetylcholine traverses the intersynaptic space and becomes attached' to molecular receptors which are situated on the postsynaptic membrane (the neuronal cytoplasm to be activated) and this causes a postsynaptic current of action in this membrane. Free acetylcholine liberated is hurriedly destroyed by the acetylcholinesterase. The mitochondrion transmits energy necessary for these processes.

The neuro-transmitter substances are probably synthesised in the region of the axonal terminals and stored there in the synaptic vesicles. At rest these transmitter substances are also slowly liberated from these vesicles at a very slow amount which is incapable producing any propagated impulse. However, when the NAP reaches axon terminals, there is synchronous release of several quanta of transmitter substance. There is no proper explanation of the mechanism underlying the release of the transmitter substance from the synaptic vesicles following activation of the synaptic knobs by the propagated action potential. It is claimed that for the adequate release of transmitter substance, proper ionic concentration of extracellular Ca^{++} which may enter the extra axonal medium and in turn activate the discharge of the contents of the vesicles to the exterior.

Transmitter substances thus released, diffuse across a distance of 100-500 A° of synaptic cleft and combine with the hypothetical receptor substance of the postsynaptic membrane causing increase permeability of membranes. It has been postulated that there are two types of permeability changes in the postsynaptic membrane. One is the generalised increased permeability of all types of ions causing a localised depolarization of the membrane and excitatory postsynaptic potential (EPSP). Other possibility is the selective increase in permeability of the membrane to only the smaller ions like K^+ and chloride ions, causing hyperpolarization of the membrane, and that constitutes that inhibitory postsynaptic potential (IPSP).

If the EPSP exceeds threshold value, then it initiates the propagated NAP in the postsynaptic neuron or muscle action potential (MAP) in most skeletal and cardiac muscles.

During the development of the EPSP, simultaneously IPSP may be developed at the same site by the incoming NAP from the other sources. The propagation of nerve impulse by the EPSP is dependent upon the intensity of this postsynaptic potential.

As soon as the impulse is transmitted, the transmitter substance is immediately destroyed by the specific enzymes present to the rim of the synaptic gutter. As for example, AChE (acetylcholinesterase) in the cholinergic junction (Fig. 9.9).

Neuro-transmitters

A special group of chemical substances known as neuro-transmitters are involved in the process of synaptic transmission. They are present in the vesicles that are generally observed aggregated at the terminals of the presynaptic neurons. Many types of neuro-transmitters, also called as neuro-humours, have been identified from the nervous system of vertebrates and invertebrates. They are of two types, excitatory and inhibitory. The effect of an excitatory neuro-humour is physiologically antagonistic to that of the inhibitory neuro-humour on the target which may be a neuron or a effector like gland or muscle.

A neuro-transmitter after its release from the presynaptic membrane diffuses through the synaptic cleft and reacts with specific receptor sites on the subsynaptic membrane. It is this interaction between a neuro-humour and subsynaptic receptor site that triggers the permeability changes in the postsynaptic membrane thereby generating or inhibiting the action potentials in the postsynaptic effector. The synaptic delay is the fraction of a second required for release, transmission and attachment of a neuro-humour from the presynaptic membrane to the subsynaptic membrane.

More than 30 different chemical substances have either been proved or postulated to be synaptic transmitters, most are listed in Table 9.1.

Table 9.1 : Neuro-transmitters.

Class I:

- Acetylcholine

Class II : The Amines

- Norepinephrine
- Epinephrine
- Dopamine
- Serotonin

Class III : Amino Acids

- γ-Aminobutyric acid (GABA)
- Glycine
- Glutamate

Class IV : Peptides

A. Hypothalamic-releasing hormones
   - Thyrotropin-releasing hormone
   - Luteinizing hormone-releasing hormone
   - Somatostatin (growth hormone-inhibitory factor)

B. Pituitary peptides

ACTH

β-Endorphin

α-Melanocyte-stimulating hormone

Vasopresslin

Oxytocin

C. Peptides that act on gut and brain

Leucine enkephalin

Methionine enkephalin

Substance P

Cholecystokinin

Vasoactive intestinal polypeptide (VIP)

Neurotensin

Insulin

Glucagon

D. From other tissues

Anglotensin II

Bradykinin

Carnosine

Bombesin

Some of the most common neuro-transmitters are described here:

(A) *Acetylcholine* : It is secreted by neurons in many areas of the brain, but specifically by the large pyramidal cells of the motor cortex, by many different neurons in the basal ganglia, by the motor neurons that innervate the skeletal, muscles, by the preganglionic neurons of the autonomic nervous system, by the postganglionic neurons of the parasympathetic nervous system, and by some of the postganglionic neurons of the sympathetic nervous system. In most instances acetylcholine has an excitatory effect; however, it is known to have inhibitory effects at some of the peripheral parasympathetic nerve endings, such as inhibition of the heart by the vagus nerves. Generally, neurons releasing it are called as *cholinergic neurons*. Coenzyme A is involved in the synthesis of acetylcholine and the neuro-humour after its action is generally destroyed by a hydrolysing enzyme, *acetylcholineestarase. Noradrenaline (Norepinephrine)* is secreted by many neurons whose cell bodies are located in the brain stem and hypothalamus. Specifically norepinephrine secreting neurons located in the *locus ceruleus in* the Pons send nerve fibres to widespread areas of the brain and help to control the overall activity and mood of the mind. In many of these areas it probably causes excitation, but in others inhibition. The chatecholamines are synthesized from tyrosine.

(B) *Dopamine*, the immediate precursor of norepinephrine is also suspected to act as transmitter in certain motor functions of the CNS. The effect of dopamine is usually inhibition.

(C) *Serotonin* is secreted by nuclei that originate in the median raphe of the brain stem and project to many brain areas, especially to the dorsal horns of the spinal cord and to the hypothalamus. It acts as an inhibitor of pain pathways in the cord, and it is also believed to help control the mood of the person, perhaps even to cause sleep.

(D) *Gamma-aminobutyric acid (GABA)* is secreted by nerve terminals in the spinal cord, the cerebellum, the basal ganglia, and many areas of the cortex. GABA is synthesized only in the CNS from glutamic acid by a specific decarboxylase. It is believed always to cause inhibition.

(E) *Glycine* is secreted mainly at synapses in the spinal cord. It probably always acts as an inhibitory transmitter.

(F) *Glutamate* is probably secreted by the presynaptic terminals in many of the sensory pathways as well as in many areas of the cortex. It always causes excitation.

(G) *Peptides : Substance* P is probably released by pain fibre terminals in the dorsal horns of the spinal cord. And it is also found in the basal ganglia and hypothalamus. In general, it causes excitation.

Histamine : This amine is also present in the highest concentration in the hypothalamus. Some histamine has also been extracted from the synaptosomal fractions of centrifuged brain homogenates. Enzymes required for synthesis and catabolism are also present in the CNS.

Enkephalins are probably secreted by nerve terminals in the spinal cord, in the brain stem, in the thalamus, and in the hypothalamus. These probably act as excitatory transmitters to excite other systems that inhibit the transmission of pain.

(H) *Fatty acid derivatives-Prostaglandins* are also present in high concentration in the brain. These are also released from cerebral cortex, cerebellum and spinal cord. It is suggested that prostaglandins may take part in central synaptic transmission. Definite role is not known.

Motor Unit : In an organism, excitation of skeletal muscle is under the control of nervous system. In man hundreds, or even thousands of nerve fibres innervate each muscle, each fibre dividing further into many branches. Thus, all the muscle fibres are controlled by a single neuron constituting *motor unit*. The number of muscle fibres forming a motor unit varies from 2 to 6 as in eye muscles to several hundreds in the limb muscles of the mammals. The motor units are usually smaller where the movements are delicate. Though all the muscle fibres are controlled by single motor unit, however, there is no protoplasmic continuity between the neuron and muscle fibre. There remains a potential space between the two cell membranes called *myoneural junction*. The portion of the muscle membrane directly under the end of the axon is called a *motor end plate*, motor end plate invaginates into the muscle fibre but less entirely outside the muscle fibre membrane. At the tip of the many nerve branches in the end plate are *sole feet*. The invagination of the muscle fibre membrane is called the *synaptic gutter*, and the space between the sole foot and the fibre membrane is called the *synaptic cleft* or *subneural cleft*. The synaptic cleft is filled with a gelatinous "ground" substance through which diffuses extracellular fluid.

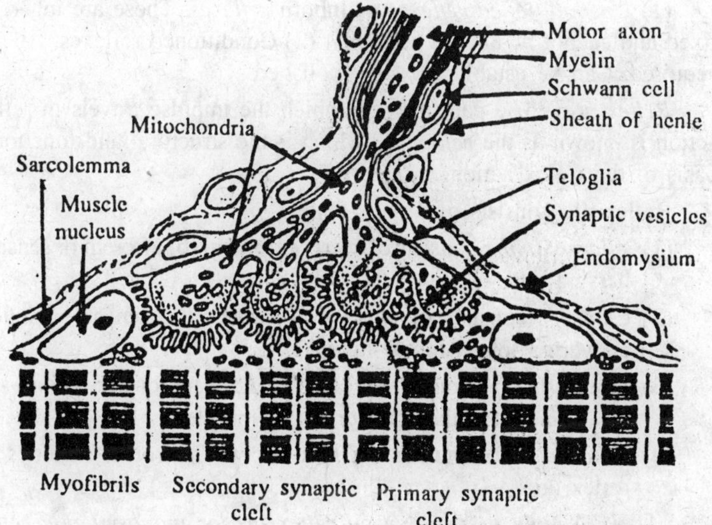

Fig. 9.10 : Diagram of the structure of the motor end plate of mammalian skeletal muscle.

Stored in the nerve terminals of the motor end plate are many small vesicles containing the neuro-transmitter *acetylcholine*, which is synthesized by the cytoplasm of the nerve terminals.

When a nerve impulse reaches a motor end plate, calcium ions diffuse from the extracellular fluid into the nerve terminals causing the vesicles to rupture and release acetylcholine into the synaptic cleft. The acetylcholine, which acts at specific receptor sites in the muscle membrane, causes depolarization of the underlying sarcolemma and initiates contraction of the muscle fibres. Almost immediately after depolarization of the muscle fibre the acetylcholin is destroyed by the enzyme *cholinesterase*, which is present in the synaptic cleft.

REFLEX ACTION

Reflex action is a quick and involuntary (automatic) response to the stimulus, irrespective of the intelligence and deliberations. It is so called because, the action is so quick as if the stimulus reflected back in the form of response. It is the basic physiological unit of integration in the neural activity.

Varieties of reflexes : There are mainly two types of reflexes :

(1) *Unconditioned reflexes* or Inborn *reflexes*. These are inherent, fixed and cannot be altered normally. (2) Conditioned reflexes. All are acquired. Can be established and abolished.

Reflex arc : The path through which the impulse travels in reflex action is known as the *reflex arc* which is the structural and functional basis of the reflex action.

Reflex are consists of 4 parts :

(1) *Afferent limb :* consists of (a) receptor and (b) afferent or sensory nerve fibre.

(2) *Centre :* consists of nerve cells where the sensory stimulus converted into a motor impulse.

(3) *Efferent limb :* consists of (a) efferent or motor nerve fibre and its endings, (b) the effector organ muscle.

(4) *Synapse :* communicating link of two neurons. Varieties of reflex arcs :

1. *Simple or two-neuron reflex arc or monosynaptic reflex arc :* Has two neurones only, *e.g.,* stretch reflex.
2. *Three-neuron reflex or disynaptic reflex arc :* Extension and crossed extension reflexes are the examples of this arc.

There is a connecting neuron in between the afferent fibre and the motoneuron.

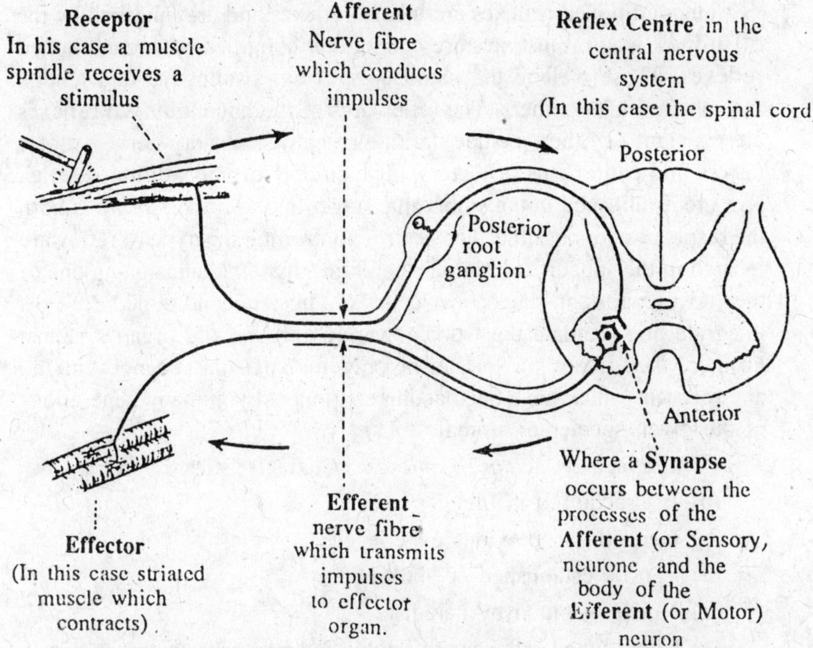

Fig. 9.11 : Showing a reflex arc.

3. *Polysynaptic or multisynaptic reflex arc :* Several neurons. One or more internuncial (intercalated) neurons are also involved. *Withdrawal reflex* is a typical polysynaptic reflex and occurs in response to a anxious and usually painful stimulation of the muscles, skin and subcutaneous tissues.
4. *Complex reflex arc :* The axon of a sensory neuron, while passing upwards, gives off collaterals at different levels, each of which may form separate reflex arcs. Thus, the same fibre will carry conscious sensations to cortex and also form multiple reflex arcs.
5. *Asynaptic reflex arc :* This reflex arc is not concerned with the synapse or nerve cell and also known as *axon reflex arc*. This is not a true reflex arc, and afferent and efferent limbs of this reflex arc are constituted by the branching of a single

nerve fibre. Because the reflex is obtainable even after section of the posterior root peripheral to their ganglia, so long as the cut nerves are not degenerated.

Unconditioned reflexes are inborn reflexes and are inherited by the offsprings. Natural instincts are nothing but complicated unconditioned reflexes. These include the papillary sucking, swallowing and tendon reflxors and many others. The reflex arcs of the unconditioned reflexes are constant *i.e.,* they include definite receptors, sensory nerves, motor nerves and end organs (effectors). The circuits of unconditioned reflex arcs are established in the embryonic stages and as the offspring is born the responses are possible. The centres controlling this type of reflex are located in the subcortical regions (cerebral), hypothalamus being one of the most important subcortical centres. Thus, unconditioned reflexes integrate and regulate the work of various organs and organ systems. Further, they adapt the organism only to particular changes in the environment which have been acting continuously on many generations of the given species of animal.

Conditioned or acquired reflexes : Characteristics :

(a) It is acquired in life.

(b) Depends on previous experience,

(c) Can be established or abolished,

(d) Not transmitted by heredity,

(e) Conditioned reflexes are established primarily upon some pre-existing unconditioned reflexes,

(f) Cerebral cortical and subcortical centres are responsible for it. Example : Food stimulates salivary secretion. This is an unconditioned reflex. Now, if a second neutral stimulus, viz, ringing of a bell or flash of light, be applied just before or during the giving of food for some days, the bell sound or flash of light itself will be able to elicit the salivary reflex, even if no food be given at all. (Fig. 9.12) such a neutral stimulus is called *conditioned* stimulus.

Pavlov (1906) had carried this experiment in the dog, the dog associates the bell sound with the giving of food and starts salivation in anticipation. A good lot of mental analysis and association is required for the establishment of this reflex. This reflex has been termed by Pavlov as conditioned reflex. The conditioning process may be represented schematically in such a way as to show the S-R relationships. Thus, before the salivary response is conditioned to a bell, the situation is as follows:

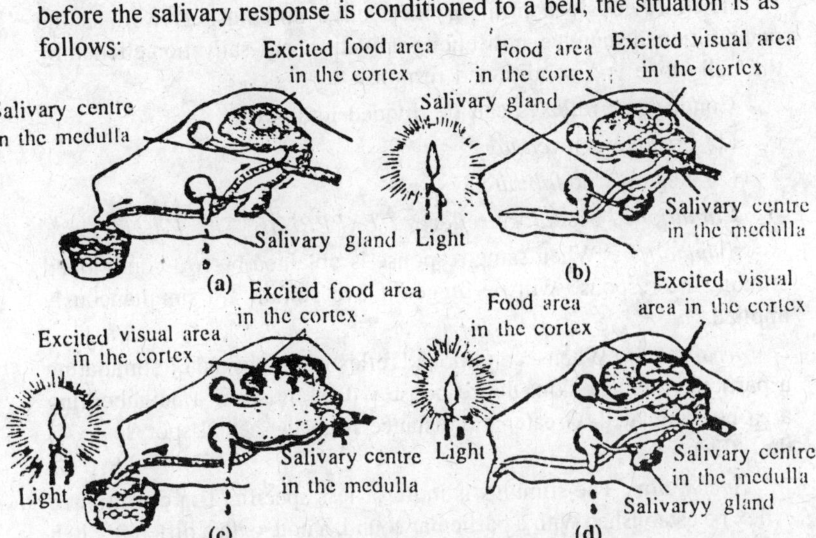

Fig. 9.12 : Diagrammatic representation of the formation of conditioned salivary reflex. (a) showing unconditioning salivary reflex (food), (b) showing application of conditioning stimulus (light) before establishment of conditioning reflex where the visual area of the cortex excited but there is no conditioned response (CR). (c) representing application of a conditioning stimulus (light) with an unconditioning stimulus (food) visual area and food area in the cortex excited simultaneously, (d) showing establishment of CR by giving conditioned stimulus (CS) (light) only and the arrow indicates resultant momentary connection between visual area and food area in the cortex.

Unconditioned stimulus (food) --------------→ Unconditioned response (salivation)

Stimulus to be conditioned (bell) --------------→ Response (pricking up ears, etc. but not salivation)

After the stimulus to be conditioned has been paired with the unconditioned stimulus a number of times, and salivation in response to it (now the conditioned stimulus) has developed, the situation is as follows :

Unconditioned stimulus (food) --------------→ Conditioned response (salivation)

Conditioned stimulus (bell).

The previously neutral or ineffective stimulus, as well as the unconditioned stimulus, now elicits salivation, *i.e.*, salivation elicited by the bell alone is a conditioned response.

Conditioned reflexes can be divided into two :

(1) Positive or *excitatory*

(2) Negative or *Inhibitory*.

Conditioned excitatory reflexes : EXPERIMENTAL FACTS :

Summation : When same response is obtained by two conditioned stimuli, the response will be bigger if two stimuli are simultaneously applied.

Irradiation : When a conditioned reflex is established by stimulating a particular area of skin, the response will be lesser if a neighbouring area be stimulated. Greater the distance from the actual spot, lesser is the effect.

Specificity : The stimulus is more or less specific. If a conditioned reflex be established with a particular sound, a note with a different pitch will be ineffective, provided the animal has the power to recognise the difference.

Decay : If a conditioned reflex be not elicited for several months it undergoes decay (unresponsive) due to disuse.

Reinforcement : A decayed reflex may be fully revived by applying the same conditioned stimulus several times. It is easily formed if the unconditioned stimulus is associated with a pleasant or an unpleasant effect. Stimulation that follows with *reward system* is called *positive reinforcement* and when it is associated with avoidance system or a painful shock-is termed *negative reinforcement*.

Trace phenomenon : Trace reflexes can be established by applying the unconditioned stimulus (food) *after an appreciable interval* following the conditioned stimulus (sound). When established, the reflex response follows the conditioned stimulus after the same interval. According to the length of the interval the trace reflexes may be *short* or *long*.

Extinction : If the conditioned stimulus be repeated several times without unconditioned stimulus, reflex becomes extinct. Repeated disappointment creates a state of cortical inhibition so that no response occurs.

Induction : A positive conditioned response induces a state of increased inhibition. Similarly, an inhibitory conditioned reflex creates a state of increased excitation. When the conditioned inhibitory stimulus, the positive effects of the former are enhanced. This is called *positive Induction*. The reverse changes are known as *negative Induction*.

Conditioned Inhibitory reflexes :

Like excitation, a conditioned reflex may also have inhibitory effects. Inhibition may be of two types: (a) external and (b) internal.

External Inhibition-Definition : A positive conditioned reflex is weakened or inhibited by a simultaneous excitatory process. *Two types*: (a) *Temporary*. A sudden noise or fear or any other emotion, distracts the attention of the subject and inhibits the conditioned reflex. Here, *inhibition arises in a part of the brain other than that where the conditioned reflex is initiated*. As soon as the distraction is off, the reflex returns. (b) *Permanent*. If the distraction or disturbance be lasting the inhibition may also last long, atleast as long as the disturbance persists.

Internal Inhibition — Definition : The stimulus sets up an inhibitory state in that part of the cerebral cortex which initiates the conditioned reflex.

Functions of conditioned reflexes :

(1) Most of our habits are conditioned reflexes. Hence, it is of immense personal and social importance. (2) It has a great applied value in clinical and psychological medicine. (3) With the help of conditioned reflexes cerebral centres can be localised.

MEMORY

Memory is a special faculty of brain which retains the events developed during the process of learning.

All of us know that all degrees of memory occur, some memories lasting a few seconds and others lasting hours, days, months, or years. Possibly all these types of memory are caused by the same mechanism operating to different degrees of fulfilment. Yet, it is also possible that different mechanisms of memory do exist. Indeed, most psychologists classify memory into two to four different types. For the purpose of the present discussion, we will use the following classification.

1. Sensory memory;
2. Primary memory;
3. Secondary memory.

The basic characteristics of these types of memory are the following:

Sensory memory : Sensory memory means the ability to retain sensory signals in the sensory areas of the brain for a very short interval of time following the actual sensory experience. Usually these signals remain available for analysis for several hundred milliseconds but are replaced by new sensory signals to less than one second. Nevertheless, during the short interval of time that the instantaneous sensory information remains in the brain it can continue to be used for further processing; most important, it can be "scanned" to pick out the important points. Thus, this is the initial stage of the memory process.

Primary memory : Primary memory is the memory of facts, words, numbers, letters, or other information for a few seconds to a few minutes at time. This is typified by a person's memory of the digits in a telephone number for a short period of time after he has looked up the number in the telephone directory. It is also typified by the ability of a person to look at a visual scene, then to turn the head away and still be able to recall for seconds or a minute or more many features of the scene.

One of the most important characteristics of primary memory is that the information in this memory store is instantaneously available so that the person does not have to search through his or her mind for it as one does for information that has been put away in the secondary memory stores. However, still another feature of primary memory is that when new bits of information .are put into the primary store, old information is displaced. Thus, if a person looks up a second telephone number, the first is usually lost. Also, if one sees a rapid succession of visual scenes, it is usually the last of these that remains most prominently in the primary memory store.

Secondary memory : Secondary memory is the storage in the brain of information that can be recalled at some later time-hours, days, months, or years later. This type of memory has been called long-term memory, fixed memory, permanent memory, and several other names. One of its characteristics is that, except when the memory is very deeply engrained, one must "search" through the memory stores for seconds to minutes before it is possible to recall the memory.

"Shot-term" and "long-term" memory : Memory is also frequently divided into either "short-term" or "long-term". However, use of these terms are extremely loose. Psychologists frequently classify short-term memory to the same as primary memory and long-term memory the same as secondary memory. However, many physiologists and clinicians include in short-term memory the early stages of secondary memory lasting for as long as several days to a week or more, and reserve the term long-term memory for memories that can be recalled weeks, months, or years after the initial experience.

It is claimed that hippocampus (most medial) portion of the temporal lobe cortex of brain is related with recent memories, as because electroshock on the hippocampus causes abolition of recent memories. Bilateral destruction of the hippocampus causes striking defects in recent memories but not of remote memories. Several drugs that affect recent memories also alter the function of hippocampus considerably.

Regarding permanent memory storage, several explanations have been put forward on the basis of structural changes. It has been suggested that activation of a synapse during learning process may induce a dendritic growth or new formation of the axonic boutous terminaux, that strengthens the connections between two neurons.

Other than structural changes, biochemical changes have been suggested in relation to the process of learning and memory. As the remote memory is not lost even after electroshock and brain concussion, it has been suspected that memory may be stored as an actual biochemical change in the neurons. This fact has come from the work on planarians.- the flat-worms having rudimentary nervous system and remarkable ability to regenerate from cut pieces. These worms can be taught to avoid certain visual stimuli. If these trained worms are cut into two pieces then the regenerated worms from either piece, head or tail can retain previous (learned) response. This has been explained on the basis of changes in RNA of cells. Through the process of learning, there is a stable change in the RNA which is presumably transferred to the new parts of the regenerated parts. It is further supported that if ribonuclease is administered into the cut pieces of conditioned planarians, then the regenerated planarians cannot retain previous condition response due to destruction of RNA. Besides this, if trained planarians are ground up into powder and fed to untrained planarians then the fed planarians become trained up more earlier than those of the control (unfed) one.

Protein synthesis has got relation with the process of memory and learning. Drugs that inhibit protein synthesis affect the memory and learning. Puromycin which inhibits protein synthesis also disrupts recent memory.

REPRODUCTION

The power of reproduction is one of the essential characteristics of life. Reproduction involves transmission to the next generation of genetic material that results in the offspring having the characteristics of the species and of an individual within the species. The genetic material is carried on *chromosomes* in specialized cells called *gametes*. Male gametes, spermatozoa, are produced in the testes, female gametes, ova, are found in the ovaries. The fusion of a spermatozoa with an ovum combines the genetic material from the father and from the mother and begins the process of development that results in the formation of a new individual.

The reproductive organs of the male and female differ in anatomical structure and arrangement, each being adapted to the functional activities they are required to perform. For a normal reproduction, both sexes have to perform some activities in a sequence. In male, this sequence requires normal libido (which depends on endocrine and psychogenic factors), the erection of the penis (dependent on vascular, nervous and psychogenic factors), penetration, and ejaculation, which involves neuro-muscular co-ordination. In the female, ova must be released regularly enough to allow conception and the secretion of the genital tract must permit the passage of spermatozoa and their access to the ovum. The lining of the uterus must be in a suitable condition to allow the newly fertilized ovum to set itself. The embryo has then to be sustained until it is ready for independent existence.

Reproductive Cycle

Together with the development of the cerebral hemispheres and complex behaviour, the mammals owe their success to the efficiency of their reproductive system. In this class of vertebrates, we find a intense parental care from embryonic development and also after the birth. Sexual cycle in mammals is more marked in female as compared to the male. On the basis of their annual reproductive activities, mammals generally exhibit two patterns of sexual behaviour (1) *Continuous breeders* that reproduce throughout the year (*e.g.*, human, mouse, hamster, guinea pig) and (2) *Seasonal breeders* in whom the reproductive events are restricted to specific seasons (*e.g.*, cattle, sheep, dog). In both continuous and seasonal animals, sexual activity show a cyclic pattern. Continuous breeders undergo several sexual *(Oestrous) cycles* in one year and therefore are called *Polyoestrous species*. Some seasonally breeding forms undergo a single reproductive cycle in one year and this condition is called the *monoestrous* (fox), while in others, show a high peak of sexual activity twice in a year, such condition is called *dioestrous species* (dog). In the cat and some rodents, the follicles develop, but ovulation does not occur (ova are not released from follicles) until after copulation. In rabbits the follicles do not develop fully before copulation and a long oestrous may occur, ripening of the follicles and ovulation are initiated by copulation. In non-primate animal like pig the oestrous cycle is of 21 days duration and if pregnancy does not occur then it continues throughout the year. The oestrous cycle is divided into several well - marked phases, those are as follows (Fig. 10.1).

(a) *Proestrous (Preparatory stage) :* It is also called the "building up" phase. During this ovarian follicle with its enclosed ovum increases in size by increasing the follicular fluid, which contains oestrogenic hormones. Uterus and vagina become congested and secrete a sanguinous (red) fluid. Vaginal epithelium proliferates. Vaginal smear shows a large number of nucleated cells, broken off from the proliferating vaginal epithelium. During this period copulation is not permitted.

(b) *Oestrous (Heat period) :* This is the period of heat, and copulation is allowed only at this time. During this period the vaginal epithelium thickens further and the superficial layers are fully keratinized. Examination of the ovaries shows that the Graffian follicles come to maturity at about the middle of this period and at that point ovulation occurs. Then after the ovum is expelled from the follicle to pass into the upper part of fallopian tube. Follicular rupture occurs spontaneously in most animal species. However, in the rabbit, mink, ferret and a few other animals rupture is possible only if coitus occurs. Apparently some nervous reaction at this time initiates the follicular rupture. If coitus does not occur in these animals, the follicle with enclosed ovum regresses. A sterile mating frequently is followed by pseudo-pregnancy.

The duration of this period varies considerably in different groups of animals, for example, in cat it lasts for 9 to 15 hours while in dog it lasts for nine days.

(c) *Metestrus (Luteal phase) :* Metestrus period of functional development of corpus luteum. This occurs shortly after ovulation and is also said to be the post ovulatory phase. During this period there is a decrease in estrogen and increase in progesterone formed by the ovary. The lining of the ruptured follicle begins to grow inwards as the blood vascular supply increases within the cavity. The cells lining the cavity which have not been expelled increase in size, multiply and become laden with fat droplets. The newly reorganized structure is called the corpus *luteum* or *yellow body*. In the absence of pregnancy, the corpus luteum degenerates and the changes of the generative organs subside.

(d) *Diestrus and Anestrus :* Diestrus (resting internal) is a relatively short period of quiescence between estrus cycle in polyestrus animals. It shows preparatory changes for the initiation of second estrus. There is a functional regression of the corpus luteum. In rat it lasts for 4-5 days.

Anestrus is the resting asexual period. In monoestrus animals up to the next mating season.

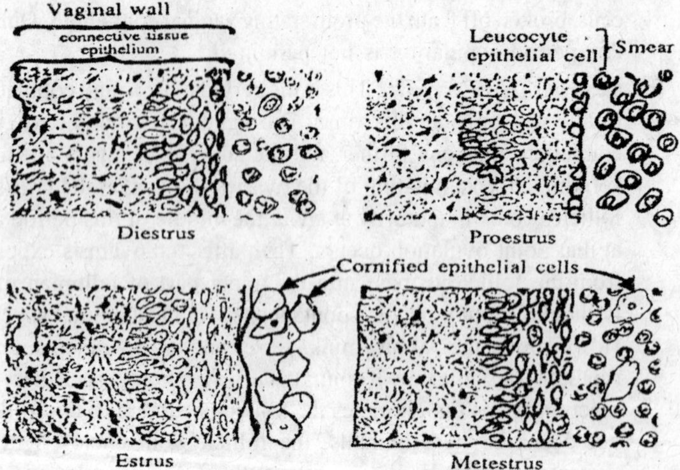

Fig. 10.1 : Diagrammatic representation of the characteristic features of vaginal cell types found the vaginal smear during oestrous cycle.

When another breeding season comes about, the ovary is again activated and a new cycle is started. Pathologic anestrus results from disease or malfunctions involving the hormonal apparatus of the female reproductive organs.

Table 10.1 : Duration of oestrous cycle and period of heat in some mammals.

Animal	Length of cycle	Duration of heat
Rat	4-5 days	9-15 hours
Guinea pig	15-16 days	6-12 hours
Ewe	16 days	30-36 hours
Goat	18-21 days	24-36 hours
Sow	20-22 days	2-3 days
Mare	20-22 days	4-6 days
Cat	15-21 days	4-10 days
Bitch	3-4 months	7-10 days

Hormonal Control of the Oestrous Cycle

This cycle is controlled by combined secretions of pituitary and ovarian hormones, and based on a feedback mechanism in which the output of follicle stimulating hormone (FSH) and leutinizing hormone (LH) depends upon the levels of oestrogens and Progesterone in blood. The factors initially activating the pituitary-ovarian axis are not known, but it has been proposed that very low levels of oestrogens coming from the immature follicles and adrenals may stimulate the release of pituitary FSH. The consequent growth of follicles causes high level of oestrogens in blood and this inhibits further FSH output and at the same time enhances the secretion of LH. Under the influence of rising amounts of LH the follicles undergo final maturation and ovulate at which time the LH has already attained a peak level. There is also an immediate fall in circulating oestrogens. The ruptured follicles are transformed into corpora lutea which become functional under the stimulus of prolactin. The secretion of LH is inhibited by rising progesterone secreted by the corpora lutea which function for only a short period unless there is pregnancy.

The Menstrual Cycle

In mammals except primates, the female receives the male only during a definite period (heat period) in heir sexual cycle. But in primates including human copulation may be performed at any time during the sexual cycle. In female primates including women, reproductive activity is also cyclical, but the cycles are termed menstrual rather than oestrous. In fact, menstrual cycle is a modified oestrous cycle.

Female puberty is signalled by the first menstruation, the *menarche (men = month, arche = beginning)*. In temperate climate, menstruation usually commences at the age of 13 to 14 years. The menstruation continues until the time of the *menopause.* The span of a women's reproductive life shows an inverse correlation between menarche and menopause. As a rule, the younger a girl is when she begins menstruating, the older she will be when she stops.

Definition : Cyclical discharge of blood, mucus and certain other substances from the uterus in the reproductive life of the females, at an average interval of 28 days (24-32 days) is called menstruation. It occurs every month from puberty to menopause. It is absent;

(a) before puberty,

(b) during pregnancy and

(c) after menopause (45-55 years).

Duration : The flow lasts for 4-6 days without any appreciable pain.

Composition : It is made up of;

(a) blood (30-40 ml),

(b) stripped of endometrium (lining of uterus),

(c) mucus,

(d) leucocytes, and

(e) an unfertilized ovum. The menstrual blood which comes out from the uterus clots promptly due to rapid formation of fibrin.

During each cycle the uterine mucosa (Fig. 10.2) gradually hypertrophies. The whole purpose is to prepare a suitable place for the reception, and implantation of the fertilized ovum. If pregnancy takes place, the proliferated mucosa becomes converted into *placenta.* If pregnancy does not take place, the hypertrophied mucosa breaks down and is discharged as *menstruation.* Menstruation, therefore, may be described as the funeral of the unfertilized ovum or as the *weeping of the uterus for the lost of ovum.*

The primary functions of the endometrium are preparation for implantation of a trophoblast, participation in implantation, and formation of the maternal portion of the placenta. The structural and functional changes in the endometrium are dependent upon the endocrine activity of the ovaries. Ovariectomy causes atrophy of the endometrium.

The fully developed endometrium is about 6 mm thick. Its inner portion is the relatively thin and juxtamyometrial basalis. This is a permanent layer. The rest of the endometrium lying above or superficial to the basalis is called the *functionalis*. It undergoes periodic changes in the menstrual cycle and is lost at menstruation and at parturition. The functionalis is distinguished into the superficial and relatively narrow *compacta*, while between the basalis and the compacta lies the *spongiosa* which forms the bulk of the endometrium. The columnar surface epithelium is a mixture of secretory and ciliated cells. This epithelium invaginates to form numerous tubular *uterine* or *endometrial glands* that extend tortuously deep into the endometrial stroma. The endometrium has a dual arterial supply. The basalis is provided with small basal *arteries* while into the functionalis pass unbranched but highly coiled *spiral arteries*. The latter ramify into arterioles that supply a rich capillary bed in the compacta. There are also thin walled veins forming an irregular anastomosing net with sinusoidal enlargements throughout the endometrium. The blood vessels play an important role in menstruation. In this process, only the basalis with its contained deeper portions of the uterine glands and arterial supply remains intact. Remainder of the endometrium is lost accompanied by bleeding.

The menstrual cycle involves the following phases (Fig. 10.2).

(1) *Proliferative phase or estrogen phase of follicular phase* : When the damage resulting the menstrual period has been fully repaired the proliferative phase begins. The estrogen is secreted in increasing quantities by the ovary. The endometrium is initially thin and consists of a ciliated columnar epithelium, dipping down into a loose stroma to form simple tubular glands. During the next 8 days or so (*i.e.,* 6th-14th day) the mucosa thickens, becomes more vascular and the glands elongate and become dilated in their deeper part. Upto the end of this phase the endometrium increases 2 to 3 mm in thickness in case of human female. The phase continues to the time of ovulation (10 days from the end of menstruation).

(2) *Ovulatory phase* : No remarkable changes have been reported in the endometrium. During this phase the ovum is expelled out

and the process is called ovulation. The temperature of the body is comparatively high and remains high until the onset of next menstrual period. Corpus luteum develops in ruptured follicle.

(3) *Secretory phase or luteal phase or progravid phase or premenstrual phase :* During this phase both estrogen and progesterone are secreted in large quantities by the corpus luteum. The endometrium progressively increases in thickness, *e.g.*, to 4-6 mm. The outstanding features are the increase in the length and diameter and the change in the outline of the glands; they are greatly distended with mucus and the lining is thrown into folds which project into the lumen giving the gland wall a saw-edge, tufted appearance. The lipid and glycogen deposits of the stroma cells increase.

The whole purpose of all these endometrial changes is to produce and store, highly secretory endometrium and large amount of nutrients that can provide appropriate conditions for implantation of a fertilized ovum respectively. This phase lasts for about 13 to 14 days.

(4) *Menstruation phase :* This phase is characterized by bleeding and shadding of the superficial part of the endometrium, leaving the basal layer intact. The mechanism is obscure. It is suggested that the spiral arteries close down for hours and the walls of the contained capillaries are weakened. When the spasm passes away and the circulation is restored, blood leaks out through the destroyed areas of the capillary was into the stroma, under the superficial epithelium and into the lamina of the glands. The necrotic endometrium, together with exuded blood and much mucin, is cast off into the lumen of the uterus, whence it passes to the exterior.

Endocrine Regulation of the Female Sexual Cycle

The ovarian hormones, estrogens and progesterones regulate the female sexual cycle. On one hand, they exert a negative feedback on the pituitary thereby controlling the release of gonadotropins and on the other hand, modify the reproductive tract to maintain the pregnancy if at all fertilization occurs. However, if ovum is not fertilized, their circulating level drops down and fresh cycle begins. That is why, during an ovarian cycle and subsequent events leading to the pregnancy, the level of these hormones fluctuates characteristically (Table 10.2). In the beginning the rising level of the estrogens suppresses the release of FSH and stimulates the pituitary to secrete LH, which in turn brings about ovulation and development of corpus luteum. During later stages, the level of progesterones increases more than estrogens. Thus, under the influence of progesterone uterine endometrium gets modified for implanting the fertilized eggs. However, if fertilization is not ensued, the corpus luteum regresses and FSH production is resumed thus again a fresh ovarian cycle begins. An accurately balanced relationship between hypophysial gonadotropins and ovarian hormones in this way regulate the female sexual cycle.

Male Sexual Cycle

Sexual cycle is of most common occurrence in females. Males also show a tendency towards activity of sexual cycle. Testicular activity in the majority of mammals is a seasonal event, as is associated period of sexual excitement known as *rutting period.* At such time the males may develop very special secondary sexual characters such as the antler of the musk-deer, as well as great irritability and desire for combat with other males. In seasonal breeders an annual period of spermatogenesis is followed by an intervals of inactivity. Man, who is a polybreeder, does not show rut cycle.

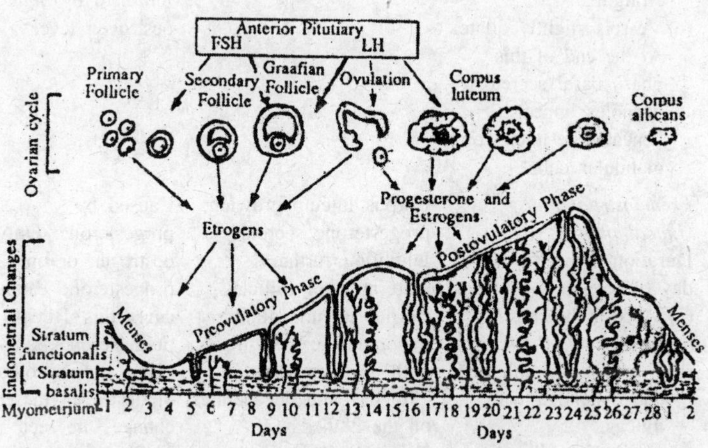

Fig. 10.2 : Menstrual and ovarian cycles.

Table 10.2 : Short Summary Explaining Phases of Menstruation.

Phases and Uterine Changes	Ovarian Change and Excretion of Ovarian Hormones in the Urine	Cause and Control
1. *Resting phase* (*Follicular phase*). Duration - 1 st-5th day (about 1 week) Endometrium heals and becomes normal. Slow proliferative changes begin.	Corpus luteum has degenerated. Inhibitory action of progesterone absent, hence, follicles slowly maturing and oestrogen secretion rising. Urine-oestrone and oestriol rising.	Proliferative changes are due to the action of oestrogens from the maturing follicles. Controlled, by FSH of the anterior pituitary.
2. *Proliferative phase* (Duration-6th-appx. 14th day, *i.e.*, until ovulation. (a) Mucosa thickens (from less than 1 to more than 2 mm) and becomes more vascular. (b) Endometrial glands become longer, tortuous, narrow and straight. (c) Vessels slightly dilate. At the end of this phase basal secretory vacuoles appear beneath the nuclei of glandular cells.	Graafian follicle maturing and oestrogen secretion rising, on the 14th day ovulation occurs and corpus luteum formation starts. Urine-maximum oestrogen excretion.	Caused by further action of oestrogens. Injection of oestrogens in immature or ovariectomised animals produces same changes. Controlled by FSH of anterior pituitary, which is finally inhibited by high oestrogen level.
3. *Premenstrual phase* (*Luteal phase*) Duration-15th-28th day (2 weeks). (a) Mucosa thickens further. (b) Glands more enlarged and distended with mucus. (c) Capillaries dilated like sinus. (d) Exudation of clear or blood-stained fluid.	Corpus luteum growing; progesterone secreted inhibiting further maturation of follicles. Corpus luteum attains maximum size on the 19th day, lasts upto 27th day and degenerates on the 28th day. Urine-(1) Pregnanodiol appears 2-3 days after ovulation, rises to maximum about one week	Caused by progesterone. Only oestrogen or only progesterone cannot cause this. But if progesterone be given after a course of oestrogen these changes are seen. These hormones have got effect on the spiral arteries of the endomeirium.

(e) Proliferation of stroma cells (as in early placenta). (f) Secretory vacuoles containing glycogen appear above nuclei.	before the period and falls 2-3 days before the flow start. (2) Oestrogen falls.	Formation of corpus luteum and secretion of progesterone are controlled by LH and LTH of anterior pituitary. Discharge of menstrual fluid is aided by the presence of certain prostaglandins.
4. *Destructive phase* (*Menstrual stage*) Starts on the 28th day. Duration- 4-6 days. During this period capillaries rupture and haemorrhage occurs. Superficial endometrium, with psedodecidual stroma and tortuous glands is sheded; basal layer remains intact.	Corpus luteum degenerates because placental gonado-tropins are essential for the further growth of corpus luteum. In absence of pregnancy no placenta forms, hence, corpus luteum degenerates.	Lack of progesteron is the cause. If a course of progeste-rone, be given after a course of oestrogen, typical premenstrual changes occur in the endometriun. If then progesterone be suddenly witheld, bleeding takes place, identical with menstrual discharge

Pregnancy

From the instant that fertilization (conception) takes place until parturition (the process of birth) is the period of *gestation* or *pregnancy*. Normally, it lasts for 280 days (viz, ten menstrual cycles).

Fertilization usually occurs in the ampulla of the uterine tubes within 12 hours of coitus and the early embryo then passes along the tube into the uterine cavity, undergoing cleavage as it goes (Fig. 10.3). It is thought to implant in the endometrium at the blastocyst stage 5 days after fertilization, progress along the uterine tube is facilitated by peristaltic contractions, ciliary activity and epithelial secretions, all of which increase around the time of ovulation.

When an ovum is fertilized, the corpus luteum persists instead of degenerating and menstruation does not occur. This ensures a continuous production of progesterone to maintain the secretory changes in the endometrium and prevent it from breaking down in menstruation. It is likely that the corpus luteum is maintained by human chorionic gonadotrophin (HCG) produced by the blastocyst as it embeds in the endometrium. Little is known of the factors that control the process of implantation but HCG produced by the embryo is probably important.

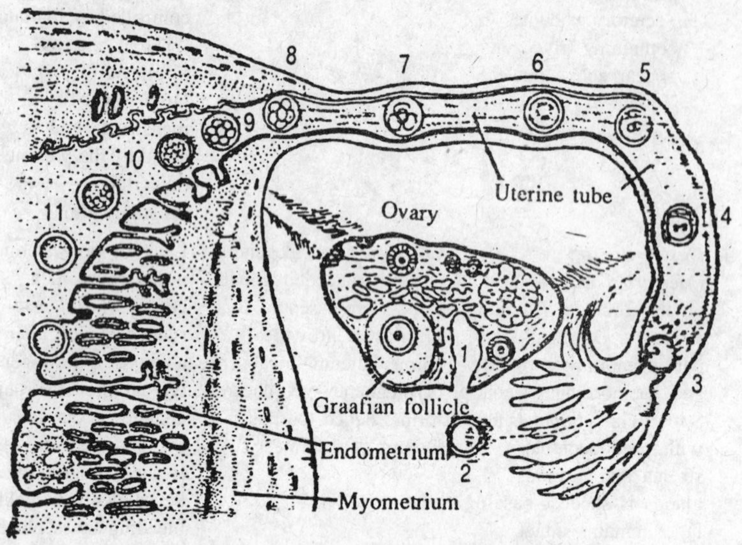

Fig. 10.3 : process of implantation.

The endometrium continues to grow during pregnancy since there is no menstrual degeneration and it may eventually reach 10 mm or more in thickness. The superficial layer of the stroma becomes compact and the greatly enlarged stromal cells are known as decidual cells; the function of these cells is not clear since it occurs a considerable time after implantation. It may protect the uterus against invasion by the trophoblast.

In the decidua basilis under the developing embryo the maternal blood vessels dilate and small finger like outgrowths of the outer layer of the blastocyst, the *chorionic villi*, grow into them. This penetration by the villi is helped by obliteration of small arteries of the decidua, causing necrosis and the formation of large spaces in the decidua that fill with maternal blood. The villi are soon invaded by mesoderm carrying foetal blood vessels and so the foetal and maternal circulation are brought very close to one another; and in this way placenta is formed (Fig. 10.4).

Placenta : A functional connection between the embryo and the uterus is necessary in animals in which development of the foetus occurs within the uterus, and in which nutrients for the foetus come directly

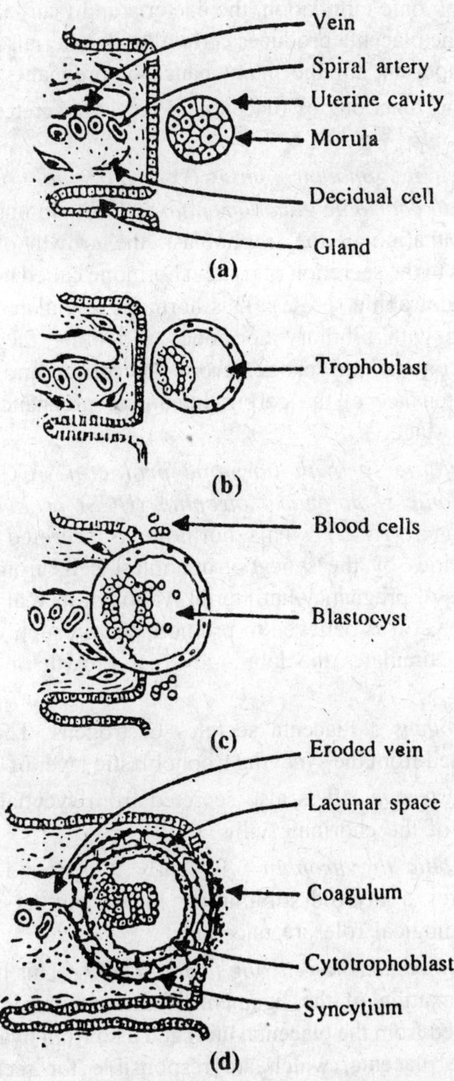

Fig. 10.4 : Steps in the implantation of the embryo into the uterine wall.

from the uterus rather than from the yolk stored in the ovum. This connecting structure, the placenta, allows for nutritional, respiratory and excretory interchange of material by diffusion between embryonic and uterine tissues. The placenta also functions as a barrier that excludes from the embryonic circulation, the bacteria and many large molecules. In addition, the placenta produces certain food materials and synthesizes hormones important for the maintenance of pregnancy.

Endocrine functions of placenta : Placenta secretes the following hormones :

(a) *Chorionic gonadotrophin (CG) or placental gonadotrophin or human chorionic gonadotrophin (HCG)* : In human, soon after implantation of the trophoblast, the growth of chorion cells leads to the secretion of protein hormone called human chorionic gonadotrophin (HCG). This hormone stimulates the ovary and along with pituitary hormones and other factors, maintains oestrogens and progesterone secretion and helps in the maintenance of the corpus luteum of pregnancy atleast at an early stage.

(b) *Chorionic 'growth hormone prolactin' (CGP) or human chorionic somatomammotrophin (HCS) or human placental lactogen (HPL.)* : This hormone is secreted in increasing quantities by the syncytiotrophoblast cells from the first few weeks of pregnancy until term. Although its real function is not clear, yet it is believed to promote energy supply to the foetus. HCS stimulates the lobulo-alveolar growth of the mammary gland.

(c) *Oestrogens* : Placenta secretes oestrogens. This hormone is secreted from the syncytial trophoblastic layer of chorionic villi.

(d) *Progesterone* : It is also secreted from sycytial trophoblastic layer of the chorionic villi.

(e) *Chorionic thyrotrophin* : Recently it is found that placenta secretes a thyroid-stimulating factor but its structure and physiological role are uncertain.

(f) *Relaxin or uterine-relaxing factor (URF)* : This hormone helps in relaxation of the ligament of the symphasis pubis and is secreted from the placenta, uteri and also from ovaries. The cells of the placenta, which are responsible for secretion of this hormone are not yet clear.

In addition to this, placenta in some unknown *way, inhibits lactation.* It is claimed that high titers of oestrogen and progestarone during pregnancy inhibit the secretion of milk. Because milk secretion is increased after parturition when the titers of oestrogen and progesterone become low.

Thus, with the help of its hormones, placenta;

(a) stimulates the growth of mammary glands,

(b) inhibits lactation,

(c) stimulates the growth and persistence of corpus luteum,

(d) inhibits ovulation,

(e) controls anterior pituitary,

(f) stimulates growth of uterus and placenta itself, etc. In other words, all the important changes during pregnancy are carried out with the help of placenta.

Physiological changes during pregnancy : Main changes are :

(1) *Uterus and birth canal* : (a) Uterus enlarges due mainly to hypertrophy but partly to hyperplasia of uterine muscle fibres. The individual muscle fibre becomes wider by 6 or 7 times and longer by 10 or 11 times than non-pregnant uterus. Connective tissue in between the muscle fibres also increases. Weight of the uterus increases.

Causes : (i) Progesterone inhibits movement and facilitates growth. (ii) Oestrogen stimulates growth directly, (iii) Mechanical tension and irritation caused by the growing foetus also act as an important stimulus.

(b) Development of placenta.

(c) Enlargement of the birth canal and relaxation of the pelvic ligaments.

(2) *Breast* : Mammary glands proliferate and development of breasts is completed. Lactation begins after parturition. Pigmentation of the areola and nipple occurs. The pigmentation may be due to ACTH or MSH (melanocyte-stimulating hormone).

(3) *Ovaries* :

(a) Formation and growth of corpus luteum in the early months and its degeneration in the later months,

(b) Cessation of ovulation.

(4) *Blood* :

(a) Blood volume and blood cholesterol are increased.

(b) Plasma fibrinogen level also increases.

(5) *Circulatory system* : Cardiac output is increased. Heart may be enlarged. It may be due to enlarged uterus pressing the diaphragm and causing the change of position of the heart. There is slight

fall of systolic blood pressure and greater fall of diastolic blood pressure. Blood flow in the forearm and hand is increased.

(6) *Respiration* : Vital capacity is increased. Tidal volume and pulmonary ventilation are increased.

(7) *Digestive system* : Nausea and vomiting occur in the early months of pregnancy.

(8) *Excretory system* : There is an increased glomerular blood flow and glomerular filtration. Sometimes glycosuria is found. Excretion of the following sex hormones occurs in the urine

(a) oestrogen,

(b) pregnanediol, and

(c) placental gonadotrophins.

(9) *Endocrine system* :

(a) Thyroid gland is enlarged and increased thyroid hormones secretion occurs,

(b) Adrenal cortex is enlarged especially the zona fasciculata. Secretion of cortisol is increased

(c) Parathyroids are enlarged. Secretion of parathormone is increased.

(10) *Metabolism* :

(a) Carbohydrate-Renal threshold may be lowered and as a result glycosuria may occur during pregnancy.

(b) Protein-There is positive nitrogen balance and more nitrogen is retained in the body provided there is intake of balanced diet.

(c) Lipid-Lipaemia often occurs,

(d) Water-Increased water retention usually occurs in later months of pregnancy. Water is retained in the amniotic fluid, placenta. foetus, breast, uterus, blood and other tissues. There is increased blood volume. The retention of Na and H_2O is probably due to effects of female sex hormones.

Parturition

Parturition in its simplest sense is a process by which an offspring is born and takes place normally, at about 280 days from the beginning of the last menstrual period. At the termination of pregnancy the uterus becomes progressively more excitable until finally it begins strong rhythmic contractions with such force that the embryo is expelled out.

Completion of this process is due to number of factors that work in combination, these are progressive hormonal changes that cause increased excitability of the uterine musculature, and second, progressive mechanical changes (Fig. 10.5)

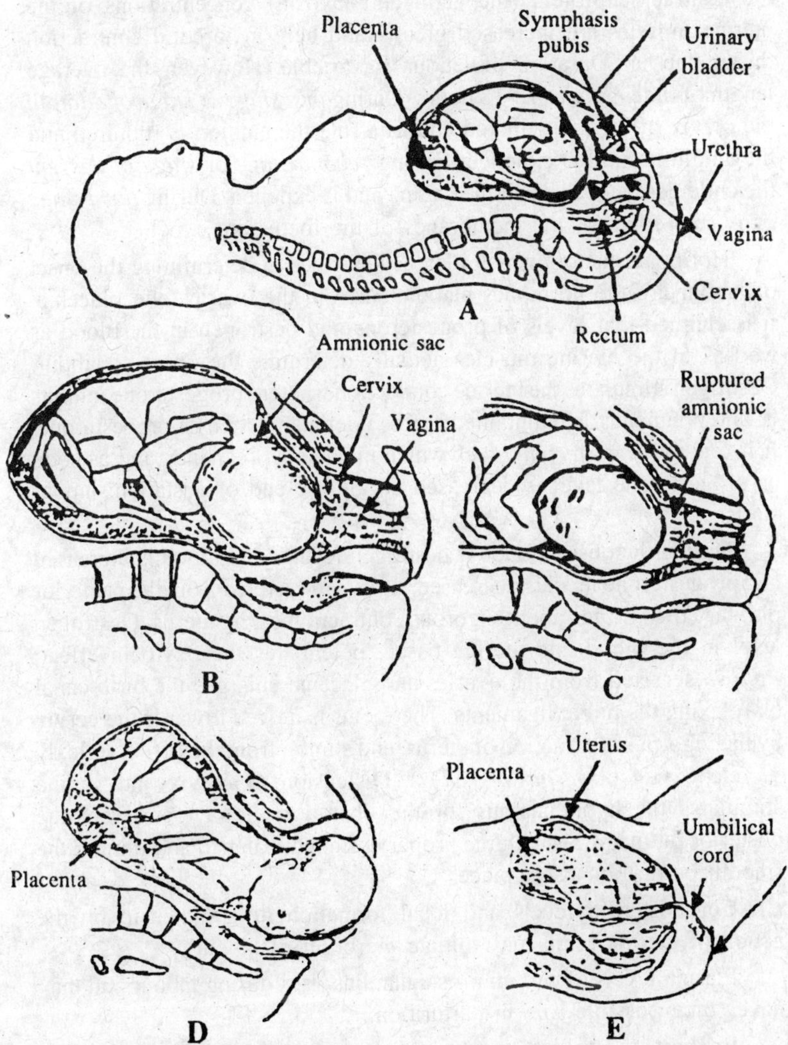

Fig. 10.5 : Parturition.

Parturition starts with a long series of involuntary contractions of the uterus called "labour pains". During gestation the placenta remains in a quiescent state but as the labour approaches the uterine myometrium becomes irritable and excitable. It is claimed that at the end of gestation, the contractile protein (the actin and myosin) concentrations of the uterine muscles are increased greatly and help in forceful contraction during labour. Duration of labour is variable. However, the average length of time is about 12-18 hours. During *first stage* or *stage of dilation* the cervix of uterus is dilated and as a rule the amnion is ruptured and the amniotic fluid is expelled. During *second stage* or *stage of descent* the child descends through the vagina and is expelled. During *third stage* or *placental stage*, the membranes of the foetus are expelled.

Hormonal factors which play as key roles in determining the onset of labour are the hormones elaborated from the ovaries and placenta. It is claimed that levels of progesterone and oestrogen in the blood as well as in the uterine muscles actually determine the onset of labour. Oestrogen stimulates the uterine contraction whereas progesterone inhibits it; and pregnancy is maintained by the dominant action of progesterone. It is due to *progesterone block* which maintains pregnancy and as soon as progesterone level is decreased during the end of gestation, labour starts.

During the onset of labour oestrogen level in the blood is increased and progesterone level is decreased. *Oxytocin* secreted from the posterior pituitary then brings about vigorous contraction of the uterus. Oestrogen level in the blood and uterine tissue, potentiates the oxytocin effect. *Relaxin* secreted from the ovaries and placenta enlarges the birth canal by relaxing the pubic ligaments. The foetus is moved towards the cervix by the vigorous contraction of uterus, and stimuli from the cervix reflexly secrete oxytocin (*ferguson reflex*). Distension of cervix and vagina stimulates the hypothalamus for the liberation of oxytocin from the posterior pituitary. So with the proper hormonal balance and timing, the smooth parturition takes place.

Corticosteroid levels and local formation of angiotensin by the action of uterine renin may initiate the onset of labour.

Plasma levels of certain prostaglandins rises during labour and may have some possible role in parturition.

In short, the following factors helps expulsion of the foetus :

(1) Oestrogen rises the content of uterine actomyosin.

(2) An increasing stretch tends to make the uterus contract like all smooth muscles.

(3) Oxytocin tends to cause contraction of the uterus.

(4) Relaxin softens birth canal and relaxes the ligament.

Progesterone may be the only factor which opposes uterine contraction.

Involution : It is the process of rapid decrease in the size of the uterus. It is brought about by a gradual autolysis or self-digestion of the uterine wall and requires from 6-8 weeks. During this period the uterus again resumed its original position in the pelvic cavity and approximately its original size.

Lactation

The breasts (mammary glands) : The breasts are accessory glands of the female reproductive system. In childhood and in the mate they

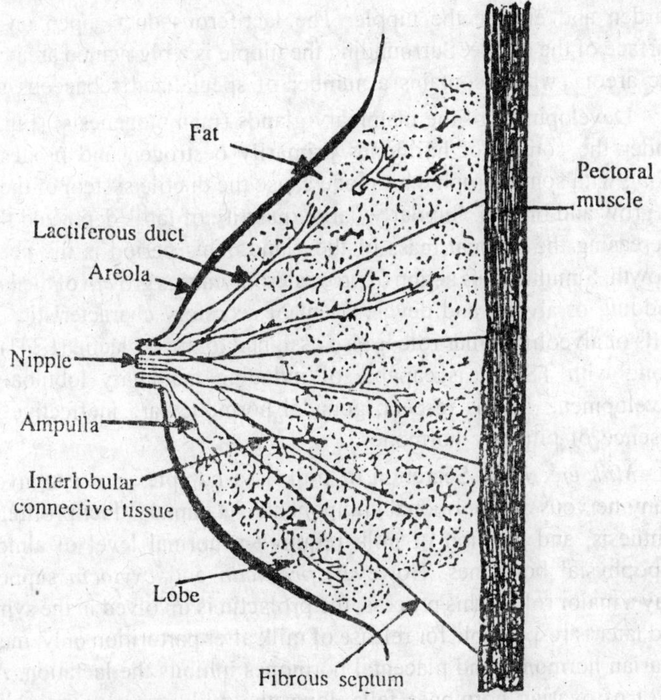

Fig. 10.6 : Section of the breast.

are present in a rudimentary form only in the female, the breasts begin to develop at puberty due to the influence of the ovarian hormones. Each breast lies over the pectoralis muscles, extending from the second rib downwards to the sixth rib, and horizontally from the margin of the sternum to the mid-axillary line. The size and shape of the breasts of mature women vary considerably.

Structure : (Fig. 10.6). The breast consists of 15 to 20 lobes separated by fibrous tissue, which also acts as a supporting framework by forming suspensory ligaments. Each lobe is divided into numerous lobules by delicate connective tissue containing fat cells. Embedded in the lobules are clusters of alveoli the secretory cells of the gland. The alveoli are drained by minute ducts, which unite to form one lactiferous duct for each lobe. The lactiferous ducts pass towards the nipple, and close to their termination widen to form *ampullae* or *lactiferous sinuses*.

The nipple is composed of erectile tissue covered by pigmented epithelium containing smooth muscle fibres, which when contracted harden and elevate the nipple. The lactiferous ducts open on to the surface of the nipple. Surrounding the nipple is a pigmented area of skin, the areola, which contains a number of specialized sebaceous glands.

Development of the mammary glands (mammogenesis) (Fig. 10.7) under the control of hormones primarily oestrogen and progesterone along with somatotrophic hormone cause the ductile system of the gland to grow and branch. Similarly, large quantity of fat is deposited thereby increasing the stromal mass of the gland. This period is the period of growth. Simultaneous action of progesterone causes growth of the lobules, budding of alveoli and development of secretory characteristics of the cells of alveoli. Similar role is also assigned to the prolactin (LTH), thus, along with TSH it is capable of inducing mammary lobuloalveolar development. In this respect, gonadal hormones are ineffective in the absence of pituitary hormones.

Milk ejection : Secretion of milk is a complex process involving many nervous and hormonal components. Mammary duct proliferation, synthesis, and ejection of milk required a normal level of almost all hypophysial hormones. However, *prolactin* and *oxytocin* suppose to play a major role in this process, the prolactin is involved in the synthesis and later is responsible for release of milk after parturition only, meaning ovarian hormones and placental hormones inhibits the lactation. As the level of ovarian hormones falls down the milk secretion is initiated.

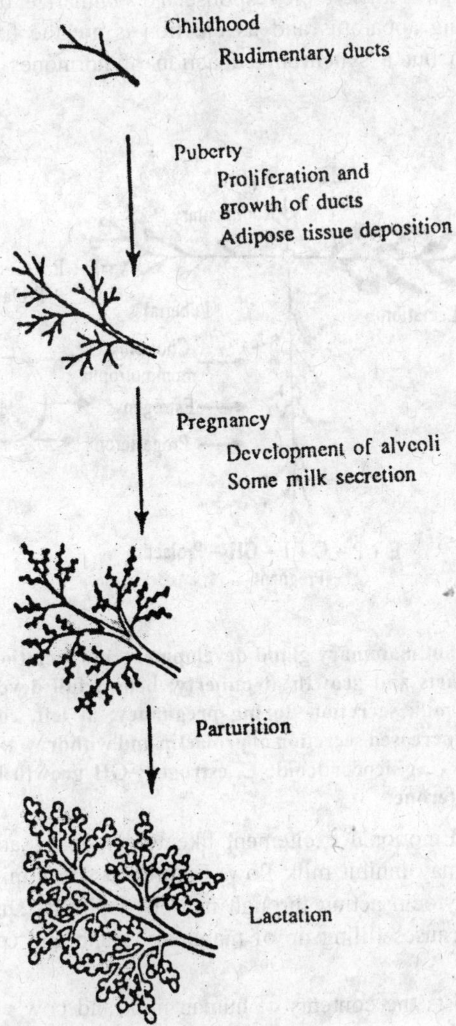

Fig. 10.7 : Stages in the development of a lobule of breast.

The secretion of oxytocin is in part a response to the tactile stimulus of the baby suckling but also occurs in many mothers in anticipation of suckling in response to the baby crying or becoming restless.

In addition, maximum response is also dependent on the action of growth hormone thyroxine, insulin, paratharmone and frequent removal of the milk that initiates oxytocic response. To summarize, development of milk producing apparatus and its ejection is not the function of a hormone or two but a synchronized action of hormones from many endocrine sources.

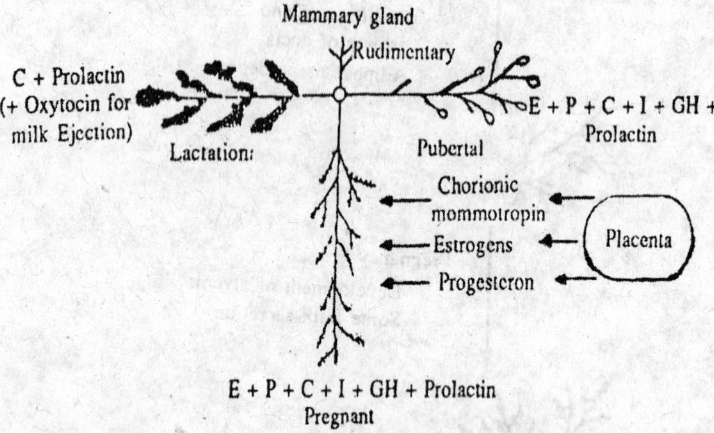

Fig. 10.8 : Control of mammary gland development and lactation. At right, proliferation of ducts and growth at puberty; below, full development of alveoli and some milk secretion during pregnancy; at left, copious milk production due to increased secretion of prolactin and withdrawal of estrogen and progesterone. C, glucocorticoid; E, estrogen; GH growth hormone; I insulin; P, progesterone.

Inhibition : Emotional excitement like worry, fear, sadness, etc., during lactation may inhibit milk flow. Emotional stress might inhibit the release of oxytocin acting through neurohypophysis. Disturbances in milk ejection causes filling up of mammary gland and cessation of lactation.

Table 10.3 lists the contents of human milk and cow's milk. The concentration of lactose in human milk is approximately 50% greater than that in cow's milk, but on the other hand the concentration of protein in cow's milk is ordinarily two or more times as great as that in human milk.

Table 10.3 : Percentage Composition of Milk.

Water	88.5	87
Fat	3.3	3.5
Lactose	6.8	4.8
Casein	0.9	2.7
Lactalbumin and other protein	0.4	0.7
Ash	0.2	0.7

Endocrine Control of Reproduction

Reproductive cycles in both the sexes not only under the control of a single hormone or two, but a combined action of hormones from many endocrine sources.

Pituitary hormone : If the pituitary is removed from an immature male and female animal, the gonads remain infertile and the development of the secondary sex organs is also restricted. The secondary sex organs atrophy after removal of the ovaries and testis in adult female and males respectively in spite of the presence of the pituitary gland; it is clear therefore that the gonadotrophins produced by the anterior pituitary have no direct influence on the secondary sex organs, but only an indirect one through the gonads. In both sexes, two gonadotrophins, FSH and LH, are produced by the anterior pituitary and another gonadotrophin is produced by the placenta in pregnancy (*human chorionic gonadotrophin*, HCG, for details see placenta). The release of the pituitary gonadotrophins is controlled by the hypothalamic peptide hormone *gonadotrophin releasing hormone* (GnRH).

Gonadotrophic hormone (GTH) or *gonadotrophins* are of two types, which are secreted by the cyanophils of adenohypophysis and control the action of gonads.

(a) *Follicle stimulating hormone (FSH)* : It is a water soluble glycoprotein with molecular weight, ranging between 30,000 and 67,000. It contains galactose, glucosamine, galactosamine, mannose, etc.

Functions : In female, it stimulates the development and maturation of the ovarian follicles upto the point of ovulation.

In males, it excites the epithelium of the seminiferous tubules and thereby process of spermatogenesis and sperm formation.

During childhood it is not manufactured, and due to its action on both male and female gametes, FSH is also called as gametokinetic factor.

(b) *Luteinising hormone (LH) or Interstitial cell stimulating hormone (ICSH)* : Biochemically it is a conjugate protein with a molecular weight ranging between 26.000 and 30,000.

Functions : In female, it is essential for final maturation of ovarian follicles, ovulation and transformation of the empty follicle to corpus luteum that in turn secretes *progesterone* which maintains the pregnancy.

In male, LH is known as interstitial cell stimulating hormone (ICSH). It stimulates the interstitial cells or cells of Leydig of testes to secrete *testosterone* or *male sex hormone*. It is involved in the maintenance of accessory reproductive organs and secondary sexual characters.

The secretion of LH is under the control of hypothalamus. It is also regulated by stimuli like light, temperature, genital stimulation, etc.

Ovarian Hormones

The ovarian hormones, estrogens and progesterones regulate the female sexual cycle, apart from this, these are also responsible for the maintenance of the female reproductive tract and the development of the secondary sexual characters.

The Estrogens : In the normal non-pregnant female, estrogens are secreted in major quantities only by the ovaries. In pregnancy, tremendous quantities are also secreted by the placenta.

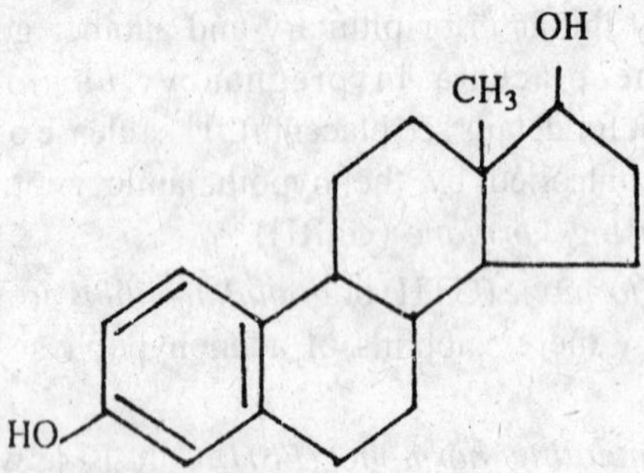

OH
CH_3
HO

Fig. 10.9 : B-oestradiol.

In women, the principal ovarian oestrogen in reproductive life is *oestradiol-17 B*, which is produced by the granulosa cells (Fig. 10.9). The other oestrogens are oestrone, which can arise from a follicle or from peripheral conversion of oestradiol or androgens in adipose tissue, and oestriol, produced by the foetus and by the placenta. Oestriol is the principal oestrogen in pregnancy.

Functions of Oestrogen

1. *Responsible for all the puberty changes*, such as
   - (a) growth of uterus, vagina, stratification of vaginal epithelium;
   - (b) increased contractility, secretion and ciliary movement of the Fallopian tube;
   - (c) development of breasts chiefly by proliferation of ducts;
   - (d) menstrual changes;
   - (e) appearance of secondary sex characters.
2. Responsible for the proliferative stage of menstruation.
3. *Causes growth of uterus during pregnancy.* The enormous growth of uterus is believed to be due to oestrogens aided by the mechanical stimulus of the growing embryo.
4. *Exerts synergistic action with oxytocin* (causes onset of parturition). It has been shown that oestrogens increase the sensitiveness of the uterine musculature to the action of oxytocin, while progesterone depresses it. At full term, progesterone level falls-due to degeneration of corpus luteum and to some extent, of the placenta. But oestrogen level still remains high. This enhances oxytocin effect and thus parturition starts.
5. *Relation with progesterone and corpus luteum :*
   - (a) Oestrogen and progesterone often act synergistically, viz.

     (i) *Menstrual changes :* Progesterone can cause the premenstrual changes in the endometrium only after the proliferative changes has been already done by oestrogen. Progesterone alone will have no effect,

     (ii) *Breast formation-Glandular* (lobulo-alveolar) development of breasts, as seen during pregnancy, only occurs by their combined action.
   - (b) They may antagonists-in large doses, oestrogen antagonises the actions of progesterone and prevents the progestational changes in the uterine mucosa.
   - (c) Oestrogen is also necessary for the maintenance of corpus luteum during pregnancy. Probably this is brought about through the action of anterior lobe of hypophysis.
6. Inhibits the secretion of anterior pituitary, particularly the FSH. In this way, anterior pituitary and ovaries maintain a reciprocal relationship. Due to this inhibitory action, administration of large doses of oestrogens may cause atrophy of the ovaries,

arrest menstruation and produce sterility. Oestrogens have no direct action on the gonads. They work by inhibiting the follicle-stimulating hormone (FSH) of anterior pituitary.

7. *Inhibits thymus* : Oestrogens depress thymus and causes its involution at puberty.
8. *Exerts synergistic action with androgen* : In males, oestrogen in physiological dosage acts synergistically with androgen and helps in the development of secondary sexual characters.
9. *Stimulates oestrous* in female animals.
10. *Stimulates the secretion of ACTH* from anterior pituitary and causes hypertrophy of adrenal cortex.
11. *May help water balance* : Administration of oestrogens causes water, sodium and chloride retention, increase of blood volume and of the water content of muscles.
12. *Effect on protein synthesis* : Oestrogens increase total body protein as indicated by positive nitrogen balance. The effect is however much less than that of testosterone.
13. *Effect on bone growth* : Oestrogens induce positive calcium balance and thus increases skeletal growth. However, oestrogen (like androgen) hastens closure of epiphysis and thus stops growth.
14. *Effect on fat deposition* : Oestrogens cause increased deposition of fat in subcutaneous tissue and also in other particular regions to make a typical feminine body.
15. *Effect on cholesterol metabolism* : Possibly by its action on lipoproteins, oestrogens lower plasma cholesterol level.
16. The oestrogens are responsible for the development of the female secondary sexual characteristics that distinguish the female from the male, *e.g.*, formation of narrow shoulders, broad lips, thighs that converge, etc., the larynx retains its prepuberal proportions and voice stays high-pitched; there is less body hair and more scalp hair, etc.

Progesterone : This hormone is secreted by the corpus luteum and in pregnancy, by the placenta. Its main action during the menstrual cycle is on the oestrogen-stimulated endometrium, the glands of which develop further and begin to secrete. Progesterone prevents bleeding from the endometrium and a fall in progesterone secretion is probably the signal for the start of menstruation.

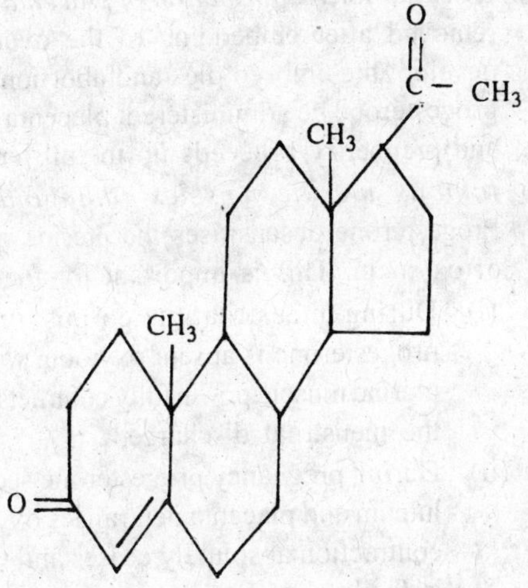

Fig. 10.10 : Progesterone.

Progesterone is a sterol derivative with a side chain at the 17 C position. Its structure is shown in Fig. 10.10. It is found in two crystalline forms, *e.g.*, α and β.

Functions of Progesterone

Progesterone is essential for the maintenance of pregnancy and various other changes associated with it. It also takes part in menstruation. Its functions are briefly summarised below :

1. *Responsible for premenstrual changes of uterine mucosa- Evidence :* In ovariectomised animals, if progesterone be injected after a course of oestrogen, typical premenstrual changes will take place in the uterus. If then progesterone be discontinued, bleeding will take place, identical with menstrual bleeding. Progesterone alone fails to cause these changes. It must be preceded by a course of oestrogens. The latter produces the initial change on which only progesterone can work.
2. *Takes an essential part in pregnancy, for instance :*
   (a) *Embedding of ovum :* Progesterone secreted by the corpus luteum is responsible for the premenstrual hypertrophy of the endometrium which is essential for the reception and embedding of the fertilized ovum.

(b) *Essential for the formation of placenta :* If corpora lutea be removed after embedding of the ovum, placenta fails to develop, the embryo dies and abortion takes place. If then progesterone be administered, placenta formation continues and pregnancy proceeds up to full term.

(c) *Inhibits uterine muscles (antagonistic to oxytocin):* Progesterone desensitises the uterine muscle to the action of oxytocin. This is important for the following :

(i) During menstruation corpus luteum degenerates, progesterone is absent oxytocin works unopposed and uterine muscle powerfully contracts. This helps to expel the menstrual discharge,

(ii) During pregnancy progesterone secreted by the corpus luteum and placenta neutralises oxytocin action uterine contraction absolutely ceases and the growth of uterus is facilitated,

(iii) At full term corpus luteum dies and placenta also degenerates to some extent. Hence, progesterone secretion falls. Oxytocin acts unopposed and parturition starts.

3. *Development of breasts.* Breasts develop further during pregnancy-chiefly due to the proliferation of the glandular elements. Experimentally, it is seen that progesterone alone fails to cause this change. But if progesterone and oestrogens be given simultaneously, typical pregnancy changes are seen in the breasts. During actual pregnancy, both hormones are present in the body and are responsible for the breast changes.

4. *Inhibits oestrous or menstrual cycle and ovulation:* During pregnancy, maturation of follicles, ovulation, oestrous or menstrual cycle are inhibited also. The production of pituitary luteinising hormone (LH) is inhibited by large doses of progesterone. Experimentally, injected progesterone prevents ovulation. Its purpose is to prevent formation of further embryos (superfoetation) during pregnancy. Probably it acts by inhibiting FSH.

5. *Causes enlargement of birth canal :* At full time birth canal enlarges due to growth of vagina and relaxation of pelvic ligaments. The same effect can be experimentally produced by giving progesterone along with oestrogens, but not with the former alone.

6. *Protein catabolic activity* : Progesterone has slight protein catabolic activity.
7. *Water and salt metabolism* : In animals progesterone causes mild salt and water retention, but administered to men or women it causes salt loss. On the other hand, the synthetic progesterones have a mild sodium-retaining effect.
8. Progesterone stimulates respiration and this is confirmed by the fact that in women during the luteal phase of menstrual cycle, the alveolar PCO_2 is lower than in males.

Relaxin

Relaxin is a water-soluble polypeptide hormone present in pregnant mammalian ovary, placenta and uterus. This non-steroidal hormone of pregnancy has not been isolated from blood of either non-pregnant women or men. Relaxin level of blood reaches maximum at the terminal stages of pregnancy.

Testicular Hormones : The testis perform two important functions: the proliferation of spermatozoa and secretion of certain steroid hormones. Formation of sperms occur in the germ cells in the epithelium of the seminiferous tubules and synthesis and secretion of hormones by

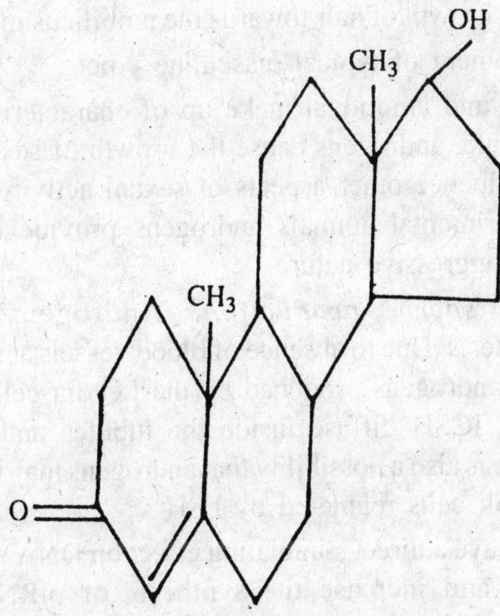

Fig. 10.11. Testosterone.

the interstitial cells of Leydig, which are found interspread in groups between the seminiferous tubules.

The male sex hormones are usually referred to as *androgens. Testosterone, dihydrotestosterone*, and *androstenedione* are the main androgens produced by the testes. The plasma of normal man contains about 0.5μg of testosterone per 100 ml of plasma while in normal women the value is about 0.1 μg/100 ml plasma. Androgens develop and maintain the male sex characters and their normal circulating level is essential both for the control of secondary sexual characters as well as for the functional competence of the accessory reproductive ducts and glands.

All androgens are steroid compounds, illustrated by the formula in Fig. 10.11 for testosterone, and can be synthesized either from cholesterol or directly from acetylcoenzyme A.

Functions of Androgens

1. Growth of accessory male sex organs, the seminal vesicles, prostate, epididymis, vas deferens, penis, etc.
2. *Normal development of male secondary sex characters.* These are the following :
   (a) the growth of hair on the face in the axillae, include on the chest and in the pubic region at puberty, responsible for the upward growth of hair towards the umbilicus in the midline,
   (b) development of typical masculine voice,
   (c) activity and emotional make up of characteristic man. In the female, androgens cause the growth of sexual hair and may influence other aspects of sexual activity and libido. In experimental animals androgens provide boi-oestrous and of aggressive nature.
3. *Effect on sperm production.* Androgens facilitate spermatogenesis. Due to absence of blood vessels at the germinal epithelium, androgens produced by the Leydig cells under the influence of ICSH diffuse inside the tubules and exert their action. There is also a possibility that androgens may be produced by the Sertoli cells regulated by FSH.
4. Androgens have a direct stimulating effect on DNA and on RNA polymerase and increase the synthesis of mRNA and the incorporation of amino acids into protein.
5. *Protein anabolic action.* Testosterone is a protein anabolic hormone (nitrogen-retaining effect). It causes increased passage

of amino acids inside the cell and positive nitrogen balance. This effect is a direct one, independent of the presence of endocrine organs.

6. *Muscular development*. Selective stimulation of certain muscles by androgens indicates that the hormone has myotrophic effect.
7. *Effects on growth of bone*. Due to the protein anabolic nature of testosterone it causes increase in bone matrix and thus increases deposition of calcium salts. It also leads to closure of epiphyses of long bones, thus arrests growth.
8. *Effect on BMR*. Testosterone increases BMR. This effect might also be secondary to the protein anabolic nature of the hormone.
9. *Effect on RBC*. Total number of RBC in males is higher than in females. Castration causes reduction of RBC which comes back to control level on androgen treatment.
10. Effect on water and mineral metabolism. Testosterone causes retention of sodium, potassium, calcium, phosphate and water to some degree. This is probably related to increased protein anabolism.

Castration : It is the removal of testes in males. It shows the following effects :

(i) Before Puberty

(a) Accessory organs of reproduction do not develop.
(b) Ossification of epiphysis of long bones is retarded.
(c) There is no growth of hairs on face, trunk and axillae.
(d) Pubic hair is female type, the outline being concave upwards.
(e) There is abdominal deposition of fat on the buttocks, hips, pubis and breast.
(f) Larynx is not prominent and the voice remains high pitched.
(g) Muscles are soft and poorly developed.

(ii) After Puberty

(a) Secondary sexual characters and accessory organs of reproduction remain depressed.
(b) Seminal vesicles and prostate atrophy.
(c) Sexual desire and erection may be absent.
(d) There may be a peculiar mental state, but this is due to psychological trauma produced by castration.

Endocrine regulation of testicular function : Hypophysectomy usually within few days brings about functional degeneration of the testes; the epithelial lining of the seminiferous tubule becomes disorganized and spermatogenesis is completely stopped. Testes become soft and decreased in size and even regress into the abdominal cavity in certain species. Apart from these degenerative changes in the testes, hypophysectomy also results in an atrophy of the reproductive tract and genital organs. Thus, normal secretion of pituitary gonadotropins is an essential factor for the maintenance of gonads, reproductive tract and secondary sexual characters.

There are two phases in the testicular cycle; one is spermatogenesis simultaneously followed by the production of certain hormones grouped as testicular androgens. The functional significance of hypophysial gonadotropins in the second phase is well-established by many experimental evidences. However, their role in spermatogenesis is still a matter of controversy.

FSH, a hypophysial gonadotropin, on administration into a hypophysectomized animal brings about significant increase in the diameter of the seminiferous tubules so also growth of sertoli elements; however, there is no effect on the primordial germ cells. For promoting the growth of seminiferous tubules and accessory elements, the role of LH is still a matter of doubt. Whether LH acts along with FSH to bring about these changes or through inducing the production of androgens by the cells of Leydig is not conclusively proved.

The second testicular function, *i.e.,* production of androgens is one of the best understood phenomenon of pituitary-gonadal relationship. Testicular regression on hypophysectomy is followed by degeneration of seminiferous tubules and interstitial cells of Leydig leading to the degenerative changes in the secondary sexual characters.

LH or ICSH (interstitial cell stimulating hormone) secreted by the adenohypophysis stimulates the cells of Leydig to secrete the androgens that complete spermatogenesis, keep reproductive tract functional and maintain secondary sexual characters. Thus, the endocrine portion of the testis is interstitial cells of Leydig, which is under the influence of LH secretes the androgens.

The Adrenal Androgens

Several moderately active male sex hormones called adrenal androgens (the most important of which is *dehydroepiandrosterone*) are continually secreted by the adrenal cortex, especially so during foetal life. Also, progesterone and oestrogens, which are female sex hormones, are secreted in very minute quantities.

PUBERTY IN MALE

Between the ages of 13 and 16 years Testicular tissue becomes rsponsive to stimulation by

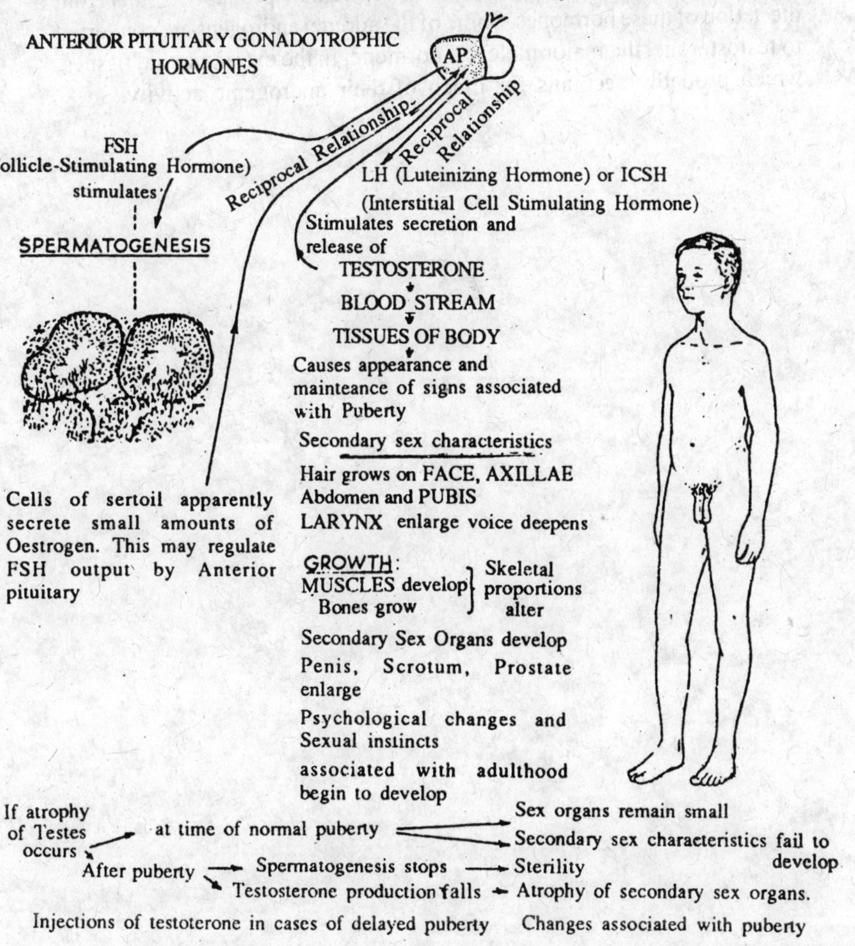

Fig. 10.12 : Changes during puberty in male.

In normal physiology of human being, the adrenal androgens have almost insignificant effects. However, it is possible that part of the early development of the male sex organs results from childhood secretion of adrenal androgens. The adrenal androgens also exert mild effects in the female, not only before puberty but also throughout life. Much of the growth of the pubic and axillary hair in the female probably results from the action of these hormones. Some of the adrenal androgens are converted to testosterone, the major male sex hormone, in the extra- adrenal tissues, which probably accounts for much of their androgenic activity.

11

SENSE ORGANS

Life of animal depends on a constant flow of information from the environment, the collection and integration of this into meaningful and purposive instructions for the effectors, and the relay of the instructions to the appropriate glands, muscles etc., and other organs concerned with activity. The first link communicating an animal with its environment is the sensory receptor system, specialized to transfer chemical, radient, electrical or mechanical energy into a chain of action potentials which are the only data transmitted to the computing centres of the brain.

Receptor are specific as far as detection of a particular form of energy is concerned; thus, gustatory and olfactory receptors are sensitive to chemicals; photoreceptors to different wavelengths of the electromagnetic spectrum; thermoreceptors to radiations and so on. Again, a receptor is generally sensitive to particular range of that energy form and its reception power has always got a limit. Thus, a sensor must operate in a particular range of an energy form that is sufficient to excite it by activating molecules involved in the process of transduction.

VISION (Photoreception)

Human eye can be the best example for generalized morphological discussion of a typical vertebrate eye. Eyes are a pair of visual organs situated bilaterally in the protective bony orbits in the skull.

Eye consists of essential organs like *eyeball*, the *optic nerve* and visual centres in the brain, there are certain accessory organs which are necessary for the protection and functioning of the eye. A horizontal cross-section of the eye is shown in Fig, 11.1.

The acccessory organs of eye include:

(1) the eyebrows;

(2) the eyelids;

(3) the conjunctiva;

(4) the lacrimal apparatus; and

(5) the muscles of the eye.

(1) *The eyebrows* : These are formed by the skin covering the orbital process of the frontal bones, which in its natural state is plentifully supplied with short thick hairs. Their main function is protective and by their shape prevent the sweat of the brow from pouring into the eye:

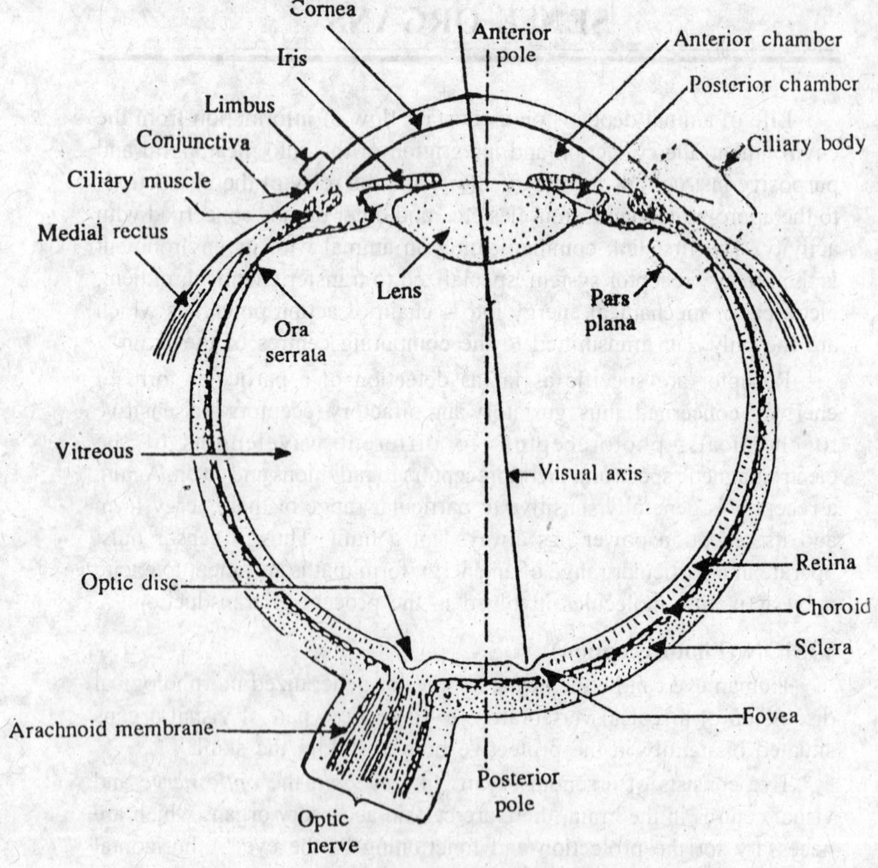

Fig. 11.1 : Horizontal section of the eye.

(2) *The eyelids* : These are two movable folds, upper and lower, which form the anterior protection for the eye. The upper is the larger and more mobile of the two and is provided with a muscle which elevates it. The eyelids are covered externally with skin and their inner lining consists of mucous membrane, the conjunctiva. Between these layers is a dense plate of fibrous

tissue called tarsus. Into the tarsal plate of the uppper lid the muscle which raises it is inserted (elevator palpebrae superioris). Surrounding both lids is a circular sphincter muscle (orbicularis oculi) which closes them and, when fully contracted, 'screws them up'.

The space between the two lids is the palpebral fissure. Its lateral angle is also called the lateral canthus and its medial angle the medial canthus.

The eyelids blink every few seconds. This movement keeps the front of the eye free from dust and helps to move the tears across the conjunctival sac. In addition to protecting the eyes from the entrance of foreign bodies fhe eyelids also prevent the entry of excessive light.

(3) *The eyelashes :* A row of short thick hairs project from the free margin of each eyelid. Arranged immediately behind the eyelashes are the openings of the *tarsal (Meibomian) glands*, which are modified sebaceous glands and are sometimes the site of small cysts. Infection of the hair follicles of the eyelashes results in the common condition known as stye.

(4) *The conjunctiva :* This is a delicate mucous membrane which lines the inner surface of the eyelids and is then reflected on to the outer surface of the eyeball. The space between the two layers is called the conjunctival sac.

(5) *The lacrimal apparatus :* This is concerned with formation of tears and consists of the following structures :

(1) the lacrimal glands;

(2) The lacrimal canaliculi; and

(3) the lacrimal sac and nasolacrimal duct.

(6) *The lacrimal glands :* These are situated in the orbital cavity immediately above the lateral angle of the eye. Each is almond shaped and lies in a depression in the orbital plate of the frontal bone. A number of small canals leads from it to the lateral angle of the conjunctival sac.

(7) *The lacrimal canaliculi :* If the medial end of each eyelid is carefully examined the orifice of a minute duct can be seen. From this opening the lacrimal canaliculus passes inwards to enter the lacrimal sac.

(8) *The lacrimal sac and nasolacrimal duct :* The lacrimal sac may be regarded as the upper expanded portion of the nasolacrimal

duct which passes downwards inside the bony wall of the nasal cavity to open into the inferior meatus of the nose.

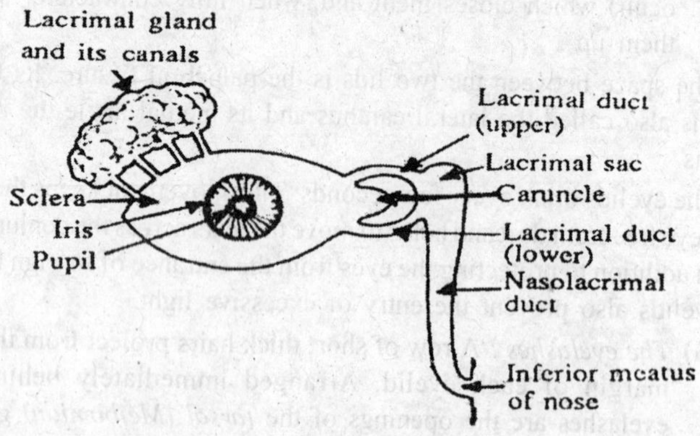

Fig. 11.2 : The lacrimal apparatus.

Tears are slightly alkaline watery fluid containing a small amount of sodium chloride which give them a salty taste. Normally there is a constant secretion from the lacrimal glands just sufficient to keep the interior of the conjunctival sac moist and free from dust. By the frequent movement of the eyelids the tears pass across the front of the eye from the lateral to the medial side, where they pass through the openings of the lacrimal canaliculi and are drained into the nose by the nasolacrimal duct to mix with the secretions of the nose.

Having observed tne minute openings of the lacrimal canaliculi at the medial corners of the eyelids it is clear that any excess of tears must overflow from the conjunctival sac and run down the cheek.Some of the excess, however, does pass down the ducts and accounts for the excess of watery secretion from the nose after crying which, if severe, requires the use of a handkerchief, although in these circumstances its place is frequently taken by 'sniffing'.

The secretion of tears is increased by the presence of foreign bodies and inflammation caused by bacteria or irritating vapours. Irritation of the nasal mucous membrane and very bright light provoke reflex lacrimation, while emotional states and path also result in the flowing of tears.

The functions of the tears may be summarized as:

(1) keeping the eyes moist, thereby allowing free movement of the lids;

(2) removal of dust and foreign bodies, including bacteria;
(3) acting as a mild antiseptic;
(4) expression of emotion or pain.

The extraocular muscles of the eye (Fig. 11.3) : Each eyeball is moved by muscles which arise from the posterior wall of the bony orbit close to the entrance of the optic nerve and are inserted into the outer fibrous coat (sclera) of the eye. There are four straight and two oblique muscles in addition to the muscle elevating the upper lid (levator palpebrae superioris).

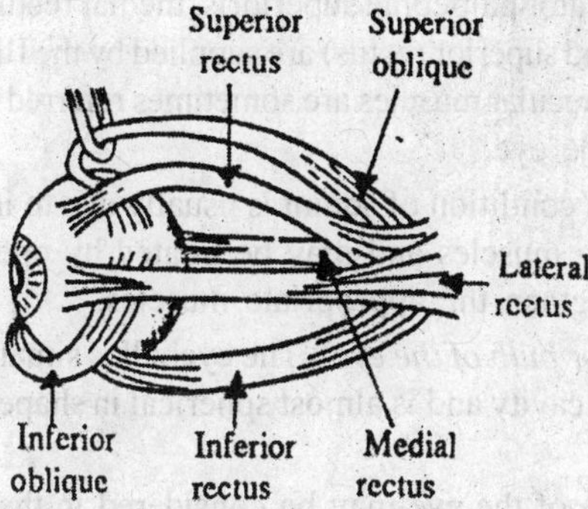

Fig. 11.3 : Diagram of eye muscles. Left orbit (lateral aspect).

The straight muscles are the superior rectus, inferior rectus, medial rectus and lateral rectus. Their position in relation to the eyeball is indicated by their names. The action of these muscles is not too difficult to follow if two facts are remembered.

(1) If one eye alone is considered, contraction of the superior rectus turning the eye upwards will be associated with relaxation of the inferior rectus, and vice-versa. The medial and lateral recti move the eye to one side or the other respectively and work together in the same way. This action is similar to the opposing action of the flexor and extensor muscles of the forearm. When one set contracts the opposite set relaxes.

(2) In normal vision both eyes move together (conjugate deviation). Therefore, if the eyes are turned upwards both right and left superior recti will contract and both inferior recti will relax. On the other hand, if both eyes are turned to the right it follows that the right lateral rectus and the left medial rectus will contract while the right medial rectus and left lateral rectus will relax.

The converse is true if the eyes are turned to the left. This is quite simple, and with a little thought the individual can work it out for herself or himself.

Of the two oblique muscles, the superior oblique is so arranged as to direct the eye downwards and outwards. The inferior oblique muscle turns the eye upwards and outwards.

The muscles of the eyes are supplied by the cranial nerves (IIIrd, IVth and VIth). The lateral rectus is supplied by the^VIth or abducens nerve. The superior oblique is supplied by the IVth or trochlear nerve. All the others (levator palpebrae superioris, medial rectus, inferior rectus, inferior oblique and superior rectus) are supplied by the IIIrd or oculomotor nerve. These extraocular muscles are sometimes referred to as the extrinsic muscles are of the eye.

The common condition of squint is usually due to imperfect balance between opposing muscles and may be treated by operations designed to shorten or lengthen the appropriate muscles.

The eyeball or bulb of the eye : The eyeball is situated in the anterior part of the orbital cavity and is almost spherical in shape. It is surrounded by a pad of fat.

The structure of the eye may be considered in the following way :

A. Three tunics or layers :

(1) Fibrous:
   (a) sclera.
   (b) cornea.

(2) Vascular:
   (a) choroid.
   (b) ciliary body.
   (c) iris.

(3) nervous retina.

B. The light transmitting mechanism :

(1) aqueous humor.
(2) the lens.
(3) the vitreous body.

(1) *The fibrous coats :* (a) The *sclera* (or sclerotic coat). The posterior five-sixths of the outer coat of the eyeball consists of strong, opaque fibrous tissue and is called the sclera. It is protective in function and helps to maintain the shape of the eyeball. When viewed from the front it is that portion which is referred to as the 'white of the eye' and, in this position, is covered by the conjunctiva. Posteriorly, the optic nerve passes through it to reach the retina inside the eye, and in the orbit the nerve is protected by a sheath of fibrous tissue continuous with the sclera.

(b) The *cornea* occupies the anterior one-sixth of the external surface of the eyeball and, being transparent, allows light to enter the interior of the eye. The cornea is sometimes described as the 'window of the eye' and its anterior surface can be seen to be slightly curved or convex. Over the cornea, the conjunctiva becomes very thin and is only represented by a few layers of epithelial cells. The cornea has no blood vessels but derives its nourishment from the aqueous humor.

(2) *The vascular coat* : This is the middle layer of the eye. It contains many blood vessels and capillaries, which are derived from the opthalmic branch of the internal carotid artery, and is pigmented. The choroid, ciliary body and iris together form the uveal tract.

(a) The *choroid*. This is a thin pigmented membrane, dark brown in colour, which lines the posterior compartment of the eye. It is situated between the inner surface of the sclera and the retina.

(b) The *ciliary body*. This is a circular structure, continuous with the anterior part of the choroid, which surrounds the periphery of the iris immediately behind the outer margin of the cornea where it joins the sclera. It contains muscle fibres (the ciliary muscle) and to it is attached the ligament which helps to suspend the lens in position.

(c) *The iris*. This is the pigmented membrane which surrounds the pupil of the eye. It arises from the margin of the ciliary body and forms a diaphragm with a black central opening (the pupil) immediately in front of the lens. The colour of the eye is dependent on the pigment in the iris. In the dark eyes the pigment is plentiful, but in blue eyes it is scanty.

The iris contains two sets of muscle fibres. Those comprising the *sphincter pupillae* encircle the pupil. The fibres of the other muscle, *the dilator pupillae*, pass in a radial direction from the outer margin of the iris to the edge of the pupil. It will be clear that the circular muscle, acting as a sphincter will reduce the size of the pupil when it contracts. Contraction of the radial fibres, on the other hand, increase its size and they are, therefore, dilators. These, with the ciliary muscle, are the intrinsic muscles of the eye. The function of the iris is to regulate the amount of light entering the posterior part of the eye. Thus, when a bright light shines on the retina the pupil contracts.

The iris is under the control of the autonomic nervous system, the effect of sympathetic stimulation being pupillary dilatation (mydriasis) and that of parasympathetic stimulation being pupillary constriction.

(3) *The Retina* : It is the layer at the back of the eye, and most sensitive to light. It is formed of ten layers of cells, which in turn made up of nerve cells and nerve fibres lying on pigmented epithelial cells which attach it to the choroid. The important ones are the layers of pigment epithelium, layers of photoreceptor cells, a layer of neurons and the innermost layer of the ganglions—the central body of nerve cells. There is a small depression in the posterior part of the retina called *macula lutea*. In the centre of this area lies its most sensitive part called *fovea contrails*. A sharp visual image can be formed only by this part.

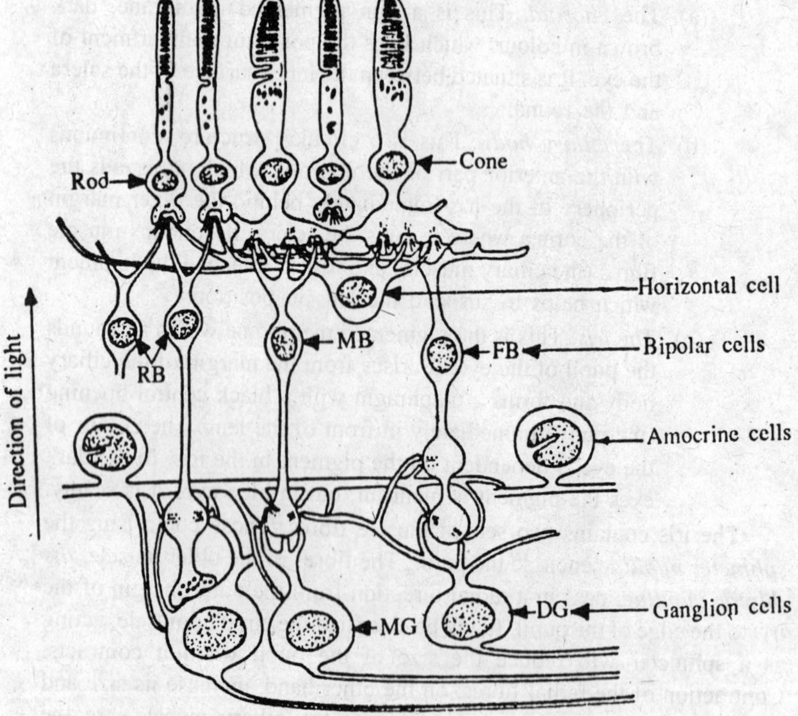

Fig. 11.4 : Ultrastructural organization of the vertebrate retina. DG, diffuse ganglion cell; FB, flat bipolar cell; MB, midget bipolar cell; MG, midget ganglion cell; RB, rod bipolar cell.

Photoreceptor cells are of two kinds, viz, *cone cells* and *rod cells.* There are approximately 5-15 million cone cells and about 100-120 million rod cells in each human eye. Generally, the function of daylight vision is performed by the cones which are colour sensitive and are concentrated in the fovea centralise, while the rods are concentrated in the retinal periphery and function as movement detectors in low light conditions; they are responsible for night vision.

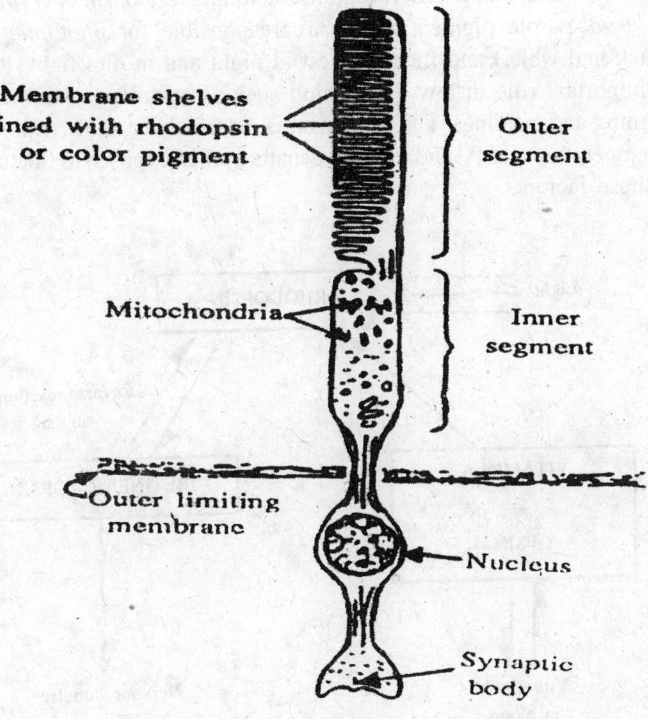

Fig. 11.5 : Schematic drawing of the functional parts of the rods and cones.

Both cone and rod cells are elongated in shape and can be divided into four morphological regions, (Fig.11.5) viz,

(1) an outer segment containing photopigment (in rods it is narrow and elongated, while in cones it is short and cone-shaped);

(2) an inner segment with mitochondria and other organelles;

(3) a nuclear zone; and

(4) a synaptic-zone.

Photopigments : Rods and cones are actually the modified cilia of sensory cells and both rod and cone cells contain photopigments which contain two types of compounds viz, *retinal* (retinene), a derivative of vitamin A; and *opsin.* a protein. Opsins are different in rod and cone pigments.

The rods are dark light receptors containing *rhodopsin* or *erythropsin* or *visual*-purple pigment. They are responsible for *photoptic vision* (black and white) and function best at night and in dim fight. It plays an important role in low-light vision such as at dusk and dawn (early morning and evening). The rhodopsin is extremely unstable with respect to temperature and P^H and tends to denature when exposed to fluctuations in these factors.

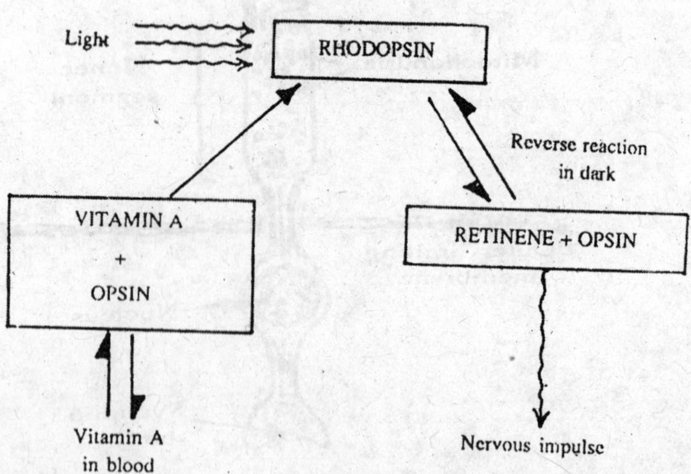

Fig. 11.6 : Flow diagram showing the changes which occur when light fall on rhodopsin.

When light strikes, the rhodopsin molecule becomes energized and undergoes a series of changes. First it splits into two fragments-the pigment *retinene* and a protein *opsin.* It is this change that generates the electric potential in the cell and sends a nerve impulse to the brain, where it is analysed and generates a sensation of vision. If the light is continually present, the retinene will be changed to vitamin A and this vitamin A (in its different isometric form) combines with opsin to regenerate rhodopsin. The regeneration of rhodopsin in the dark is responsible for the dark adaptation (*scotopic vision*) and its non-regeneration may be the cause of night blindness.

One of the constituents of rhodopsin is vitamin A which comes into our blood from a variety of diet (carrots, eggs, etc.). So what would happen if supply of vitamin A from the diet is cut off? The answer is night blindness. It is an obvious fact, because of lack of vitamin A means there will be low or almost nothing of rhodopsin present in our eyes and in the absence of this we lose the ability to sense low intensity lights.

It is a common experience that we see an object better in dark by not looking directly at it. For example, sailor stand watch at night, looking for the light of other ships. But they don't look along the horizon. Instead, they took just above the line where the ocean and sky meet. In such cases our eye lens is adjusted so as to focus on the side of retina, where most rod cells are concentrated and thus, even a trace of light is easily detected. Seeing through the corners of eyes in dim fight gives a better vision.

We have much less information about cones and their working. But it is known that cones are receptors containing *iodopsin* or visual-violet pigment and there are three types of cone cells (Young-Helmholtz theory), each sensitive to one of the three primary colours-the *green, blue* and *red.* They are responsible for *phototopic vision* or *vision in bright* light and colour vision.

The normal fovea in their cones contains a type of pigment called *chlorolabe* with a maximal absorption at 540 mμ and respond best to green light rays. This green absorbing pigment is missing in the eyes of *deuteropes* (green colour blind). Another pigment is *erythrolabe* with a maximum absorption at about 570 mμ and respond best to red light rays. It is lacking in the eyes of *protanopes* (red colour blind). In presence of third blue absorbing pigment, *cyanolabe* is still debated but blue blinds are generally called *tritanope* are very rare, only one in every 65,000 and previous two are very common. It is not known whether each visual element posseses the pigment singly or in the mixture of three. Red green confusion is of practical importance, as coloured signals must be recognised by railway and marine employees and to certain extent by motor driver too. Think of the situation when a red blind can't distinguished a red signal and tries to cross a traffic island !

Generally, rods are more sensitive to light than the cones, it is due to fact that cones act individually while rods act in large clumps. Each cone is connected with the brain by a single fibre of optic nerve. In contrast large clusters of rods are connected to a single optic fibre nerve. Since rods operate in chunk (group), the image conveyed by them is coarse and is a mosaic much like constructing a complete picture by some broken pieces of porcelain. That is why during night or in light of low intensity when rods help us to see, we may not be sure that a cat is a cat !

The point at which the optic nerve fibres all coverage, contains no nerve cells and no rods and cones. It is, therefore, insensitive to light and is called *blind spot* or *optic disc*. The retina is supplied with blood by a branch of the opthalmic artery which enters the eye with the optic nerve and is called the central artery of the retina.

Interpretation of visual impulses : Image of an object once focussed on the retina, a series of nerve impulses are set on by the visual receptor cells. These impulses are first conveyed to the lateral genaculate body situated behind the thalamus. It is a sub-cortical visual centre. From here for further fine discrimination impulses are conveyed to the occipital lobe of the cerebral cortex, where final interpretation is brought about. Thus vision of an object in front of the eyes is a complex process involving superior cortical centres. In other words, vision actually happens in the brain and not in the eye.

The Light-transmitting Mechanism

(1) *The aqueous humour* : Situated between the cornea in front and the iris and ciliary body behind,is the anterior chamber of the eye which contains a clear watery fluid (Protein-free, iso-osmotic with plasma) called aqueous humour. It is formed continuously by the ciliary epithelium at a rate of 2 to 3μ 1/min and its function is to maintain the shape of the eyeball and thereby the refracting surfaces and to provide nutrition for the lens and posterior surface of the cornea. Aqueous humour may be secreted by ciliary glands.

(2) *The lens* : This is a firm transparent structure, convex in shape, which is suspended in its capsule by a ligament attached to the ciliary body. It is composed of ribbon - like fibres arranged in concentric laminae. It is placed immediately behind the iris and pupil of the eye. Its function is to focus rays of light entering the eye through the pupil on to the retina. Although the lens has

no blood supply it is a metabolically active tissue that continues to grow throughout life.

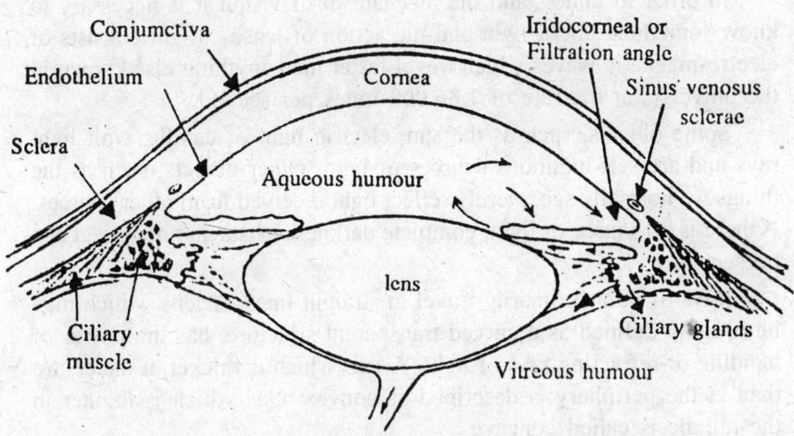

Fig. 11.7 : The probable source ot the aqueous humour in the ciliary glands and the routes of absorption into the circulation. The ciliary glands lie in the ciliary body, which is a ring-like structure. The suspensory ligaments of the lens are shown.

(3) *The vitreous body :* This is a colourless, transparent jelly-like substance which fills the posterior cavity of the eye. It helps to preserve the spherical shape of the eyeball and to support the retina.

The presence of fluid and semi-fluid material or gel in the interior of the eye maintains its shape by keeping up a constant pressure on its walls. This is referred to as the Intraocular tension.

In certain conditions drainage of the fluid may be impaired and there will be a consequent increase in the intraocular tension, a serious effect which may disturb the nutrition of the retina and lead to blindness. This is known as glaucoma.

Image formation In the eye : From a structural point of view the eye may be compared with a camera. The eyelids act as a shutter and there is an entrance window for light-the cornea; a diaphragm to regulate the aperture and therefore the amount of light entering - the iris; a lens to focus the image; a darkened interior formed by the choroid, and a light-sensitive plate which receives the image-the retina.

The optic nerve and its connections convey the details of the image to the occipital region of the cerebral cortex where they are processed before reaching consciousness.

In order to understand the mechanism of vision it is necessary to know something about light and the action of lenses. Light consists of electro-magnetic waves which travel faster than anything else known in the universe, at the rate of 1,86,000 miles per second.

Some objects, such as the sun, electric light or candle, emit light rays and are self-luminous sources of light. Other objects, such as the things we normally see, merely reflect light received from other sources. If there is no source of light, complete darkness exists and no object can be seen.

Rays of light ordinarily travel in straight lines. A lens, which may be roughly defined as a curved transparent structure, has the power of bending or refracting rays of light. A lens which is thicker at the centre than at the periphery is described as convex. One which is thinner in the middle is called concave.

A convex lens has the power of bending rays of light so that they coverge and meet at a point of focus behind the lens. The stronger the lens, *i.e.*, the greater the degree of curvature of its surfaces, the nearer is the focal point. A concave lens, on the other hand, bends the light rays so that they diverge and do not focus behind the lens. The lens of the eye is convex and focuses the rays of light passing through it on to the retina.

Actually, the image reaching the retina is inverted but this is turned the right way up by the visual cortex in the brain.

Accommodation : Rays of light from distant objects are for all practical purposes parallel and therefore strike the vertical axis of the lens at right angles. The eye is so adjusted that such rays are bent by the lens to focus exactly on the retina, forming a sharp image. Rays of light from a near object (say 25 cm or 10 in) are divergent and strike the lens obliquely. In order that such rays may be accurately focussed on the retina the lens must be made more powerful (of greater focusing power) by increasing its curvature *i.e.*, making it more convex. This is accomplished by the action of the ciliary muscles. At the same time the clearness of the image is increased by cutting down the nurnber of rays entering the eye by contraction of the iris. The process of altering the shape of the lens is called *accommodation* and operates every time a near object is looked at. The nearest point at which an object can be brought clearly into focus by accommodation is called the *near point*. For a normal child of 10 years it is about 9 cm (3.5 in) but it recedes throughout life and by the age of about 45 may become so distant that reading is difficult without spectacles.

When an object is placed near the eyes, in order to obtain a clearly focused picture on both retinae the eyes turn slightly inwards towards each other. This is called *convergence*. The extreme of convergence is illustrated by "squinting down the end of the nose". The triple response of accommodation, convergence and pupillary constriction is called the *near response*.

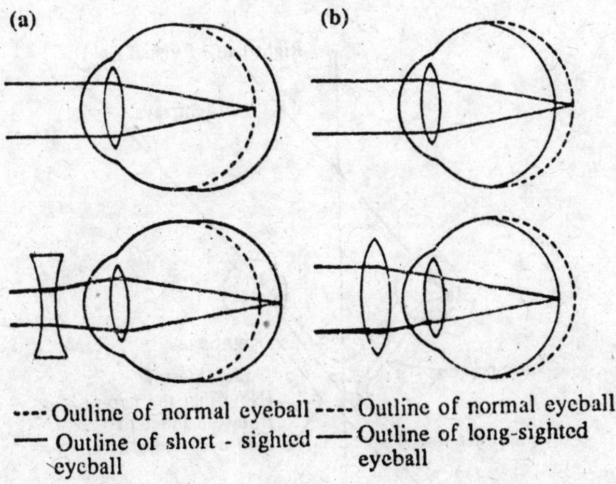

Fig. 11.8 : (a) Myopia (short sight) and its correction, (b) Hypermetropia (long sight) and its correction.

It is of interest at this point to note some of the common defects of vision requiring the use of spectacles. Whereas the normal eye is practically spherical, in some people it tends to be slightly elongated and in others flattened. In other words, in the former case the distance from the lens to the retina is increased and in the latter it is decreased. It follows, therefore, that the lens will not naturally focus the image accurately on the retina in these conditions. In the former, elongated or myopic eye (short sighted), the image will tend to fall in front of the retina, while in the shortened or hypermetropic eye (long sighted) it will fall behind the retina, in both instances the objects seen will be blurred and out of focus.

These defects can be compensated by using additional lenses in the form of spectacles. By placing a concave glass lens in front of a myopic eye the rays of light will become divergent before reaching the lens, so that its point of focus is shifted back on to the retina. A convex lens in front of a hypermetropic eye will bring the image nearer the front of the eye by increasing the convergence of the rays so that they are focused on the retina.

Astigmatism is due to unequal curvature of the surfaces of the cornea, *i.e.*, it may be curved more vertically than horizontally. This also may require correction with spectacles (cylindrical lenses).

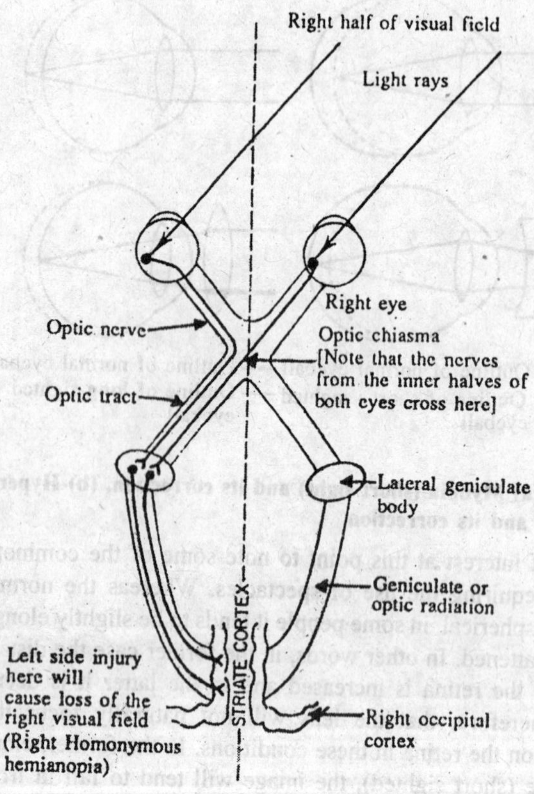

Fig. 11.9 : The visual pathways.

Binocular vision : In considering the sense of sight it must be remembered that although we can see with each eye separately, normal stereoscopic vision is obtained by the simultaneous use of both eyes.

Rays of light strike the retina from all directions. Those coming from the left-hand side of the body will fall on the nasal side of the retina of the left eye and the temporal side of the retina of the right eye. These images produced by objects on the left side of the body are eventually received by the occipital lobe on the right side of the brain. This explains the crossing of certain fibres of the optic nerve in the optic chiasma and is part of the principle that one side of the body is controlled by the cerebral hemisphere of the opposite side. These facts are easily appreciated from Fig. 11.9.

Summary of the Sense of Sight

Light waves → cornea → aqueous humour → lens → vitreous body → retina → optic nerve → optic chiasma → occipital lobe of brain.

Hearing

Hearing is one of the perceptual processes by which animals are continually being informed about their environment. In man, the general information from the ears, such as the proximity of a source of sound, is augmented by the more specific information contained in speech. Speech and hearing must be regarded as two complementary activities that subserve the function of communication. If the complete deafness occurs in infancy before vocalisation has reached the stage of speech the child fails to develop ability to speak.

In mammals the auditory apparatus consists of (1) the external ear, (2) the middle ear, (3) The internal ear.

(1) *The external ear* : This consists of (a) the auricle or pinna (b) the external acoustic meatus. (i) cartilaginous portion (ii) bony portion.

The auricle or pinna is attached to the side of the head about midway between the forehead and the occiput. It has a deep shell like cavity called the concha. Beneath the skin, the auricle is composed of yellow elastic cartilage, apart from the lobule or ear lobe which is soft because it is composed of fibrous and adipose tissues (Fig. 11.10). The function of the auricle is to collect sound waves and conduct them to the external acoustic meatus. This function is more marked in many animals than man and in consequence their auricles are relatively larger and more mobile. Although, there are several small muscles attached to the human ear, in only a few people is a limited amount of movement possible.

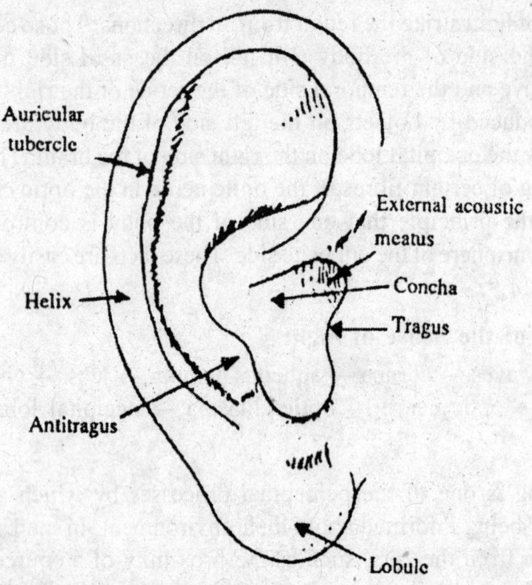

Fig. 11.10 : The pinna.

The *external acoustic* (auditory) *meatus* leads from the pinna to the tympanic membrane or ear drum. It is tubular passage about 2.5 cm long. Its path is not straight but shows a slight double or S-shaped bend, being directed at first medially, forwards, and slightly upwards, and then medially and slightly backwards. Structurally the external acoustic meatus consists of two parts : the outer *cartllagenous* portion which is continuous with the cartilage of the pinna; and the *inner bony* part in the temporal bone.

The meatus is lined by skin which is continuous with that covering the pinna, but is characterized by special glands, the *ceruminous glands*, which secrete a yellow greasy substances called cerumen or wax. They are modified sweat glands and their secretion helps to prevent the entry into the meatus of foreign bodies, especially insects. A few hairs are present which also assist in this function.

The middle ear : The middle ear or tympanic cavity is a small irregular cavity situated in the petrous portion of the temporal bone. It contains a chain of small bones or *ossicles* by which the sound waves are transmitted from the *tympanic membrane* to the internal ear. Roughly speaking, it is a narrow oblong box having anterior, posterior, medial and lateral walls with a roof and a floor.

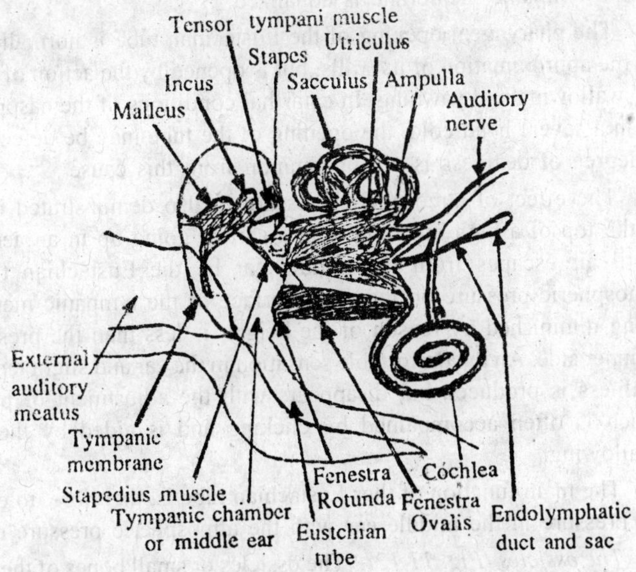

Fig. 11.11 Section through the ear.

Its walls are both bony and membranous in structure. The outer or lateral wall is formed by the tympanic membrane. Its medial wall, though mainly consisting of bone, has two openings which are covered by membrane, namely the *fenestra vestibull* (f. ovalis)or oval window of the vestibule above, and the *fenestra cochleae* (f. rotunda) or round window of the chochlea below.

In addition to these membranous defects in its outer and inner walls, both the anterior and posterior walls have openings. Entering the middle ear in its anterior wall is the outer or lateral end of the *auditory (Eustachian) tube* which communicates with the nasopharynx. Posteriorly the middle ear communicates with the mastoid antrum and the mastoid air cells which occupy the mastoid process of the temporal bone.

The whole of the cavity, of the middle ear is lined by mucous membrane which, therefore forms the inner lining of the tympanic membrane and is continuous with the mucous lining of the Eustachian tube and with that of the mastoid antrum and cells.

The auditory tube connects the nasopharynx with the middle ear and is less than 4 cm (1½ in) in length. There is thus a connection between the middle ear and the outer air so that the pressure of air on each side of the tympanic membrane is equalized.

The pharyngeal opening of the Eustachian tube is normally closed by the approximation of its walls, but is opened by the action of muscles in swallowing and yawning. In catarrhal conditions of the nasppharynx, as in a severe head cold, the opening of the tube may be defective and a degree of deafness is not uncommon from this cause.

The effect of atmospheric pressure is also demonstrated in going to the top of a high hill rapidly in a car, or going up in an aeroplane. Until air escapes from the middle ear by the Eustachian tube the atmospheric pressure on the outer surface of the tympanic membrane, being diminished by reason of the height, is less than the pressure on its inner side. An uncomfortable sensation in the ear and slight temporary deafness is produced but disappears with the adjustment of pressure, which is often accompained by clicking and is aided by the act of swallowing.

The main function of ther Eustachian tube is, therefore, to equalize the pressure in the middle ear with the atmospheric pressure outside.

The ossicles (Fig. 11.12) : The ossicles or small bones of the middle ear are three in number, the *malleus*, the *incus* and *stapes*. They stretch from the tympanic membrane to the fenestra vestibuli or oval window of the vestibule.

The *malleus* or hammer bone consists of a head which articulates with the incus and a handle which is attached to the tympanic membrane. The *incus* or anvil is the middle of the three bones and consists of a body and two short legs, one of which articulates with the roof of the middle ear, the with the stapes. The *stapes* or stirrup bone is the smallest of the three. Its head articulates with the incus while its base or foot-plate is attached to the membrane covering the fenestra vestibuli.

These three bones act as a series of levers transmitting the movements or vibrations of the tympanic membrane, caused by sound waves impinging upon it, to the membrane covering the fenestra vestibuli. It will be seen later that from the fenestra vestibuli the vibrations are passed on to the internal ear.

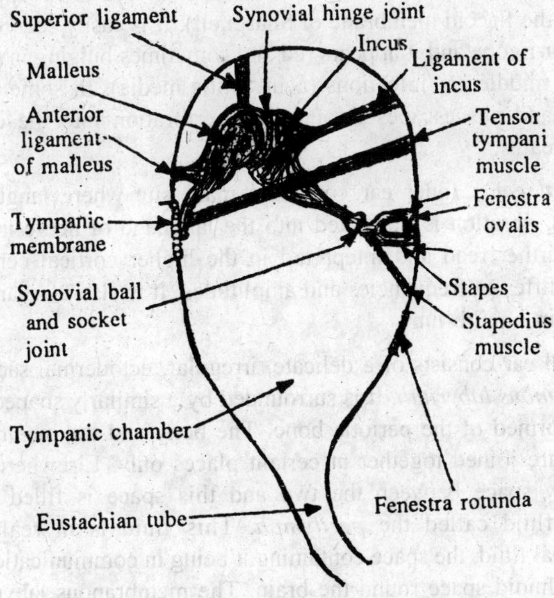

Fig. 11.12 : Middle ear of mammal.

The movement of the ossicles are controlled to some extent by two tiny muscles, the *tensor tympani* inserted into the handle of the malleus, and the *stapedius* muscle inserted into the neck of the stapes. These muscles act as dampers to prevent excessive movement of the ossicles in response to loud noise. They also attenuate low frequency components of sound so that weaker high frequency components are not masked. This improves the perception of sounds obscured by background noise.

The tympanic memrane : The *tympanic membrane* (tympanum, or eardrum) is situated at the deepest part of the external acoustic meatus which it separates from the middle ear. It lies obliquely so that its upper part is nearer the exterior than its lower part. In structure, its outer surface consists of epithelium continuous with the skin lining the external acoustic meatus, while its inner lining is mucous membrane continuous with that of the middle ear. Between these two layers is a small amount of fibrous tissue. Firmly attached to its inner wall (and passing downwards and slightly backwards from its upper edge to a point Just below and behind its centre) is the handle of the malleus.

It appears as an almost circular structure tightly stretched between the walls of the bony meatus except for a small area in its upper part (known as the flaccid membrane of Sharpnell). It is easily seen with the aid of an auriscope and it appears red and sometimes bulging in patients with acute middle ear infections (acute otitis media). In some cases it perforates and pus escapes through the perforation into the external acoustic meatus.

Internal ear : Inner ear constitute main site where language of mechanical vibration is translated into the language of nerve impulses which is further read and intepretad in the higher cortical centres as sounds of different frequencies and amplitudes. It is also a organ which is helping in equilibrium.

Internal ear consists of a delicate, irregular, ectodermal sac called the *membranous labyrinth.* It is surrounded by a similarly shaped bony/ *labyrinth* formed of the periotic bone. The bony and the membranous labyrinths are joined together at certain places only. Elsewhere, there is a narrow space between the two and this space is filled with a lymphatic fluid called the *perilymph.* This fluid is in reality the cerebrospinal fluid, the space containing it being in communication with the subarachnoid space round the brain. The membranous labyrinth is also filled with a similar fluid, the *endolymph*, having viscosity 2 or 3 times that of the water.

The bony labyrinth includes : (1) the vestibule, (2) the bony *semi-circular canals*, and (3) the cochlea. Vestibule and semicircular canals are concerned with the equilibrium sense and cochlea with sense of hearing.

(1) *Vestibule :* The vesibule is the central sac-like part of the membranous labyrinth. It is differentiated into two chambers : the upper larger *utriculus*, which communicates with the semicircular canals, and the lower small sacculus, which communicates with the cochlear duct. The two are jointed by a narrow tube, the *saculo utricular duct.* A slender tube, the *endolymphatic duct*, arises from the sacculus dorsomedially and ends blindly at a short distance from the cranium.

The vestibule bears in it two sensory spots, the *maculae*, for equilibrium. One of these lies in the wall of the utriculus and is called the *macula utricull.* The other lies in the wall of the sacculus and is named the macula sacculi (Fig. 11.14).

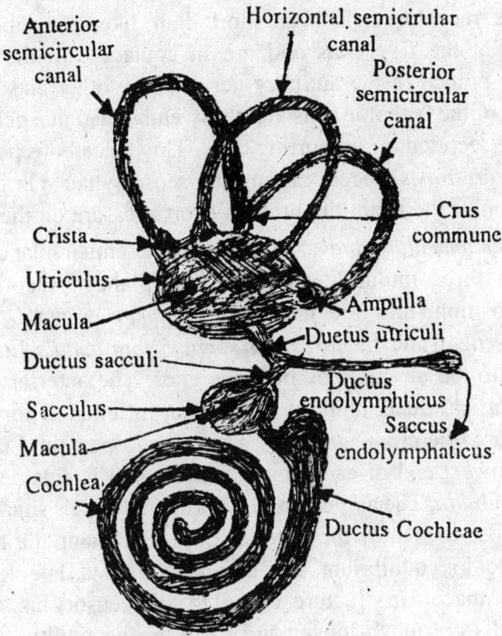

Fig. 11.13 : Membranous labyrinth.

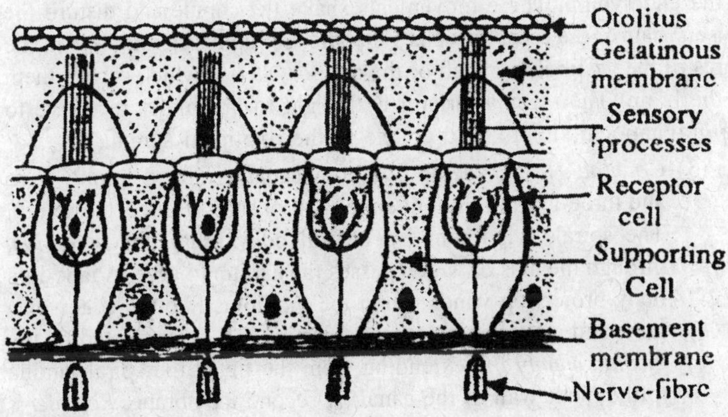

Fig. 11.14 : V. S. macculla.

Each macula consists of a group of receptor cells and supporting cells. The receptor cells bear short, hair like, non-vibratile sensory processes at the free ends and are in contact with the fibres of the vestibular branch of the auditory nerve at the other ends. The sensory processes of the receptor cells are partly embedded in a gelatinous mass, the cupule secreted by supporting cells. Tiny calcareous particles, called *otoliths* (*ear stones*), occur among the sensory hair. On any change in the position of the head, the otoliths exert pressure on the sensory hair.

(2) *Semicircular canals :* There are three semicircular ducts arranged in three mutually perpendicular planes. According to their position, they are named the *anterior vertical*, the *posterior vertical*, and the *horizontal semicircular canals*. Each duct opens into the utriculus by both the ends. The anterior and posterior vertical ducts unite by their adjacent ends to form a common duct, the crus *commune*, which then opens into utriculus. One (lower) end of each semicircular canal is enlarged to form an *ampulla*. The ampulla of the horizontal duct is situated anteriorly close to that of the anterior duct. Each ampulla has a sensory spot for equilibrium. This is called the crista. The crista resembles the macula in structure, except that the sensory hair of its receptor cells are much longer and there are no otoliths.

Equilibrium : Cristae and maculae, as mentioned earlier, act as organs of equilibrium. Any change in the position of the body (stop, or start or accelerate or decelerate, or change direction) sets up movements in the endolymph. These movements shake the cupule and disturb the sensory hair of the receptor cells. The later set up nerve impulses in the fibres of the vestibular branch of the auditory nerve, which carries them to the brain. The macula utriculi is thought to be chiefly receptive to the gravitational stimuli; and cristae to the rotational stimuli.

(3) *Cochlae :* It is made up of a bony canal, arranged spirally (two and three-fourth turns) like the shell of snail (Hence, the name). The spirals wind round a central bony pillar, the *modiolus*, through the axis of which passes the auditory nerve. A tape-like bony projection winds round the modiolus like the edges of a crew and makes an incomplete partition. It is completed by the *basilar membrane* extending from the tip of the spiral lamina to the outer wall of the canal. A second membrane, *Relssner's membrane* stretches from the upper surface of the spiral lamina to the bony wall of the canal a little above the attachment of

the basilar membrane. Though the cochlea is spiral, yet it can be regarded as a long straight tube divided down its length by a *membranous partition*, the cochlear partition. Thus, the bony cochlea is partitioned down its length by the triangular duct, the cochlear duct into two halves-(i) *scala vestibull*, and (ii) *scala tympani*. This portion is actually containing sense organs situated on the basilar membrane and other *accessory organs* and endolymph. Near the apex of the cochlea, the vestibular and tympanic scalae become continuous and this common space is known as the helicotrema that responds to the vibrations of low frequencies.

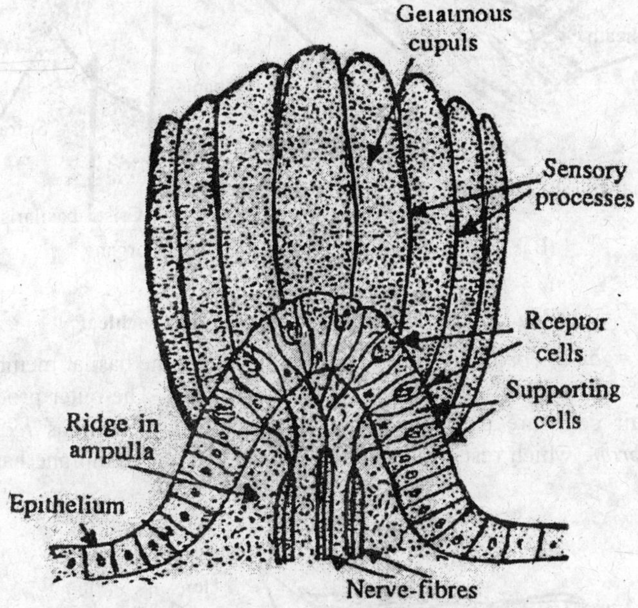

Fig. 11.15 : V. S. Crista.

Thus, the original bony canal is subdivided into three spiral canals. That below the basilar membrane is called the *scala tympany*, that between the two membranes is *scala media* (canal of cochlea), and that above Reissner's membrane the *scala vestibull*. The scala media are filled up with *endolymph*. The scala vestibuli and scala tympani are filled up with *perilymph*. On the basilar membrane lies the *organ of corti* which is the sense organ for hearing.

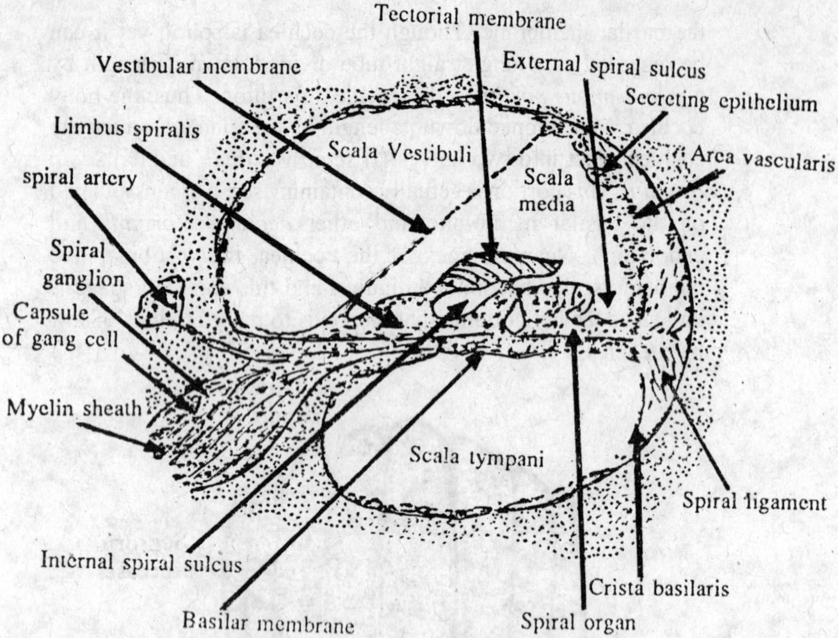

Fig. 11.16 : Structure of mammalian cochlea.

Organ of corti (Fig. 11.17) : It is situated on the basilar membrane, consists of supporting cells and sensory hair cells. The outer processes of hair cells are embedded in an overhanging gelatinous *tectorial membrane* which rests lightly upon them. Tecterial membrane has fine

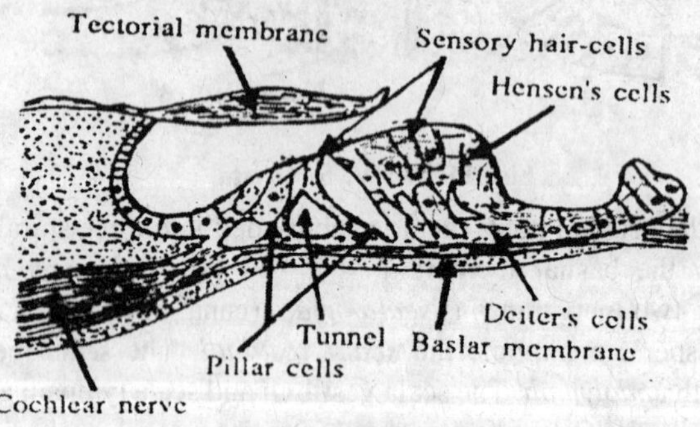

Fig. 11.17 : Organ of corti.

fibres. The axonic fibres of the hair cells are connected to the cochlear branch of the VIII cranial nerve. In the middle of the organ of corti is a *tunnel of corti* supported by cells called *pillar cells.* Supporting cells lying close to the hair cells have received different names, such as Hensen's cells and Deiter's cells.

Mechanism of hearing : The sound waves from the external environment are collected by external pinna. Sound waves travel through the external auditory meatus and cause the tympanic membrane to vibrate. The vibrations of tympanic membrane are conveyed through the chain of ear ossicles to the membrane over the fenestra ovalis to which the stapes is attached. Vibrations of the membrane of the fenestra ovalis cause alternate increase and decrease in the pressure in the perilymph filling the scala tympani, while the membrane of the fenestra ovalis moves outwards and inwards with the same frequency as that of the sound waves. Since the wall of the cochlea is made of a rigid bone the fluid under compression causes the Reissner's membrane to vibrate up and down. Scala vestibuli is connected with the scala tympani by a small aperture, the helicotrema, but this aperture is too small to allow movements of the frequency of the sound vibrations to be transmitted through it. The movements of stapes are damped by the resistance of helicotrema and fenestra rotunda. Accordingly when the pressure rises the scala vestibuli, then both Reissner's membrane and basilar membrane begin

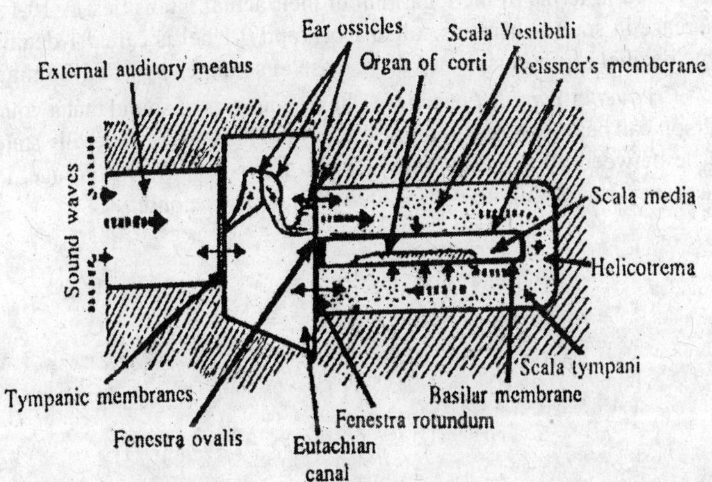

Fig. 11.18 : Diagrammatic representation of the course of sound waves in the ear.

to vibrate in unison. Vibrations of the basilar membrane and Reissner's membrane produce two effects, (1) the fluid in the scala tympani is compressed causing the membrane over the fenestra rotunda to bulge out, (2) the endolymph in the scala media is set into vibration.

Vibrations in the scala media result in the distortion or bending and stretching of the hair cells of the organ of corti, since they are embedded in the tectorial membrane. Distortions set up a train of events resulting in the production of nerve impulses in the hair cells that are conveyed by the cochlear nerve to the brain. Such impulses are interpreted as sound by the brain.

Sound is due to waves or vibrattons in the air and has three main qualities.

(1) *Pitch*-which depends on the frequency of the vibrations. The more rapid the frequency the higher the pitch of the note produced.

(2) *Intensity* or *laudness*, which depends on the amplitude of the vibrations.

(3) The *quality*, which is due to the combination of various vibrations. They may blend to produce harmony or music, or fail to unite giving rise to a discord or noise.

The decibel unit : Because of the extreme changes in sound intensities that the ear can detect and discriminate, sound intensities are usually expressed in terms of the logarithm of their actual intensities. A 10-fold increase in sound energy is called 1 *bel*, and 0.1 bel is called 1 decibel. One decibel represents an actual increase in sound energy of 1.26 times.

Frequency range of hearing : The frequencies of sound that a young person can hear, before aging has occurred in the ears, is generally stated to be between 20 and 20,000 cycles per second (CPS). In old age, the frequency range falls to 50 to 8000 cycles per second.

12

CHEMICAL MESSENGERS

The coordination and integration of various body activities is primarily the function of nervous system. However, during the evolution some neurons have secondarily become secretory and morphologically distinguishable from rest of the nervous tissue. These neurons so called *neurosecretory cells* elaborate and dispose special products known as *neurohormones*. These neurohormones are some type of chemicals (*neurotransmitters*) which excite other nerves or effector organs, while the integration of a complex physiological process such as molting in crustaceans, metamorphosis in insects, the oestrous cycle in mammals, or carbohydrate metabolism depends on the interplay of several different but very specific *Hormones* or *chemical* messengers. For present purposes, the diversity of chemical messengers will be grouped according to the tissues or cellular types from which they originate : transmitters or neurotransmitters, neurohormones or neurosecretory substances, glandular hormones of non-neural tissues, tissue hormones or hormone-like substances and the pheromones.

Neurotransmitters are produced in nerve cells relatively unspecialized for secretory purposes. They are released at the ends of the fibres and move only very short distances before being enzymatically destroyed, transmitters act on other neurons, muscles or glands that are in intimate contact with the nerve endings. Thus, they lire snort range and short-lived materials.

Acetylcholine, adrenaline, and noradrenaline are the most familiar transmitters, but this group of chemical messengers includes in addition several other amines, and a few amino acids and purines.

Neurohormones or neurosecretory substances are produced in nerve cells that are specialized for secretion rather than conduction. These messengers may be released directly into the circulation or temporarily stored in *neurohaemal organs*.

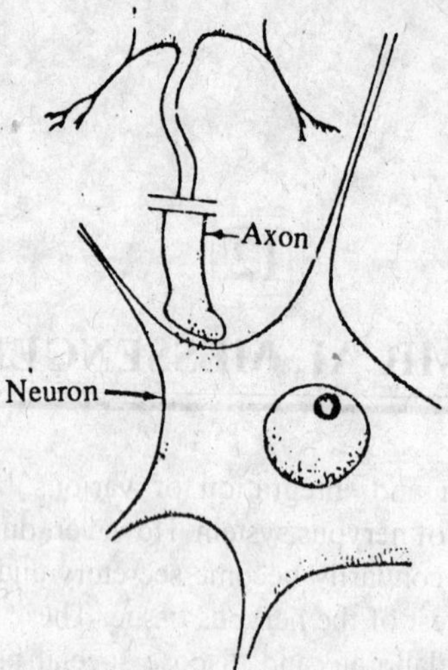

Fig. 12.1 : Discharge of secretions from neurons and endocrine cells. Neurotransmitter released from axon terminal at a synapse with another neuron.

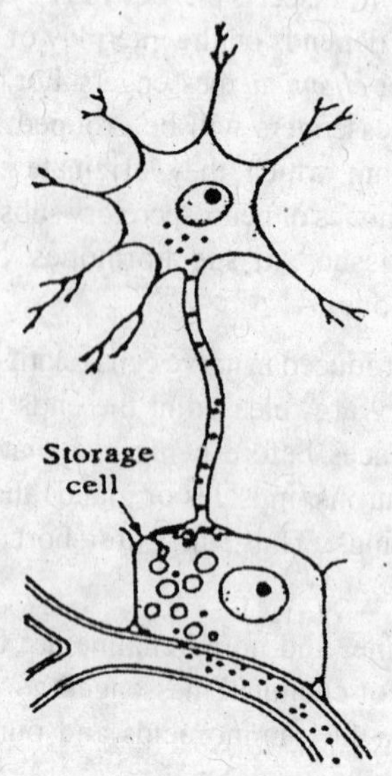

Fig. 12.2 : Neurosecretory cell of primitive sort with one-step control and neurohaemal storage.

Neurosecretory substances are true hormones and in contrast to the transmitters, these have a longer life and act on receptors located at some distance from the point of release. They may exercise their control directly on the target or act by way of a second endocrine gland of non-nervous origin. Neurohormones control such varied phenomena as molting and chromatophore activity in arthropods or water balance and milk production in the vertebrates (oxytocin, vassopressin).

Some of the arthropod and vertebrate hormones are secreted by endocrine glands of non-nervous origin. The best known examples of these epitheloid endocrine glands are the Y-organs and androgenic glands of crustaceans, the corpora allata and prothoracic glands of insects and the anterior pituitary, thyroid and adrenal cortex of vertebrates.

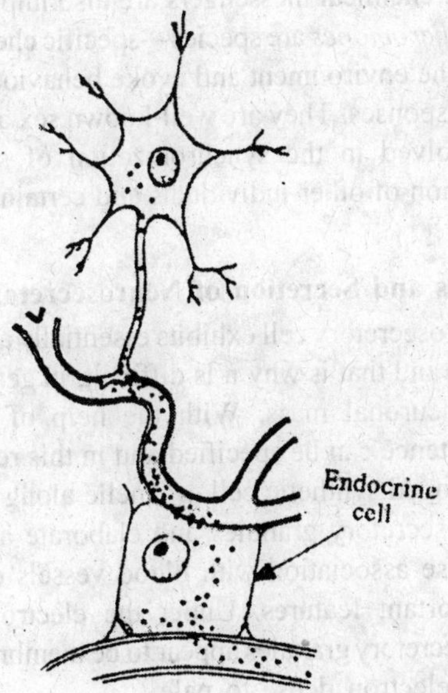

Fig. 12.3 : Two-step control, where endocrine cell is regulated by blood-borne neurosecretory substance.

Throughout the animal kingdom a measure of regulation is achieved by feedback stimuli from *tissue metabolities*. The most important is carbon dioxide, one of the universal *by-products* of metabolism. It acts directly on the cardiac and vasomotor centres in the vertebrate medulla to affect breathing and respiratory pressure. Similar reactions are also very common in invertebrates. Several other physiologically important agents are known to be formed in active tissues. The polypeptide *Bradykinin*, for example, is released by active sweat and salivary glands, it is a powerful vasodilator that enormously increases the blood flow locally and thus promotes secretion of sweat and saliva. In a comparable manner, low blood O_2 stimulates the production of more red blood cells by triggering the formation of a glycoprotein *erythropoetin* in the kidney. Other "*near hormones*" (*parahormones*) are histamine, the kinins, renin, the prostaglandins and the thymic hormone. These substances are synthesized widely in many tissue (prostaglandins) or in organs such as the kidney (renin, erythropoetin), whose obvious functions are non-endocrine. For this reason they are sometimes grouped together as *Tissues Hormones*.

Finally, some chemical messengers are also important in regulating behaviours. The *pheromones* are species—specific chemical agents which are released into the environment and evoke behavioural developmental or reproductive responses. They are well-known sex attractants, and they may also be involved in the synchronization of sexual cycles, trial marking, recognition of other individuals and certain other intraspecific reactions.

Nature, Synthesis and Secretion of Neurosecretory Cells

A typical neurosecretory cell exhibits essentially all the characteristic features of neuron and that is why it is difficult, in general to distinguish it from general neuronal mass. With the help of selective staining techniques its existence can be specified and in this respect its glandular nature, well-developed synthetic cell organelle along with the existence of stainable neurosecretory granules and elaborate axonal system as a rule ending in close association with blood vessels or haemocoels are some of the important features. Under the electron microscope the elementary neurosecretory granules appear to be membrane bound vesicles varying from the electron dense to pale.

Synthesis and secretion of neurohormones is a complex process involving in general three steps:

(a) synthesis of neurosecretory material,

(b) axonal transport, and

(c) release of secretion into the circulation.

(a) *Synthesis of neurosecretory material* : Well developed endoplasmic reticulum and Golgi apparatus clearly indicate that neurohormones, atleast in their precursor forms, are synthesized in the perikaryon of the neurosecretory cell. While concentration and fabrication of the secretory material is brought about on the Golgi apparatus, ultimately giving rise to the membrane bound vesicles containing active or precursor neurosecretory material. This view is further strengthened by the electron microscopic observations of stained neurosecretory granules in the vicinity of these cell organelles.

(b) *Axonal transport of neurosecretory material :* The synthesized material is transported from site of synthesis to the site of release by a process of axoplasmic flow. The existence of such system is further proved by many evidences such as cytological observations of stained material within axons just like a string of pearls, accumulation of secretory material proximal to a transaction of an axon and observations on moving secretions *in vivo*.

(c) *Release of neurosecretory material :* Release of neurosecretion from the axonal end bulb is again a complex process and as many as three views have been summarized by Hagadorn (Fig. 12.4). According to the first view (A) the neurosecretion someway passes out as an intact granule. Evidence in support of this idea has been obtained from earthworms and insects. Second view (B) proposes exocytosis or reverse pinocytosis as the process underlining the release of neurosecretory material. This occurs by the fusion of the granule and axonal membrane

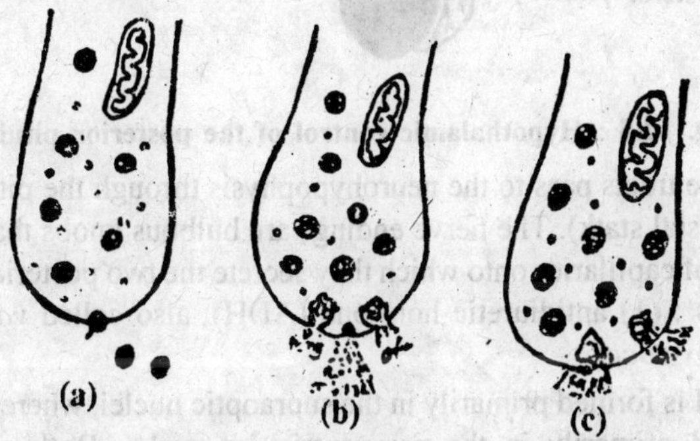

Fig. 12.4 : Mechanism of release of neurosecretory material.

followed by subsequent emptying and discharge of the hormonally active material into the intracellular space. This has been reported in the corpous cardiacum of several insects. The third possibility (C) underlines the process of diffusion. The nurosecretory material after reaching axonal end makes its way out of the granular limiting membrane and subsequently diffuses out through the neural membrane. This view is further emphasized by the occurrence of small, pale ghost granules (empty granules) in the vicinity of the supposed disrupting neurosecretory granules.

The *posterior pituitary gland*, also called the *neurohypophysis* is a neurohaemal organ where neurohormone produced in the specialized neurosecretory nuclei of the hypothalamus are stored. It is composed of mainly of glial like cells called *pituicytes*. However, the pituicytes do not secrete hormones, they act simply as a supporting structure for large numbers of *terminal nerve fibres* and terminal nerve endings from nerve tracts that originate in the supraoptic and paraventrlcular nuclei of the hypothalamus as shown in Fig. 12.5.

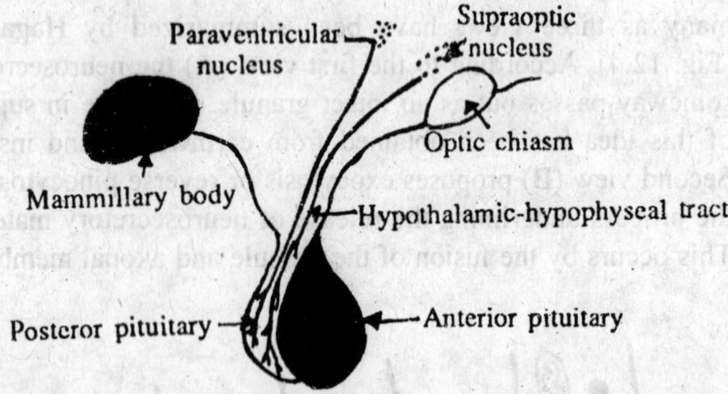

Fig. 12.5 : Hypothalamic control of the posterior pituitary.

These tracts pass to the neurohypophysis through the pituitary *stalk* (hypophysial statk). The nerve endings are bulbous knobs that lie on the surfaces of capillaries onto which they secrete the two posterior pituitarty hormones : (1) antidiuretic hormone (ADH), also called *vassopressin*, and (2) *oxytocin*.

ADH is formed primarily in the supraoptic nuclei, whereas oxytocin is formed primarily in the paraventricular nuclei. Both are proteins containing eight amino acids (octapeptide).

(1) *Antidiuretic hormone (ADH) or vassopressin* : This octapeptide is found in two types in mammalian pituitary of which arginine vassopressin is most widely distributed. Lysine vasopressin has been found in the domestic pig and hippopotamus, with molecular weight of about 1100.

The ADH plays an important role in the osmoregulation, *i.e.,* water balance of the body. It affects all the sites of water metabolism and organs concerned with water exchange. In this regard ADH has a prominent action on the kidneys. Under the influence of its higher circulating level highly concentrated urine is produced, the effect being called as antidiuretic. At cellular level, the hormone acts on epithelial cells of the distal portion of the renal tubule. It is further evident from the fact that extremely concentrated urine is produced on exogenous injection of ADH or neurohypophysial extract. The concentration is also accompanied by reduced urinary volume. Hypothalamic lesions destroying supraoptic nucleus and supraoptico-hypophysial tract produce a clinical manifestation in the laboratory animals, such as cats and dogs, known as d*iabetes insipidus*. It is characterized by the excretion of large volumes of extremely dilute urine. Such diabetic animals consume large quantities of water (polydipsia) and eliminate a large volume of urine (diuresis). This condition can be corrected by administration of vasopressin. The effect of ADH at cellular level is on the cells of the distal segment of the nephron where it selectively increases or decreases the membrane permeability for water according to the osmotic state of the body.

Some mammals like camel and kangaroo rat (Dipodomys) are adapted for desert life where problem of water conservation is very acute. Surprisingly camel can tolerate 40 per cent loss of its body water and kangaroo rat practically does not drinkwater. The desert adaptations in turn are possible as a result of metabolic and neuroendocrine adaptations. The neurohypophysis of these animals is comparatively larger in size so also turn over of ADH is considerably high. These animals thus excrete extremely concentrated urine practically without loss of water.

Physiological and pharmacological actions : Many physiologically insignificant functions have been assigned to the vasopressin. These include release of corticotrophin (ACTH) from the adenohypophysis, adrenal steroidogenesis through a direct action on the adrenal cortex and release of iodine from the thyroid,

Under the influence of ADH smooth muscles in the walls of the blood vessels undergo contractions resulting in generalized increase in the vascular resistance. In the anaesthetized animal, this effect produces a rise in blood pressure (vasopressor) and it can be used as an effective means of controlling bleeding from the gastric and oesophageal regions.

(2) *Oxytocin or pitocin :* It is also a octapeptide, with molecular weight about 1000. An oxytocic substance is one that causes contraction of the pregnant uterus-so the term oxytocin is taken from Greek word, meaning "quick birth". Two main functions have been assigned to it (i) to facilitate the ascent of spermatozoa in the female tract after coitus, thereby promoting fertilization, (ii) to stimulate uterus during parturition.

Sexual stimulation of the female during coitus increases the secretion of oxytocin, leading to uterine contraction. This is believed to promote fertilization of the ovum by causing uterine propulsion of the semen upward through the fallopion tubes.

It stimulates the myoepithelial cells of the ducts of the breasts to eject milk (*galactogogtc effect*) in response to stimuli from the nipple.

Oxytocin levels rise in labour but it is not yet clear whether oxytocin plays a part in the initiation or maintenance of labour, women with damage to the neurohypophyseal tract severe enough to cause dibetes insipidus are able to have a normal labour. Since blood levels of oxytocin are high in umbilical vein blood the foetus itself may have a role to play in its own delivery. So sometimes oxytocin or a synthetic analogue is used to induce labour or to strengthen uterine contractions in a prolonged labour. The half life of oxytocin is 1 to 4 minutes. It is metabolised in the liver and kidneys.

In addition to these above effects, it also excites the musculature of the gall bladder, uterus, urinary bladder and intestine. Its function in men is not known.

PARAHORMONES AND RELATED SUBSTANCES

Local Hormones

HIstamlne : From physiological point of view histamine is an amine, and cannot be clearly designated as hormone. But the pathological effect of histamine, when produced in excess resemble that of a hormone. It is synthesized by the decarboxylation of histamine in the most cells of the tissues or in the basophils of the blood. It is stored within the cell in granules, which are released from the cell surface.

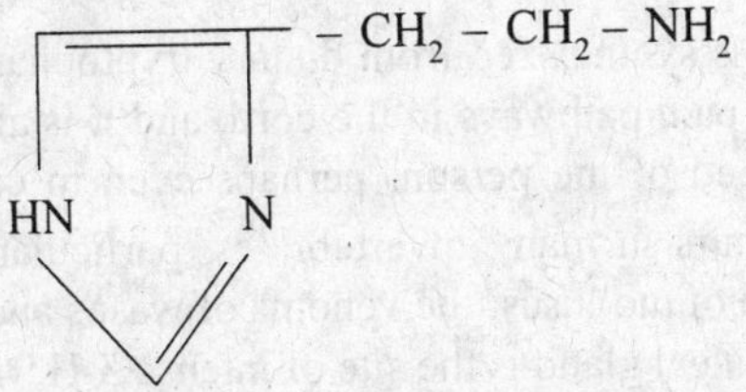

$- CH_2 - CH_2 - NH_2$

HN N

Histamine

Diagram

Histamine is formed by the decarboxylation of the amino acid histidine and destroyed enzymatically through histaminase.

Histamine increases capillary permeability and dilates the capillaries by constructing the postcapiliary sphincter and relaxing the precapillary sphincter. These effects are part of the inflammatory response to injury. It also contracts the smooth muscle of bronchi or gut and stimulates the secretion of gastric acid. Two types of histamine receptor have been identified. H_1 receptors mediate the effects of histamine on smooth muscle and on capillaries; H_2 receptors mediate the effects of histamine on gastric acid secretion.

Intravenous injection of large amounts of histamine causes "histamine shock", which has characteristics almost identical with those of anaphylactic shock (It is an allergic condition in which the cardiac output and arterial pressure often fall drastiacally), though usually less severe.

Serotonin (5-hydroxy tryptamine) : Serotonin is found in blood platelets, in the median raphe of brain stem and in the gutwall. The serum obtained from clotted blood has vasconstrictor properties due to the release of serotonin from damaged platelets.

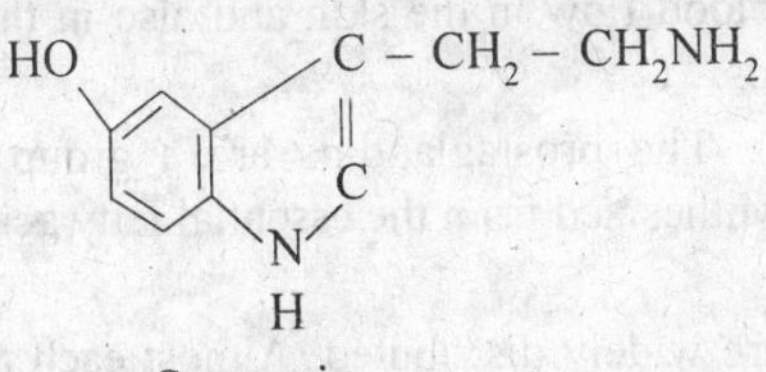

HO $C - CH_2 - CH_2NH_2$

C

N

H

Serotonin

Diagram

In the gut, serotonin is found in serotoninergic nerves and in argentaffin cells. It can cause intestinal secretion and contraction of smooth muscle.

Serotonin is synthesized from dietary tryptophan. Serotonin acts as an inhibitor of pain pathways in the cord, and it is also believed to help control the mood of the person, perhaps even to cause sleep.

It also occurs in many invertebrates, particularly abundant in the nervous system of molluscs; the venoms of wasps and scorpions are rich in 5-HT. The pineal gland is the site of intense 5-HT metabolism leading to the formation of melatonin, a harmonal substance concerned with melanophore blanching and reproductive physiology in mammals.

Kinins and bradykinin : Several substances which can cause vas odilation are called kinins and are isolated from blood and tissue fluids. One of these is *bradykinin*. Kinins cause contraction of nonvascular smooth muscle and oedema of tissue and also stimulates pain receptors.

The kinins are small polypeptides that are split away from alpha$_2$-globulins (plasma protein) in the plasma or tissue fluids. Different types of proteolytic enzymes can split the kinins from the globulin. An enzyme of particular importance is kallikrein, which is present in the blood and tissue fluids in an inactive form. kallikrein can be activated in several different ways, such as by maceration of the blood, dilution of the blood, contact of the blood with glass, and other similar chemical and physical effects on the blood. As kallikrein becomes activated, it acts immediately on the alpha$_2$-globulin to release a kinin called *kallidin*, that is then converted by tissue enzymes into *bradykinin*. Once formed, the bradykinin persists for only a few minutes, because it is digested by the enzyme *carboxy peptidase*.

Bradykinin causes very powerful *arteriolar dilatation* and also increased *capillary permeability*. It is also believed that bradykinin plays a role in regulating blood flow in the skin and also in the salivary and gastrointestinal glands.

Prostaglandins : The prostaglandins are a group of fatty acid derivatives that are synthesized from the essential fatty acid, arachidonic acid.

Prostaglandins are widely distributed. Almost each tissue contains small amount of prostaglandin. Seminal plasma and seminal vesicle, menstrual fluid, endometrium, amniotic fluid, decidua, placenta, spleen, skin, iris, lung, thyroid, thymus, submaxillary salivary gland, gastro-intestinal tracts, pancrease, kidney, adrenal medulla, cerebrospinal fluid, brain, spinal cord, phrenic nerve, vagus etc. contains prostaglandins.

Functions : The physiological functions of prostaglandins are not clear. They possess a broad spectrum of pharmacological properties including contraction and relaxation of smooth muscle, effects of levels of reproductive system and other varieties of cell function. These may be regarded as local tissue hormones that are involved in the regulation of the action of neurohormones. Possible functions of prostaglandins can be summarised as follows:

(1) (a) *Role in reproduction :* Prostaglandins have got significant role in super transport. Prostaglandins deposited in the vagina during coitus may act locally on the cervix and body of the uterus so as to help in sperm transport.

(b) *Menstruation :* There is some evidence that certain prostaglandins are related with the onset of menstruation.

(c) *Parturition :* Prostaglandin possibly takes part during labour as evident from high concentration of prostaglandin in aminotic fluid during labour.

(d) *Placental blood flow :* A umbilical cord contains high concentration of prostaglandins, it is suggested that prostaglandins may have some role in regulation of placental blood flow.

(2) *Central nerve transmitters :* There are certain evidences suggesting the role of protaglandins as neuotransmitters in the CNS. When administered by microelectpophoresis on the nerve cell, they alter the firing rates of neurones.

(3) *Lipolysis :* Prostaglandin is a potent inhibitor on lipolysis. Lipolytic effects of catecholamines, ACTH, glucagon. TSH, vasopressin, sympathetic nerve stimulation, cold stress, etc. are reduced by prostaglandins.

(4) Prostaglandins may inhibit gastric secretion.

(5) Permeability of water from tubule and bladder may be inhibited by prostaglandins.

(6) Prostaglandins are potent vasodilators.

13

ENDOCRINE GLANDS

The functions of the body are regulated by two major control systems (1) nervous system, and (2) the hormonal or endocrine system. Generally, response by the nervous system is rather localized and more rapid through the faster neural impulses and by the released of a local transmitter (neurohormone). The hormonal system is concerned, principally with control of the different metabolic functions of the body such as controlling the rates of chemical reactions in the cells or the transport of substances through cell membranes or other aspects of cellular metabolism like growth and secretion. Some hormonal effects occur in seconds, whereas others require several days simply to start and then continue for weeks, months, or even years.

The glands of the body may be divided into those with an internal secretion (endocrine glands) and those with an external secretion (exocrine glands). Examples of exocrine glands are the sweat, lacrimal and mammary glands which pass their secretion along ducts to the external surface of the body, and glands of the mouth, stomach and intestines whose secretions are passed along ducts into the alimentary canal. On the other hand, the endocrine (ductless) glands do not possess any ducts or openings to the exterior. They secrete internally and pour their secretions in the blood stream (or lymphatics). Their secretions are generally called as *hormones* that take an essential part in the life processes of the body.

Starling and *Bayliss* have defined hormone (*hormao*-to excite or arose or set in motion) as a chemical agent which is released from one group of cells and travel via the blood stream to affect one or more different groups of cells. According to Huxley (1935) hormones are information-transferring molecules, the essential function of which is to transfer information from one set of cells to another, for the good of the cell population as a whole.

The organ influenced by a particular hormone is called a *target organ.* When the target organ is an endocrine organ itself, the hormone is called a *trophic* (trophe = to nourish) hormone. All trophic hormones are secreted by the anterior pituitary alone.

Some glands are composite in nature having both internal and external secretions, (duplex glands), viz, pancrease, testes and ovaries. A gland may be temporary, lasting only for a certain period and then dying away, *e.g.,* thymus. Some glands are periodic and recurrent, *e.g.,* placenta and corpus luteum. These are provisional structures, formed to carry out functions on special occasions.

Properties of Hormones

(1) Hormones have low molecular weight, due to that, they can pass out easily through the capillaries.

(2) Since they are transferred with blood, they are soluble in water.

(3) As soon as their function is over, they are readily destroyed or in activated or excreted.

(4) They act in very low concentration like vitamins.

(5) Hormones are non-antigenic

(6) These are produced in response to specific secretory stimuli, secretion depend upon nature and intensity of the stimuli *i.e.,* low to high.

(7) In most cases, hormones are bound to specific carrier proteins while being transported in the blood (*thyroxine-binding globulin*) transporting thyroid hormone and *transcortin* transporting adrenal steroids.

(8) Every hormone acts basically by modifying some aspects of cellular metabolism, in no case does a hormone create any new biochemical process or property, for example, hormones may regulate the rate of secretion of glucose by the liver, but they do not themselves determine the ability of the liver to secrete glucose.

(9) They are organic catalysts probably acting as co-enzymes of other enzymes in the tissue.

Chemistry of Hormones

Chemically the hormones are of three basic types :

(1) *Steroid hormones :* These all have a chemical structure similar to that of cholesterol and in most instances are derived from cholesterol itself. Different steroid hormones are secreted by (a) the adrenal cortex (cortlsol and aldosterone), (b) the ovaries

(estrogen and progesterone), (c) the testes (testosterone, and (d) the placenta (estrogen and progesterone).

(2) *Derivatives of the amino acid tyroslne :* Two groups of hormones are derivatives of the amino acid tyrosine. The two metabolic thyroid hormones, *thyroxine* and *triiodothyromine,* are iodinated forms of tyrosine derivatives. And the two principal hormones of the adrenal medullae, *epinephrine* and norepinephrine, are both cotecholamines, also derived from tyrosine.

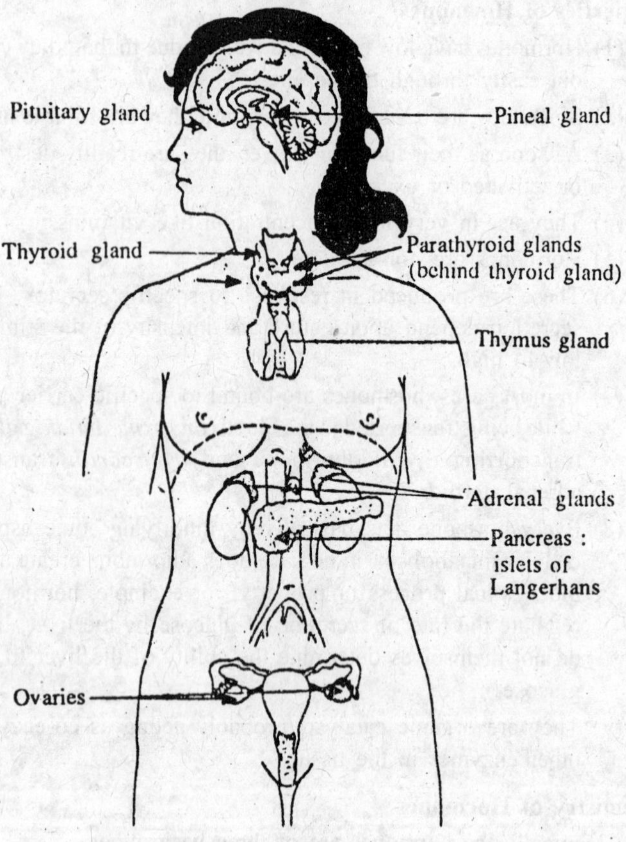

Flg. 13.1 : The anatomical loci of the principal endocrine glands of the body.

(3) *Proteins or peptides :* All the remaining important endocrine hormones are either proteins, peptides, or immediate derivatives

of these. The anterior pituitary hormones are either proteins or large polypeptides, the posterior pituitary hormones, antidiuretic hormone and oxytocin, are peptides containing only eight amino acids. And insulin, glucagon, and parathormone are all large polypeptides.

Important endocrine glands and their hormones an overview

Fig. 13.1 : Shows the anatomical position of the important endocrine glands of the body.

Anterior Pituitary Hormones

(1) *Growth hormone* causes growth of almost all cells and tissues of the body.

(2) *Adrenocorticotropin* causes the adrenal cortex to secrete adrenocortical hormones.

(3) *Thyroid-stimulating* hormone causes the thyroid gland to secrete thyroxine and Triiodothyronine.

(4) *Follicle-stimulating hormone* causes growth of follicles in the ovaries prior to ovulation, promotes the formation of sperm in the testes.

(5) *Luteinizing hormone* plays an important role in causing ovulation; also causes secretion of female sex hormones by the ovaries and testosterone by the testes.

(6) *Protactin* : promotes development of the breasts and secretion of milk.

Posterior Pituitary Hormones

(1) *Antidiuretic hormone* (also called *vasopressin*) causes the kidneys to retain water, thus increasing the water content of the body; also, in high concentrations, causes constriction of the blood vessels throughout the body and elevates the btood pressure.

(2) Oxytocin contracts the uterus during the birthing process, thus perhaps helping to expel the baby; also contracts myoepithelial cells in the breasts, thereby expressing milk from the breasts when the baby suckles.

Adrenal Cortex

(1) *Corisol* has multiple metabolic functions for control of the metabolism of proteins, carbohydrates, and fats.

(2) *Aldosterone* reduces sodium excretion by the kidneys and increases potassium excretion, thus increasing sodium in the body while decreasing the amount of potassium.

Thyroid Gland

Thyroxine and *triiodthyronine* increase the rates of chemical reactions in almost all cells of the body, thus increasing the general level of body metabolism.

(3) *Calcitonin* promotes, the deposition of calcium in the bones and thereby decreases calcium concentration in the extracellular fluid. *Islets of Langerhans in the Pancreas* :

(1) *Insulin* promotes glucose entry into the most cells of the body, in this way controlling the rate of metabolism of most carbohydrates.

(2) *Glucagon* increases the release of glucose from the liver into the circulating body fluids.

Ovaries

(l) *Estrogens* stimulate the development of the female sex organs, the breasts, and various secondary sexual characteristics.

(2) *Progesterone* stimulates secretion of "uterine milk" by the uterine endometrial glands; also helps to promote development of the secretory apparatus of the breasts.

Testes

(1) *Testoterone* stimulates growth of the male sex organs; also promotes the development of male secondary sex characteristics.

Parathyroid Gland

(1) *Parathormone* controls the calcium ion concentration in the extracellular fluid by controlling (a) absorption of calcium from the gut, (b) excretion of calcium by the kidneys, and (c) release of calcium from the bones.

Placenta

(1) *Human chrlonic gonadotropin* promotes growth of the corpus luteum and secretion of estrogens and progesterone by the corpus luteum.

(2) *Estrogens* promote growth of the mother's sex organs and of some of the tissues of the foetus.

(3) *Progesterone* probably promotes development of some of the foetal tissues and organs; helps to promote development of the secretory apparatus of the mother's breasts.

(4) *Human somatomammotropin* probably promotes growth of some foetal tissues as well as aiding in the development of the mother's breasts.

You have already studied the histology of most of the above-mentioned endocrine glands. Therefore, we will study the roles played by them in the physiology of mammals and human as base.

Pituitary Gland

The *pituitary gland*, also called the hypophysis is located at the floor of the skull just behind the optic chiasma where the optic nerves cross as they enter the underside of the brain. It lies in the sella turcica (*Turkish saddle*), a depression in the shenoid bone on the floor of the cranial cavity. It is small-about 1 cm in dtameter and 0.5 to 1 gm in weight (man), and is connected with the *hypothalamus* (part of the brain) by the *pituitary (or hypophysial) stalk.*

Physiologically the pituitary gland (Fig. 13.2), has two parts :

(a) Adenohypophysis or anterior pituitary, and (b) neurohypophysis or posterior pituitary. Between these lies a small, relatively a vascular zone called the pars intermedia which is almost absent in human being while much larger and much more functional in some lower animals.

The *hypophysis is ectodermal* in origin and embryologicaliy, the two portions of the pituitary.

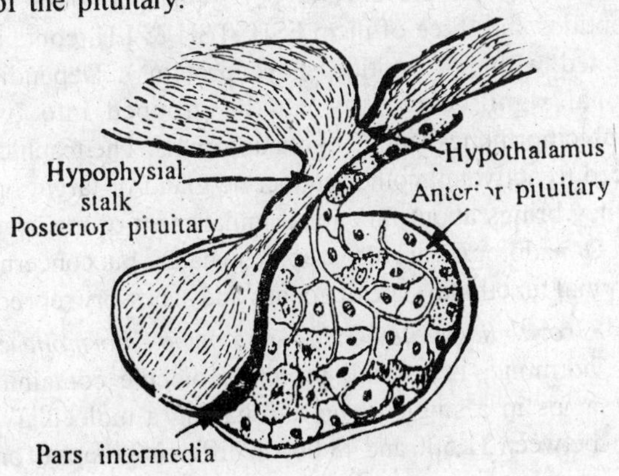

Fig. 13.2 :The pituitary gland.

Development : Thr pituitary gland is eclodermal in origin and embryologicaliy, the two portions of the pituitary originate, from different sources, the anterior pituitary from Rathke's pouch, which is an embryonic invagination of the pharyngeal epithelium, and the posterior pituitary from an outgrowth of the hypothalamus. The origin of the anterior pituitary from the pharyngeal epithelium explains the epitheloid nature of its cells, while the origin of the posterior pituitary from neural tissue explains the presence of large numbers of glial-type cells in this gland.

Adenohypophysis : Adenohypophysis is a large, compact and highly vascular structure and further, it is made up of three *parts : pars distalis;* pars tuberalis; and *pars intermedia.*

Adenohypophysis secretes six different hormones secreted by different secretory cells, and play major roles in the control of metabolic functions throughout the body, and can be listed as follows :

(1) Growth hormone GH (STH)

(2) Adrenocorticotropin (ACTH)

(3) Thyroid-stimulating hormone (TSH)

(4) Lactogenic or prolactin (LTH)

(5) Gonadotrophic hormones (GTH) or gonadotrophins.

(6) Luteinizing hormone (LH).

Acidophils and basophils or cyanophils are the hormones producing cells in adenohypophysis. The acidophils manufacture three hormones; the STH, LTH and ACTH (?). Basophils secrete FSH. TSH, and LH.

Chemically all the adenohypophysial hormones are proteins or polypeptides and three of them FSH, TSH & LH, contain carbohydrate conjugated with polypeptide (Glycoproteins). Depending upon their functional significance they can be grouped into two categories; (1) trophic hormones, and (2) gonadotropins. The trophic hormones are produced to activate another endocrine gland or target organ; and their deficiency brings about functional impairment or the specific glands or organs. Gonadotopins are also trophic in nature but concerned particularly with normal functional state of gonads and accessory reproductive organs.

1. *Growth hormone, (GH), Somatotropic hormone (STH) :* Growth hormone, is a small protein molecule containing 191 amino acids in a single chain and having a molecularweight ranging between 21,500 and 48.000 in different groups of animals (22,500 in man), it is so called because it causes growth of all (issues of the body that are capable of growing. It promotes both increased sizes of the cells and increased mitosis with development of increased numbers of cells. *Actions of Growth Hormone :*

(1) *Skeletal growth* : Stimulates the multiplication of the epiphyseal cartilage and thus increases the length of the cartilage bones. In hypophysectomised animals a membrane appears at the epiphyseal line which inhibits the growth of the cartilage cells.

(2) *Regulates' general body growth* : After administration of this hormone there is an increased body growth due to its direct effect in the tissues,

(a) *muscles* -stimulates the growth of muscles. In gigantism and acromegaly there is an increased growth of muscles.

(b) *viscera*-in hypophysectomised animal the liver cells are reduced in size, RNA and protein content from cytoplasm and nuclei reduced, and kidneys fail to function properly. After administration of GH all these defects found to be rectified.

(c) It stimulates growth of the thymus.

(d) It increases the secretion of milk during lactation.

(3) *Metabolism* : Growth hormone enhances the body proteins, conserves carbohydrate, and uses the fat stores. It is probable that the increased rate of growth results mainly from the increased rate of protein synthesis.

Growth hormone also increases the release of fatty acids from the adipose tissue and, therefore, increases the fatty acid concentration in the body fluids. This is in turn increases the use of fatty acids for supplying energy to the body. Likewise, for greater quantities of acetoacetic acid are formed in the liver and transported into the blood. Therefore, a person exposed to excessive growth hormone is much more likely to develop ketosis than in the normal person. This is called the *ketogenic effect* of GH.

GH decreases the utilization of carbohydrate for energy. Instead, glycogen is stored in the cells until the cells become saturated; thereafter, the blood glucose concentration rises above normal, for which reason it is said that GH has a *diabetogenic effect*. In addition, GH adminishes the transport of glucose into the cells, which is an effect opposite to that of insulin on the transport of glucose.

(4) *Ion or mineral metabolism* : GH increases intestinal absorption of calcium as well as its excretion. In addition to

calcium, sodium, potassium, magnesium, phosphate and chloride are also retained.

Disorders : Hypo and hyperfunctioning of the growth hormone leads to some disorders. In children, pituitary insufficiency causes *dwarfism* (midget), where there is delayed skeletal growth and retarded sexual development but alert. Intelligent, well-proportioned child. Excessive production of GH in childhood results in the rare disorder gigantism. In this there is overgrowth of all body tissues and particularly excessive bone growth. The eventual height attained may be as much as 2.6 metres (8½ feet). The growth of the limbs is relatively greater than that of the trunk, so that the tallness is largely the result of excessive growth of the legs. The internal organs are also enlarged. These patients are often mentally sub-normal and, unless treated, usually die before the age of 20.

In adults, the excessive production of GH leads to *Acromegaly* (Fig. 13.3) (gorilla-like appearance). The bones become thickened and deformed; muscles and viscera also enlarge. The most striking signs are the generalized coarsening (increase-in thickness) of the features due to

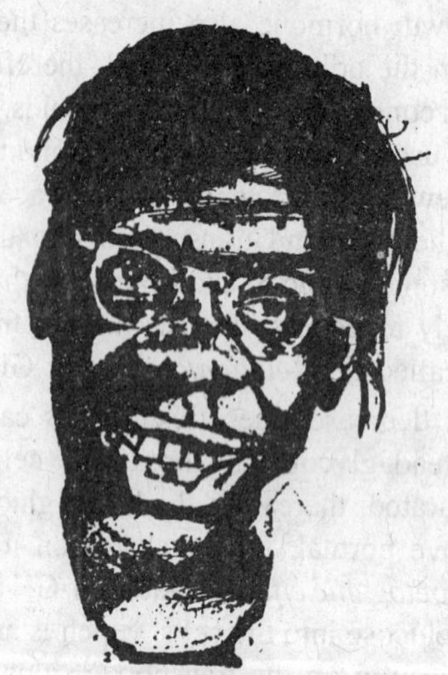

Fig. 13.3 : An acromegalic patient.

thickening of the skin and sub-cutaneous tissues and progressive enlargement of the head, hands and feet. Such patients often complain of the need for larger gloves and shoes.

Control of secretion : Little is known about regulation of secretion of GH. However, it is Supposed that hypothalamic control exists for its secretion.

2. *Adrenocorticotropic hormone (ACTH) or Adrenotrophic hormone or corticotropin* : ACTH is secreted by basophil cells and is a potypeptide composed of 39 amino acids. Its molecular weight is about 4,500.

   Action : ACTH acts on adrenal cortex influencing its synthetic activity, and are affected by a negative feedback mechanism. ACTH increases adrenal blood flow, increases the concentration of cholesterol and steroids within the adrenal cortex and increases the output of steroids, specially cortisol; into the circulation. ACTH also stimulates protein synthesis in the adrenal cortex; protonged ACTH stimulation causes hypertrophy of the adrenal cortex (*gluco-corticoids*).

   In addition, ACTH also has a lipolytic effect on adipose tissues. Another direct action of ACTH is that it possesses an intrinsic melanocyte stimutatfng activity which is due to some structural similarity with MSH.

   Disorders : Excessive output of ACTH occurs in one kind of pituitary dysfunction. It induces adrenocortical hyperplasia (cell multiplication) and hyperfunction. This pathological state is termed cushing's disease. It is a rare disorder, mainly of females. It is characterised principally by *virilism* (appearance of secondary male features in the female, obesity, hyperglycaemia) (excessive sugar in blood), glycosuria (presence of sugar in urine and hypertension).

   Control of secretion : Hypophysial secretion of ACTH is normally regulated by the hypothalamus which in turn, is influenced by blood filter of the corticosteroid. In stress, the accelerated secretion of ACTH is in part neurally effected by hypothalamus, in part by the exciting action of adrenaline on the hypothalamic centre as well as the gland itself. Median eminence of the hypothalamus appears normally involved in this regulation.

3. *Thyroid stimulating hormone – TSH or thyrotropin or thyrotropic hormone* : This is a glycoprotein with a molecular weight of about 25,000 and secreted by the basophils.

   Action : It controls various aspects of thyroid gland function including development and maintenance. It promotes accumulation of iodine and increases the quantity of intracellular colloid in the thyroid epithelial cells and induces the liberation of hormone thyroxine.

   There exists a negative feedback between circulating level of thyroxine and TSH. If the secretion of TSH is decreased due to some disease of anterior pituitary, the thyroid gland will also decrease its secretion and the animal will suffer from hypothyroidism. On the other hand, if TSH is increased, it increases the activity of thyroid gland, initiating hyperthyroidism.

   Disorders : One of the abnormalities of pituitary function is due to lack of of thyrotropin. This produces symptoms similar to those of primary hypothyroidism. This state is called *Myxoedema,* which is characterised by lethargy, apathy, skin becomes thick leathary, puffy; hairs become brittle, sparse and dry and overall slowing up of all bodily processes.

   Control : There is reciprocal regulating action of the thyroxine and TSH. The former, probably by influence upon the hypothalamus.

4. *Lactogenic hormone or prolactin or Galactin or Mammotrophic or Luteotrophic hormone (LTH)* : It is secreted during pregnancy and lactation in women by acidophil 'pregnacy cells'. It is a peptide hormone, isolated in pure form and contains tyrosine, tryptophan, cystine, methionine, arginine and sulphure. Molecular weight is about 25,000.

   Action : It exerts a lactogenic action in birds and mammals. In birds-like pigeon and doves, it enhances the production of crop milk by a process of desquamation. In mammals, usually after parturition, it brings about secretion of milk from the mammary alveoli and ductules.

   It stimulates the development of corpus luteum.

   In addition to this, prolactin also induces changes in the maternal behaviour; in some birds it promotes nesting behaviour in both the sexes.

In spotted newt, on administration of prolactin, the newt leading a terrestrial life returns to water, where it breeds or becomes sexually matured.

In short, prolactin is essential in normal circulating blood due to its role in normal breeding behaviour; pregnancy and lactation. The role of prolactin in the male is unknown.

Control of secretion : It has dual control *i.e.,* hormonal and nervous.

Hormonal control : The sex hormones and the placental gonadotropins inhibit the secretion of prolactin as is evident by the following facts; (1) Although, breasts are fully developed, yet lactation does not occur during pregnancy. It starts only after parturition and expulsion of placenta. (2) Prolactin secretion is inhibited by the injections of oestrogen, progesterone and placental gonadotropins.

Nervous control : In mammals, suckling by the baby promotes a rise in prolactin level through a reflex are whose afferent impulses arise from receptors in the nipple.

5. *Gonadotrophic hormone (GTH) or gonadotropins :* Removal of the anterior pituitary from the immature animals reduces the rate of growth and prevents the development of the gonads. Treatment with pituitary extract can correct these abnormalities. The active principle concerned with the development, maintenance and hormonal function of the gonads are the gonadotropins. The basophil cells secrete gonadotropins which control the growth and activity of the gonad and indirectly all the other processes connected with it. There are two gonadotropins (a) *Follicle-stimulating hormone* (FSH), and (b) Luteinizing hormone (LH) or *interstitial cell-stimulating* hormone (ICSH). Both the hormones are secreted by basophil cells of adenohypophysis.

   (a) *Follicle-stimulating hormone (FSH) :* It is a water soluble glycoprotein with molecular weight ranging between 30,000 and 67.000. It contains galactose, glucosamine, galactosamine, mannose, frucose etc.

   In female it stimuates the development and maturation of the ovarian follicles upto the point of ovulation. In male it stimulates the process of spermatogenesis and sperm formation. Due to its action on both male and female gametes, FSH is also known as *gametokinetic* factor.

FSH is secreted in a very small amounts only in sexually mature animals. During childhood it is not manufactured.

(b) *Luteinizing hormone (LH) or interstitial cell stimulating hormone (ICSH) :* Biochemically it is a conjugate protein with a molecular weight ranging between 26,000 and 30,000. It has the following biological actions:

In female, it results ovulation, *i.e.,* release of a mature ovum from the ovary. It works with FSH and both are responsible for the development of *corups luteum* that in turn secretes *progesterone* which maintains the pregnancy.

In males, it is known as interstitial cell stimulating hormone (ICSH). It stimulates the interstitial cells or cells of Leydig of testes to *secrete testosterone* or male sex hormone. It is involved in the maintenance of accessory reproductive organs and secondary sexual characters.

The secretion of LH is under the control of hypothalamus. It is also regulated by stimuli-like light, temperature, genital stimulation etc.

Control of Secretion of Gonadotropins

(a) *Nervous control :* The control of the secretion of the gonadotropins by nervous system is supported by the following:

(i) In the rabbit, ovulation normally takes place after 12-18 hours of mating, in presence of adenophysis intact.

(ii) Ovulation can be induced by electrical stimulation of the hypothalamic region.

It is indicated above that the act of mating in the female rabbit generates afferent impulses which are carried to the central nervous system and reflexly stimulate adeno-hypophysis. However, the exact nerve path is not known but hypothalamus seems to be involved.

(b) *Hormonal control :* The concentration of sex hormones in the blood also determines the secretion of gonadotropins. A high concentration of them inhibits, whereas low concentration stimulates the secretion of gonadotropins from adenohypophysis. Injections of estrogens and androgens for long period cause degeneration of anterior pituitary.

The functional integrity of FSH and LH : The functions attributed to FSH and LH are oversimplifications of the actual biological facts. Normal development of an egg, ovulation and maintenance of pregnancy, as a matter of fact, is the result of functional balance of these two hormones.

In males, on the other hand, the effects of gonadotropins are more clear and rather direct. In male sexual cycle FSH brings about spermatogenesis, whereas ICSH stimulates Leydig cells to function as a secondary endocrine source producing androgens.

Pars Intermedia : The pars intermedia is anatomically associated with the neural lobe and is a thin strip of tissue, separated from the anterior lobe by the *interglandular cleft.* It invests the pars nervosa and with it, forms the posterior lobe. It is prominently developed in poikilothems (fishes, amphibians and reptiles), whereas in homeotherms although it is anatomically distinguishable and possesses potential for secreting hormones, still seems to have litite functional significance.

It secretes a group of polypeptides designated as *melanophore stimulating hormones* (MSH) or intermedin. Two distinct MSH peptides are identified : α-MSH and β-MSH. The MSH peptides were named on the basis of their influence on melanophores; nevertheless, they also affect other kinds of chromatophores. They influence chromatophore system by exerting an influence on either concentration or dispersion of variously coloured granules in the chromatophores, ultimately giving them characteristic colour patterns. Thus, pars intermedia plays an important role in physiological color responses. In higher vertebrates, *i.e.,* birds and mammals chromatophores are completely absent, however, their pituitaries are capable of secreting these hormones. It is further evident from the fact that pituitary extract of these animals has got a marked chromatophorotropic effect on the chromatophore system of poikilothermic vertebrates.

Function of intermedian in man is unknown, but administration of the hormone over a period of 8 to 10 days causes intense darkening of the skin. However, this occurs in those regions of the skin which are previously pigmented; non-pigmented areas remain unaffected. *Neurohypophysis* or *Posterior Lobe* :

Anatomically the posterior lobe includes the *pars nervosa* and *pars intermedia.* But physiologically the term 'posterior lobe' commonly means the pars nervosa, which is the chief part of the neurohypophysis.

Unlike adenohypophysis, neurohypophysis is a neurohaemal organ where neurohormones produced in the specialized neurosecretory nuclei of the hypothalamus are stored. Neurohaemal nature of the neurohypophysis is further evident from the fact that its removal does not impair the normal functioning of neurohypophysial hormones.

Two hormones have been identified from the neurohypophysis; however, there is considerable overlapping in their biological actions.

The principal hormones are : *Antidiuretic hormone (ADH)* or *vasopressin*, and *oxytocin.*

For further details please see the topic *"chemical messengers"* also.

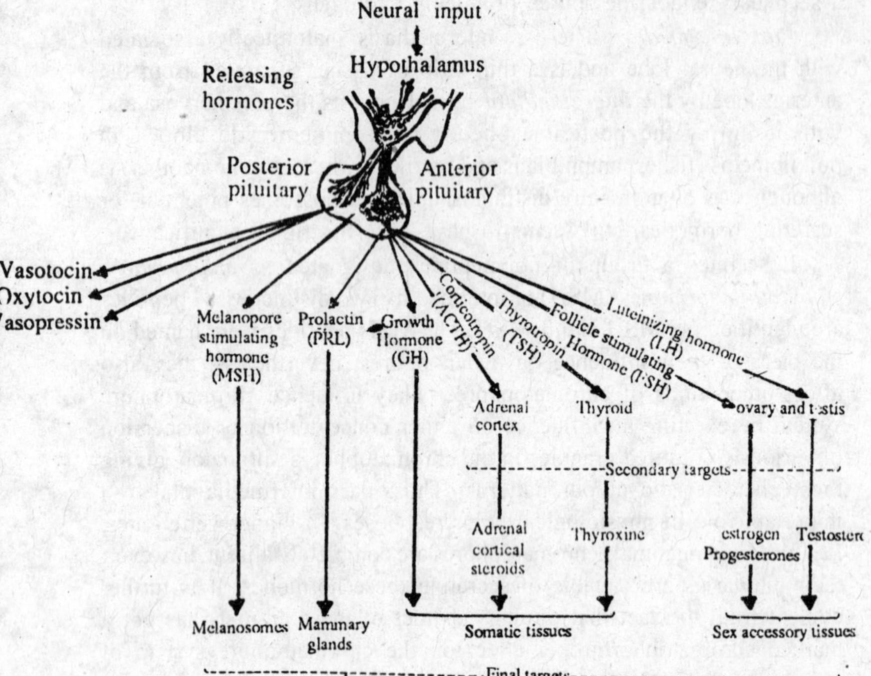

Fig. 13.4 : Hierarchial organization of endocrine control by the hypothalamus.

Thyroid Gland

The thyroid gland is situated in the lower part of the neck. It consists of *two lobes*, one on either side of the trachae, joined together by an *isthmus* which passes in front of the trachea just below the cricoid cartilage. The lobes are conical and have upper and lower poles, the upper pole extending to the side or wing of the thyroid cartilage. It receives its plentiful blood supply from the superior and inferior thyroid arteries which are respectively branches of the external carotid and subclavian arteries.

The thyroid gland develops in the floor of the embryonic mouth as a median diverticulum which grows downwards as a tubular duct with a bifurcated end that gives rise to the isthmus and part of the lateral lobes.

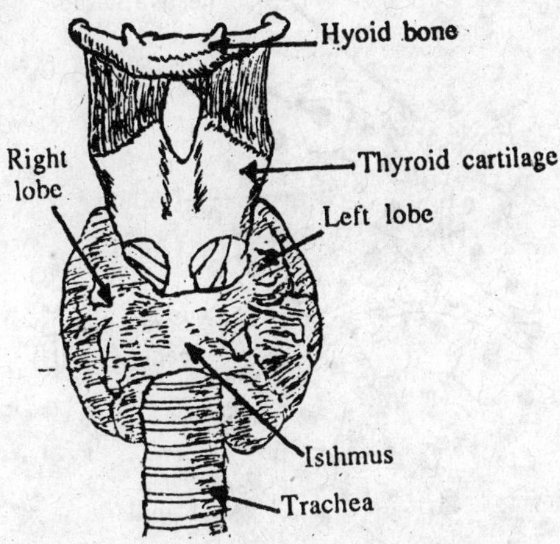

Fig. 13.5 : Anatomy of thyroid gland.

The thyroid gland, which weighs between 15 and 40 gm in a healthy adult and microscopically composed of large numbers of closed spherical follicles (150 to 300 u. in diameter) filled with secretory substance called colloid and lined with *cuboidal epitheloid cells* that secrete into the interior of the follicles. The major constituent of colloid is the large glycoprotein *thyroglobulin*, which contains the thyroid hormone called *thyroxine* and *triiodothyronine* within its molecule. Between the follicles are the *parafollicular cells* or C-cells. which produce a hormone called calcitonin or *thyrocalcitonin*.

The thyroid gland is not essential to life but it is essential for growth and for physical and mental well-being. The gland begins to synthesize thyroxine about the third month of foetal life. The secretion of thyroid hormones appears to be fairly constant throughout life but the gland enlarges and its secretion is increased at puberty and during pregnancy.

The thyroid gland contains a large amount of iodine (0.06%) almost all of which is firmly bound to protein either in the cells lining the follicles or in the colloid material within them. The characteristic protein of the colloid is thyroglobulin, on hydrolysis it gives several iodine-containing derivatives of tyrosine including mono-and di-iodotyrosine, tri-iodothyronine and tetraiodothyonine (thyroxin), as already stated. In man, dietary requirement of iodine is approximately 1 mg/week or 35 to 50 mg/yr. To prevent iodine deficiency, common table salt is iodized with one part sodium iodide to very 100,000 parts sodium chloride.

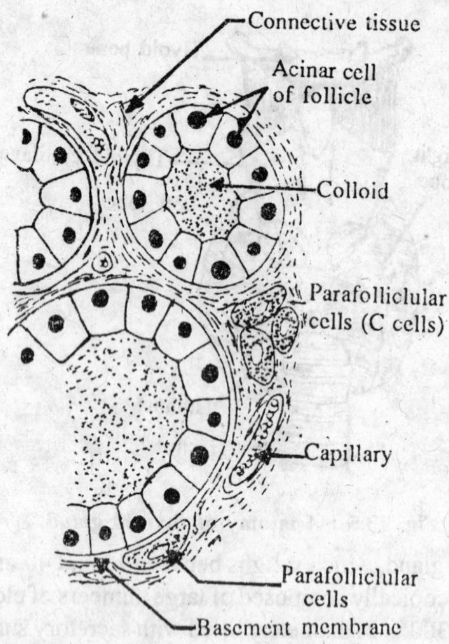

Fig. 13.6 : Histologlcal structures of thyroid gland.

Synthesis of Thyroxine

Throsine residues in thyroglobubin	Iodide (from diet) ↓ peroxidase Iodine
Mono-iodotyrosine residue ↓	Di-iodotyrosine residue
One mono-iodotyrosine and + one di-iodotyrosine residue ↓	Two di-iodotyrosine residues ↓
3,5,3-tri-iodotyronine (T_3)	Thyroxine (T_4)

Fig. 13.7 : Pathways for the synthesis of thyroxine (T_4) and tri-iodotyrosine (T_3).

Control of thyroid activity : The activity of the thyroid gland is regulated by variations in the plasma levels of thyrotrophin (thyroid stimulating hormone, TSH). The immediate action of this hormone is to release thyroid hormones from the gland. Prolonged stimulation with TSH increases the uptake of iodine from the blood and promotes hyperplasia of the gland.

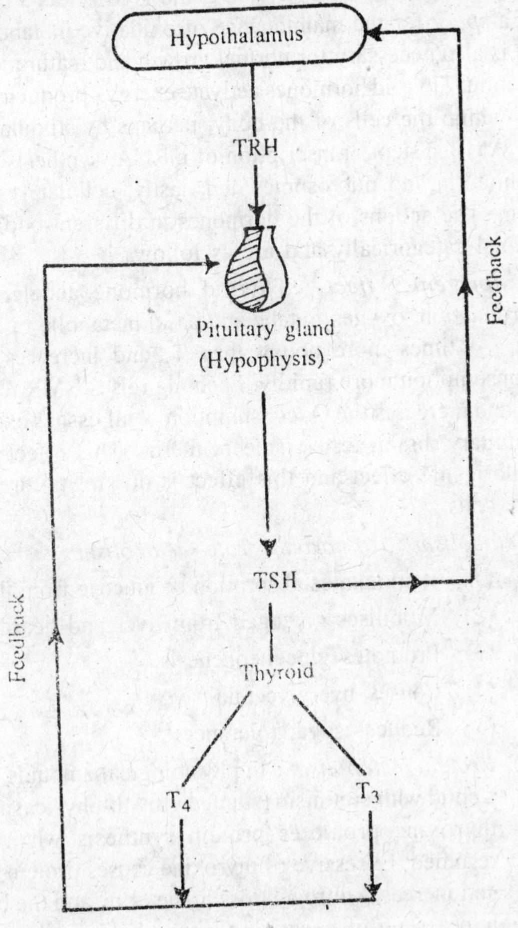

Fig. 13.8 : The hypothalamus-hypophyseal control of thyroid function.

The output of TSH from the anterior pituitary is itself governed in part by *thyrotrophin releasing hormone* (TRH), derived from the hypothalamus and in part by the plasma levels of the thyroid hormones. A fall in plasma levels of thyroxine and tri-iodothyronine increases TSH production and a rise diminishes it. There are feedback mechanisms to inhibit the secretion of TSH and TRH (Fig 13.8).

Functions of Thyroid Hormones

Principal function of the thyroid gland is to act as a catalyst of the nature of a *spark* for the maintenance of oxidative metabolism in most tissues. It is also necessary for normal growth and maturation and tissue differentiation. Thyroid hormones activate energy - producing respiratory processes within the cells of the body, perhaps by stimulating, in turn, the cyclic AMP system, transcription of mRNA, synthesis of protein in the mitochondria and microsomes and, lastly, cellular respiration and metabolism. The actions of the hormones in different bodily processes are described categorically and are as follows :

1. *Calorigenic effect :* Thyroid hormone accelerates energy production, oxygen uptake and basal metabolic rate (BMR). T_3 is 3-4 times more potent than T_4 and increases the oxygen consumption more rapidly. Each mg raises BMR to about 1000 C and increases the O_2 consumption of all tissues except anterior pituitary, brain, testes, spleen, uterus. This effect is called as calorigenic effect and this effect is due to its direct effect on the cells.
2. *Metabolism : (a) carbohydrate metabolism :*
   (1) It stimulates absorption of glucose from the intestine.
   (2) Mobilises glycogen from liver and heart.
   (3) Promotes gluconeogenesis.
   (4) Causes hyerglycemia.
   (5) Reduces sugar tolerance.

   (b) *Protein metabolism :* In physiological amounts, as when to a child with cretinism (stunted growth-physical and mental), thyroxine promotes protein synthesis when growth is resumed. Excessive of thyroxine causes protein breakdown and increases nitrogen loss in the urine and the body passes into a state of negative nitrogen balance.

   (c) *Lipid metabolism :* The concentration of most of the lipids of the serum specially cholesterol varies inversely with the level of thyroid activity. The thyroid hormone increases both the synthesis and the catabolism of cholesterol and other lipids. In hypothyroidism, the balance between the two is disrupted; there is less lipid catabolism, hence serum lipids increase.

(d) *Calcium and phosphorus metabolism* : Removes Ca and P from the bones leading to osteoporosis. Its action differs from that of parathyroid in (i) causing no rise of serum Ca, and (ii) increasing Ca loss both in faeces and urine. Similar changes are seen in Graves' disease.

3. *Kidneys* : (a) Increases nitrogen excretion, (b) Increases urine volume along with increased elimination of salt probably not by a direct effect on the kidneys but by raising the general metabolism and thus increasing nitrogenous end products which act as diuretics, (c) Increases the excretion of creatine.
4. *Growth and metamorphosis* : Thyroid is essential for normal growth and also for metamorphosis in tadpoles. In thyroidectomised animals there is retardation of growth. Growth in these animals is again initiated after administration of thyroxine.
5. *Mammary glands* : Increases the output and fat content of milk.
6. *Heart rate* : Thyroxine accelerates the rate of the normal as well as the denerated heart. It acts directly on the heart (S.A. node). The raised BMR may be an additional factor.
7. It is necessary for normal emotional responsiveness, cerebral activity, sensory activity, etc.
8. *Nerves and muscles* : Thyroid hormones influence the levels and activity of the central, peripheral and autonomic nervous systems and of the voluntary muscles. Hyperthyroid patients are nervous and irritable, and exhibit muscular tremors. Catabolism of muscles may cause wasting weakness and sometimes frank myasthenia. Autonomic stimulation causes sweating, gastro-intestinal hypermotility and vasomotor instability. In hypothyroidism, the patients are apathetic, mentally retarded. Contraction and relaxation of voluntary muscles are delayed and the gut may be sluggish.
9. It increases the tolerance to some type of drugs, *e.g.*, morphine, digitalis.
10. *Effect on respiration* : The increased rate of metabolism caused by thyroid hormone increase. The utilization of oxygen and the formation of carbon dioxide, these effects activate all the mechanisms that increase the rate as well as depth of respiration.

11. *Effect on gastro-intestinal tract :* Thyroxine increases the rate of secretion of the digestive juices, the motility of the gastro-intestinal tract and appetite. The hypertrophied patients often eat voraciously without putting on weight. Lack of thyroxine causes constipation. Diarrhoea is commonly encountered in thyro-toxicosis.
12. *Effect on the skin :* In hyperthyroidism, the temperature of the body rises. The skin becomes warm and moist, due to cutaneous vasodilation and secretion of sweat which help to promote heat loss from the body. In hypothyroidism, the skin becomes dry, pale and cool.
13. *Effect on gonads :* Under normal secretion of thyroid, the gonads functions normally. In cretins, gonadal growth is impaired and the secondary sex characters do not develop; in myxoedematous women, amerorrhoea commonly occurs. Fertility is reduced.
14. *Effect on sleep :* As already stated that the gland controls BMR. The hyperhyroidism develops extreme nervousness, feeling of constant tiredness and results increased metabolism. It becomes difficult for a person to sleep. On the other hand, extreme somnolence is characteristic of hypothyroidism.

Diseases of the thyroid : From he preceding discussion it can be concluded that thyroid gland with its hormones acts on different physiological processes, and any imbalance in its secretion causes disorders. Hyposecretion of thyroxine (hypothyroidism) produces cretinism in children and myxoedema in adults. Hypersecretion of the hormone (hyperthyroidism) causes Grave's disease or Exopthalamic goiter.

Hypothyroidism

Cretinism : Symptoms do not appear till after six months, because enough hormone is present in mother's milk. The chief features are the following:

1. The *milestones* of child's development, such as holding up the head (3 months), sitting and dentition (6-7 months), closure of anterior fontanelle (20 weeks), standing, walking, speech (12-18 months), etc., are all delayed.
2. *Skeleton :* Stunted growth, short club-like fingers, deformed bones and teeth.
3. *Skin :* Rough, thick, dry and wrinkled. Hairs scanty.

4. *Face* : Bloated, idiotic look,, thick-parted lips, large-protruding tongue. Saliva dribbling. Broad nose with depressed bridge.
5. *Abdomen* : Pot-bellied, umbilicus often protruding.
6. *Sex* : Sex glands, sex organs and secondary sex characters retarded.
7. *Mental growth* : Idiocy of varying degrees. Often deaf and dumb.

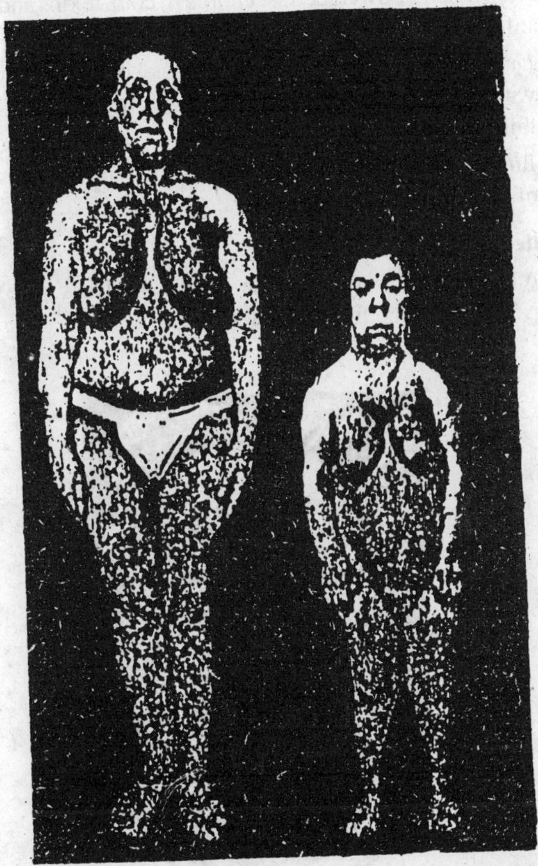

Fig. 13.9 : On the right, a cretin, aged 38 years; and on the left her normal sister, aged 48. The mental age of the cretin is about 4 years. She has a deep, croaking voice, coarse dry skin and hair.

8. *Gastro-intestinal tract and metabolism :* (a) Appetite is reduced. Motility of the gastro-intestinal tract is reduced and there is often constipation, (b) BMR lowered by 20 to 40%. (c) Low body temperature, (d) Irregular deposit of fat specially above the clavicles.
9. *Blood :* (a) Low blood sugar, (b) High sugar tolerance, (c) High serum cholesterol, (d) Low blood iodine.
10. *Resistance :* Lowered. Susceptible to cold. toxins and intercurrent infection.
11. *Urine :* Cretine excretion less. Normal output (on meat-free diet with 2g of protein per kg) is 0.6-7.8 mg daily. In cretinism it falls to 0-3.8 mg.
12. *Vitamins :* Carotene accumulates sufficiently to cause yellowing of the skin but not the sclera.

Myoxoedema or Gull's Disease

Hypothyroidism in adult human beings produces myoxoedema or Gulf's disease showing following features :

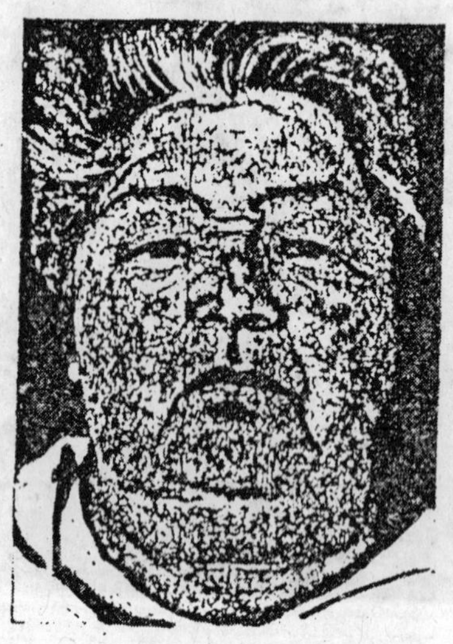

Fig. 13.10 :The face of a woman, aged 69, suffering from myoxoedema. Note the puffiness, dull expression, scanty eyebrows and dilated vessels on the cheeks.

(a) Swollen face.

(b) Mental dullness, loss of memory, slowness in thoughts, speech and actions.

(c) Lowered B.M.R. (30-40 per cent).

(d) Low temperature blood sugar and iodine.

(e) Skin is dry, nails are brittle, hairs tend to fall.

(f) Cardiovascular activity is lowered.

(g) Loss of appetite.

(h) Absence of menstruation, amenorrhoea, impotency, and failure of performance of sexual act.

Hyperthyroldism (Grave's disease or exophthalamic goiter) : In the patient with hyperthyroidism the entire thyroid gland is usually markedly hyperplastic. It is increased to two to three times normal size, with tremendous folding of the follicular cells lining into the follicles so that the number of cells is increased several time as much as the size of the gland is increased.

The chief symptoms are following:

1. Thyroid is enlarged depending upon the degree of hyperactivity of the gland.
2. B.M.R. is increased and the body temperature is increased.
3. Eyeballs protrude, with a staring look and there is less twinkling of the eyelids.
4. Body weight is reduced due to depletion of stored fats.

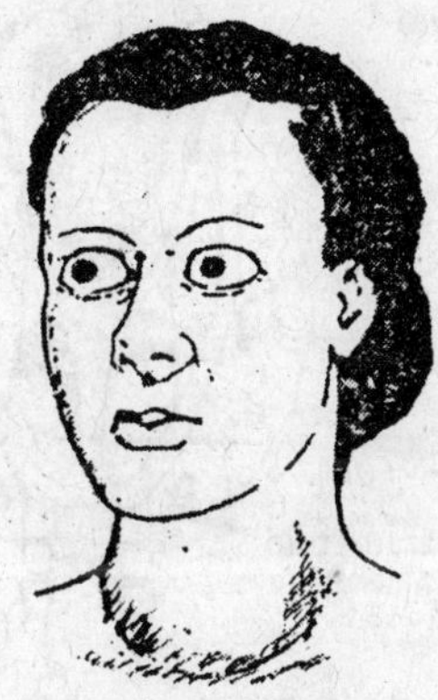

Fig. 13.11 : A patient of exophthalamic goiter.

5. The victims are mentally emotional and restless.
6. Osteoporosis results due to the excessive loss of calcium and phosphorus from bones.
7. Skin is soft and moist and is subjected to vasodilation which helps the loss of heat from the body.
8. Blood sugar and iodine are increased while calcium is decreased.
9. Heart beat rate increases. Cardiac output is increased and the victims are subjected to high or low blood pressure at different stages.
10. Due to high B.M.R. vitamin requirement is increased.

Thyrocalcitonin : This hormone is secreted by the parafollicular cells of the thyroid gland. It is a hypocalcemic, hypophosphatemic hormone. It is a protein having thirty-two amino acids. It lowers the blood calcium but increases the calcification of bones. Its effects are most striking in young animals.

Parathyroid Gland

Four small oval bodies embedded in the posterior surface of the thyroid one pair arranged vertically behind each tobe. Total weight about 140 mg. Highly vascular. Blood supply derived from paired superior and inferior thyroid arteries. Nerves supply same as the thyroid probably purely vasomotor. Upper pair of parathyroids are formed from the 4th and the lower pair from the 3rd branchial pouch.

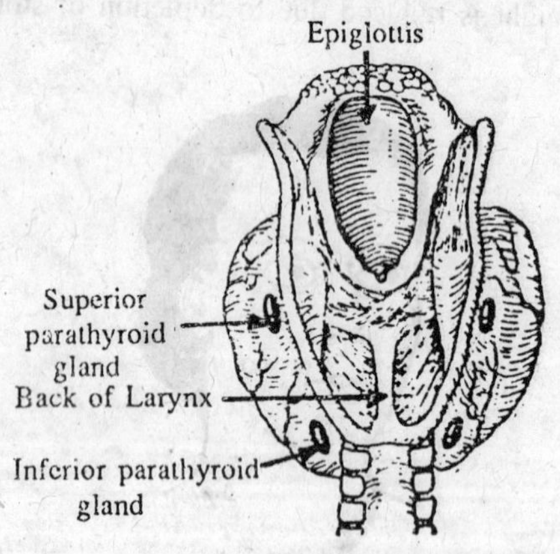

Fig. 13.12 : Anatomy of parathyroid gland.

Histology : Masses or columns of epitheloid cell, with large blood sinuses in between them. There are two types of cells-chief cells or principal cells small faintly staining non-granular cells, with clear cytoplasm and possess numerous cytoplasmic vacuoles; the cells contain glycogen. Majority in number, remain throughout the life.

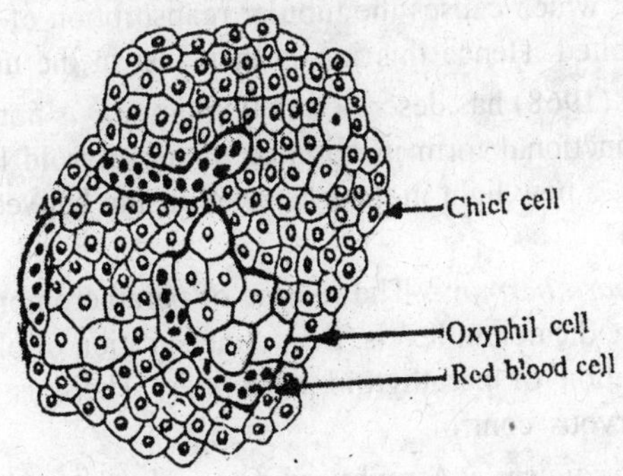

Fig. 13.13 : Histological structure of a parathyroid gland.

Oxyphil cells or eosinophil cells–These are large polyhedral granular cells and with acidophilic cytoplasm. Granules stain with eosin. These are few in number.

On the basis of cytochemical analysis chief cells are further categorised into : the *light chief cells* rich in glycogen and poor in secretory granules, and *dark chief cells* are poor in glycogen and rich in secretory granules. They are the main source of parathormone or *parathyroid hormone* (PTH). This hormone is a large polypeptide having molecular weight 9500. It consists of 84 amino acids. It is inactivated by proteolytic enzymes and cannot be taken or given orally.

Functions of Parathyroid Gland

1. The parathyroids are essential for life, as they are important for the regulation of the concentration of calcium ions in the body fluids. After parathyroidectomy the blood calcium level falls and causes a neuro-muscular irritability-the *tetany*.
2. The active principal of the parathyroid is parathormone (PTH) and acts in response to lowering of blood calcium by stimulating the osteoclasts to resorb bone and free calcium ions from the reserve skeletal depots. After administration of the hormone, blood calcium level rise due to mobilisation of calcium from the bones. With continued administration there is increase of osteoclastic activity in the bones.

3. It regulates the excretion of inorganic phosphate in the urine. After administration of parathormone there is increased phosphate excretion in the urine and serum phosphate level falls. This effect is most probably mediated by an action of PTH on the kidneys, which causes the tubular reabsorption of phosphate to be inhibited. Hence this ion is then lost in the urine.
4. DeLuca (1968) has described that vitamin D is not metabolised to its functional form in absence of parathyroid hormone. He provides a new light in the interrelationship between vitamin D and PTH.

Control of parathermone–The release of paratheromone is directly controlled by blood calcium levels. Low concentration of blood calcium causes the secretion of parathyroid hormones. There is possibly no endocrine or nervous control.

Hypoparathyroidism : Atrophy or removal of parathyroid tissue causes a fall in blood calcium level and increased excitability of neroeumuscular tissue. This leads to severe convulsive disorder called *TETANY*. This is characterised by twitching of the muscles and spasms of the hands, feet and face called *cespo-pedal* spasmar. Hypoparathyroidism increases the phosphorus level in the blood. So during the abnormality the amount of calcium is decreased and amount of phosphorus is increased in urine. Hypoparathyroidism is of rare occurrence.

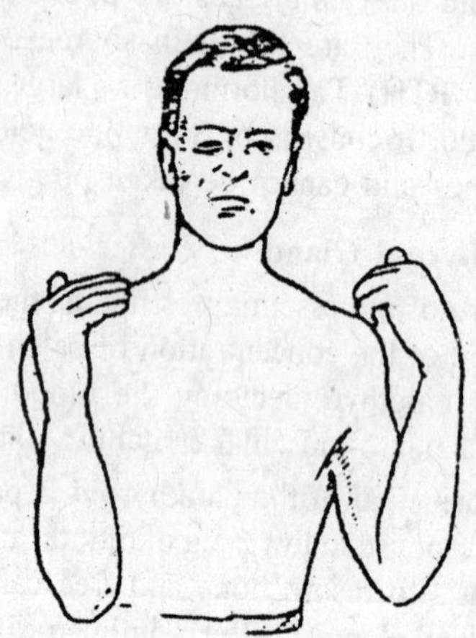

Fig. 13.14 : Tetany.

Hyperparathyroidism : It is a condition caused either by over activity of the gland or when PTH is given. In this condition, the serum calcium level rises, while serum phosphorus level falls. *Osteoclasts* become over active so that there is an excessive destruction of bone, resulting the formation of fibrous cysts called *osteitis fibrosa cystica.* It also causes extensive decalcification that may lead to bony deformities and fractures (osteoporosis). The muscles are less irritable than normally, and may become atrophied and painful. Normal calcium excretion is about 100 mg daily which is increased to 180 mg in hyperthyroidism (hypercalciurea). Sometimes, the precipitation of calcium salts occurs in kidney and results *kidney stone.*

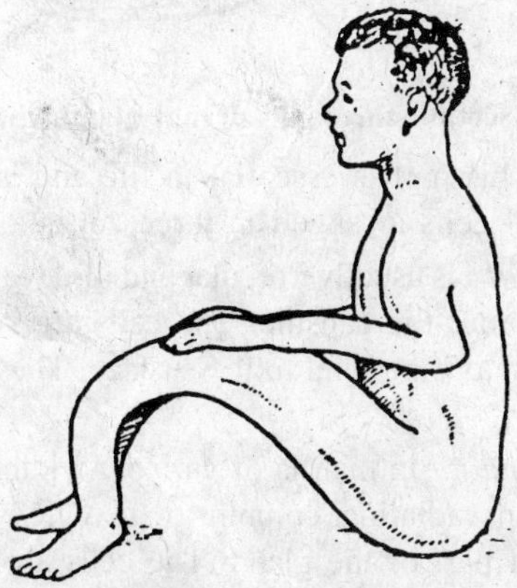

Fig. 13.15 : Osteitis fibrosa cystica.

Adrenal or Supra Renal Gland

In human beings, there are two adrenals, roughly triangular, situated on the upper pole of each kidney (hence, the name supra renal). The right gland is smaller and looks like a cocked hat; and the left one is roughly cresentric and usually larger. Each gland in the adult usually measures about 50 × 30 × 10 mm. The average weight of each gland is about 5-9 g in adults.

Adrenal gland consists of two parts : (A) outer part-the *cortex* (B) Inner part-the *medulla.* Whole enclosed in a capsule. The two parts are structurally, functionally and embryologically different. Cortex is derived from mesoderm while the medulla from ectoderm or neural crest.

Histology : The parenchyma consists of polyhedral epitheloid cells arranged in cords, generally two cells thick that run radially from capsule to medulla. Capillaries form an anastomotic network around the cords, assuring each cell of direct contact with a vessel.

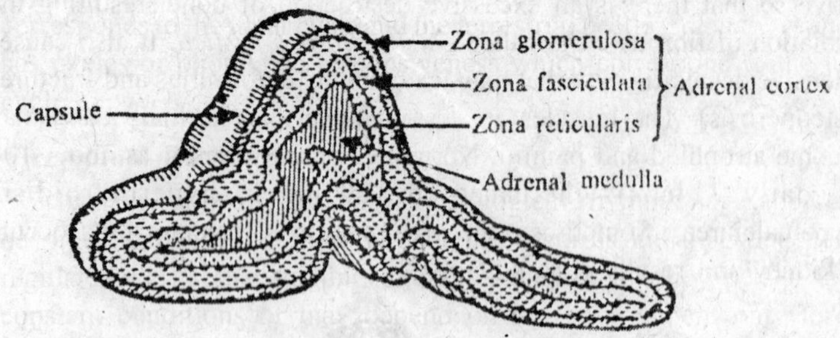

Fig. 13.16 : It shows section through adrenal gland (diagrammatic).

Adrenal cortex : This part is essential to life and is composed of large, fat rich epithelial cells arranged in three zones:

Outer *zona glomerulus* is usually irregular and ill-developed, forming islands of cells lying under the capsule. The cells are smaller, thickly set and lie with the long axis parallel to the surface. These cells secrete *aldosterone.*.

Middle *zona fasciculata* in man is of variable width. It consists of larger cells arranged in radiating columns which lie vertical to the surface. It is the widest part of the gland. The cells are rich in lipids. This zone secrete mainly *gluco-corticoids.*

Inner *zona reticularis* where the cells are arranged irregularly leaving wide blood spaces. The cells are relatively poor in lipid. This zone synthesizes mostly *sex hormones* (androgens).

The cells of the cortex have a high lipid content, the chief constituent is cholesterol, mainly in the ester form, which is the precursor of the adrenal cortex hormones.

Adrenal medulla : The adrenal medulla consists of masses of polyhedral cells separated by large blood sinuses. The cells contain granules stained blue by ferric chloride or brown by salts of chromic acid. The adrenal medulla is richly supplied by a plexus of sympathetic filaments.

The adrenal medulla secretes *adrenaline* (epinephrine) and *nor-adrenalin* (nor-epinephrine) which are often referred together as *catecholamines*. The ratio of adrenaline to nor-adrenaline in fresh human adrenals is 4:1. (80% adrenaline and 20% nor-adrenaline).

Hormones of the adrenal cortex : The hormones secreted by various layers of the adrenal cortex are commonly steroids. Nearly fifty different cortical steroids have been extracted from various animal adrenal glands, but probably not more than half a dozen are normally active and only three appear chiefly responsible for the multitudinous effects of these hormones, they are as follows :

(1) Mineralocorticoids,

(2) Glucocorticoids,

(3) Androgens.

Synthesis of adrenal steroids : Within the adrenal gland cholesterol is the precursor of all adrenal steroids. It may be synthesized there from acetate and the adrenal stores, under circumstances of high steroid output, may be replaced from circulating cholesterol. Cleavage of the

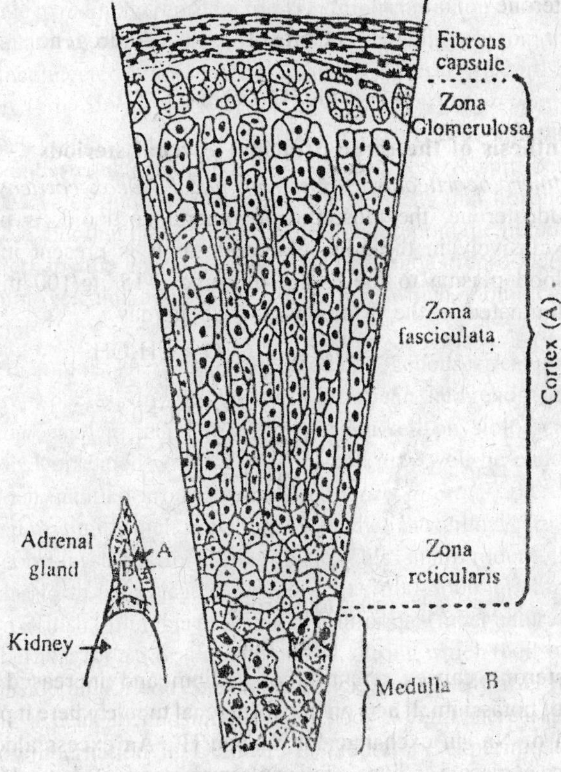

Fig. 13.17 : Section through adrenal gland.

cholesterol side chain by the enzyme, *desmolase*, produces pregnenolone. This compound in turn, under the action of the various enzyme systems present in the adrenal cortex, gives rise to the active hormones secreted by the adrenal.

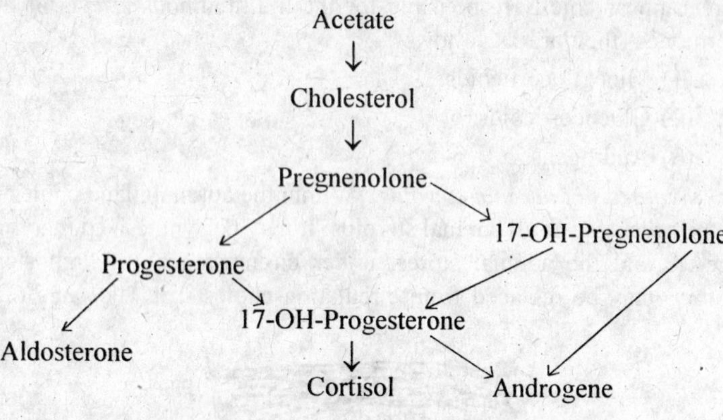

Fig. 13.18

Major synthesis of the three principal adrenal steriods

1. *Mineralocorticolds (Aldosterone and 11-Deoxycorticosterone :* Aldosterone, the most potent mineralocorticoid, is produced exclusively in the zona glomerulosa. It is present in normal blood plasma to the extent of some 2-15 μg/100 ml and is eliminated in the urine about, 5-25 μg/day.

O CH_2OH

CH C=0

HO

CH_3

O

Aldosterone

Diagram

Aldosterone causes retention of sodium and increased urinary excretion of potassium. It acts on the distal renal tubule where it promotes absorption of Na^+ in exchange for K^+ and H^+. An excess aldosterone causes a rise in plasma sodium, a fall in plasma potassium, *hypochloraemic alkalosis*, increased extracellular fluid volume and hypertension. In excess aldosterone also lowers the sodium content of sweat, saliva and gastro-intestinal secretions. The low potassium ion concentration in the body fluids (*hypokalemia*) sometimes lead to muscle paralysis. Some compounds known as spironolactones act as specific aldosterone antagonists and block the sodium-potassium exchange in the distal tubule by competitive enzyme inhibition. Lack of aldosterone leads to sodium loss, potassium retention, dehydration and circulatory collapse. Total lack of aldosterone can cause toss of as much as 12 gms of sodium in urine in a day, an amount equal to one-seventh of all the sodium in the body and, causes death within three days to a week.

Without mineralocorticoids, the sodium and chloride concentrations of the extracellular fluid decrease markedly and the total extracellular fluid volume and blood yolume also become greatly reduced. The person soon develops diminished cardiac output, which proceeds to a shock-like state followed by death. This entire sequence can be prevented by the administration of aldosterone or some other mineralocorticoid. Therefore, the mineralocorticoids are said to be the 'life saving hormones.

Cellular mechanism of aldoseterone action : Although for many years, we have known the overall effects of mineralocorticoids on the body, the basic action of aldosterone on the tubular cells to increase transport of sodium is still only partly understood. The sequence of events that leads to increased sodium reabsorption seems to be the following :

First, because of its lipid solubility in the cellular membranes aldosterone diffuses readily to the interior of the tubular epithelial cells.

Second, in the cytoplasm of the tubular cells aldosterone combines with a highly specific cytoplasmic *receptor protein*, a protein that has a stereomolecular configuration that will allow only aldosterone or extremely similar compounds to combine.

Third, the aldosterone-receptor complex diffuses into the nucleus where it may undergo further alterations, and then it induces specific portions of the DNA to form a type or types of messenger RNA related to the process of sodium and potassium transport.

Fourth, the messenger RNA diffuses back into the cytoplasm where operating in conjunction with the ribosomes, it causes protein formation. The protein formed is one or more enzymes or carrier substances required for sodium transport, possibly a specific ATPase that catalyzes energy transfer from cytoplasmic ATP to the sodium transport mechanism of the cell membrane.

Thus, aldosterone does not have an immediate effect on sodium transport but must await the sequence of events that leads to the formation of the specific intracellular substance or substances required for sodium transport. Approximately 20 to 30 minutes are required before new RNA appears in the cells, and approximately 45 minutes are required before the rate of sodium transport begins to increase; the effect reaches maximum only after several hours.

Regulation of aldosterone secretion : The regulation of aldosterone secretion is so deeply interwined with the regulation of extracellular fluid electrolyte concentrations, extracellular fluid volume, blood volume, arterial pressure, and many special aspects of renal function that it is not possible to discuss the regulation of aldosterone secretion independently of all these other factors.

(a) *Direct stimulation of the adrenal cortex* : This involves K^+ concentration. An increased K^+ concentration in extracellular fluid directly stimuates aldosterone secretion by the adrenal cortex and causes the elimination of excess K+ by the kidney. A decreased K^+ concentration in extracellular fluid decreases aldosterone production, and thus less K^+ than usual is eliminated by the kidney.

(b) *The renin-angiotensin mechanism* : A decrease in blood volume from dehydration or Na^+ deficiency brings about a drop in blood pressure. The low blood pressure stimulates certain kidney cells, called *Juxtraglomerular cells*, to secrete into the blood an enzyme called *renln*. In this pathway, renin converts *angiotensinogen*, a plasma protein produced by the liver, into *angiotensin* I, which is then convened into *angiotensin* II. Angiotensin II stimulates the adrenal cortex to produce more aldosterone. This brings about increased Na^+ water reabsorption, increase in extracellular fluid volume and a restoration of blood pressure to normal.

(c) *Neuro-secretory control* : ACTH of pituitary is primarily meant to regulate the glucocorticoid secretion. This hormone also increases aldosterone secretion to a slight extent but perhaps not enough to have major significance.

(d) *Haemorrahage stimulation* : It has been reported that haemorrhage also stimulates the adrenal cortex to produce aldosterone.

Deoxycorticosterone(cortexolone) has about one-thirtieth of the sodium retaining potency of aldosterone but causes relatively greater potassium loss.

2. *Glucocorticoids (cortisol and corticosterone)* : At.least 95% of the glucocorticoid activity of the adrenocortical secretions results from the secretion of *cortisol*, known also as hydrocortisone. In addition to this, a small amount of glucocorticoid activity is provided by *corticosterone* and a minute amount by *cortisone.*

In normal adult, it is secreted at a rate of between 10 and 30 mg/day. The rate may be considerably higher during times of stress. The half life of cortisol in the blood stream is 60-100 minutes.

The important physiological functions of adrenal cortex are briefly described below:

Table 13.1

Active Principles	**Chief Physiological Functions**
1. Adrenal Corticoids	1. On carbohydrate metabolism-Chief action. Hence, called *glucocorilcolds*-(a) stimulate formation of glycogen in the liver and muscles (b) Increase gluconeogenesis in the liver (Specially from proteins), (c) depress glucose uptake and oxidation by tissues , the enzyme hexokinase helps in the phosphorylation of glucose to glucose 6-phosphate. Glucocorticoids together with STH interfere with the phosphorylation of glucose, (d) help absorption of sugar from the intestine and possibly from renal tubules, (e) cortisol raises the blood pyruvat level and helps in the synthesis of glucose from pyruvate in the liver, (f) deficiency of cortisol proudces hypoglycaemia and increases sensitivity to insulin. Excess of cortisol produces hyper-glycaemia and depresses sensitivty to insulin.
1. GLUCOCORTICOIDS Steroids	2. On protein metabolism-Glucocorticoids (a) increase the rate of deamination and breakdown of tissue proteins to amino acids. Body proteins are lost, increasing nitrogen excretion. They also decrease protein synthesis which might be due to interference in nucleic acid metabolism, (b) Increase gluconeogenesis in the liver, (c) excess of cortisol causes wasting of muscles, osteoporosis, dissolution of lymphoid tissue and increased excretion of cretins and uric acid in the urine.

3. On lipid metabolism-Glucocorticoids (a) stimulate lipid absorption from the intestine. (b) mobilise lipid from the depot and disintegrate to form ketone bodies in the livsr. (c) excess of cortisol causes redistribution of lipid in the body, increased lipid and cholesterol level in the blood. (d) depress the synthesis of lipid from carbohydrate.

Cortisol

4. On mineral metabolism-Minimum action. There may be some retention of NaCI and water, and the increased excretion of K and PO_4.

Cortisone

5. On muscle-Cortisol and cortisone relieve muscular weakness found in hypofunction of adrenal cortex.

Corticosterone.

6. Blood-Anti-lymphocytic and anti-eosinophilic acion-causes dissolution of lymphocytes in blood and lymphoid tissues, producing (a) lymphopenia in blood; (b) involution of thymus, lymph gland, spleen, etc., (c) eosinopenia in blood.

11-Dehydrocorticosterone.

7. Blood pressure-Hypotension found in deficiency of the adrenal cortex is rectified after administration of cortisol.
8. Protect the body against stress (fright, temp, bleeding etc.)
9. Bones-Excess of cortisol causes osteoporosis due to decalcification and interference in formation of protein matrix.
10. Central nervous system-In hypofunction of the adrenal cortex, *e.g.*, in Addison's disease, the function of the central nervous system is deranged. It is rectified after administration of cortisol.
11. Cortisone-has a special action in curing certain types of arthritis.
12. Anti-inflammatory effect-At high concentrations; glucocorticoids decrease cellular protective reactions and in particular, retard migration of leucocytes into traumatised areas.

	13. Exocrine secretory effect-Chronic treatment with glucocorticoids causes increased secretion of HCI and pepsinogen by the stomach and trypsinogen by the pancreas.
2. MINERALOCORTICOIDS	1. On mineral and water metabolism - Greatest action. Hence, called mineralocorticoids : (a) retention of NaCI and water, (b) increased excretion of K. and (c) intracellular K lowered and Na raised. (a) Steroid
(a) Steroid	2. On carbohydrate and protein metabolism-Little action.
	3. More effective in protection against stress.
Aldosterone.	4. Does not inhibit the secretion of ACTH.
Deoxycorticoid	1. On mineral and water metabolism-Pronounced action, but less than Aldosterone. Also named as *mineralocorticoids* : (a) retention of NaCI and water, (b) increased plasma volume, (c) increased excretion of K, and (d) intracellular K lowered and Na raised.
Deoxycorticosterone or	2. On carbohydrate and protein metabolism - Action much, less than glucocorticoids.
Deoxycortone.	3. Regulates renal function.
	4. Most potent in maintaining life of adrenalectomised animals.

Control of glucocorticoid secretion : ACTH of adenohypophysis stimulates the adrenal cortex to secrete increased quantities of glucocorticoids cortisol and corticosterone. An elevated concentration of cortisol in the blood causes negative feedback to the adenohypophysis to reduce the productions of corticotropin (ACTH).

3. *Androgens* : Small quantities of sex-hormones, androgens and oestrogens are produced by the supra renal gland. These influence sexual development and growth. They cannot maintain secondary male characteristics after castration even when the gland is fully stimulated by ACTH. In females the supra renal glands are the principal source of androgens, which are required by both sexes for normal pubertal and skeletal development.

Adrenal medulla : Adrenal medulla consists of irregular masses of polyhedral granular cells, surrounded by blood sinuses. Granules represent stored adrenaline, disappearing during secretion and reappearing after rest. They stain black with osmic acid and brown with chromic acid. For the last property, they are called chromaffin (ganglion) cells. This region is richly supplied by a plexus of sympathetic nerves.

The adrenal medulla secretes adrenaline (epinephrine) and nor-adrenaline (nor-epinephrine) whichare combinely called as catecholamine.

Chemistry and synthesis of adrenomedullary hormones :

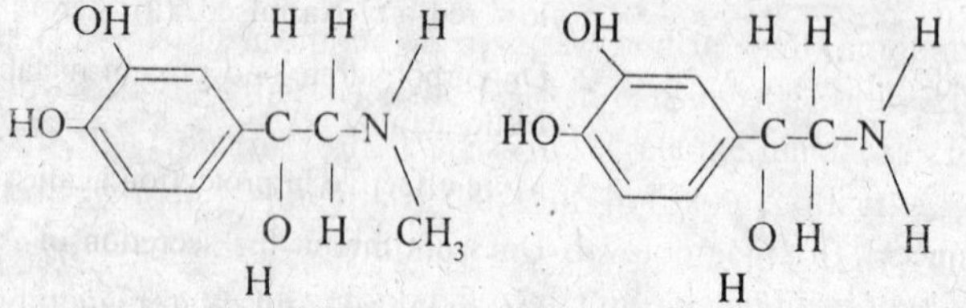

OH, HO–(benzene ring)–C(H)(OH)–C(H)(H)–N(H)(CH_3)

Adrenaline

OH, HO–(benzene ring)–C(H)(OH)–C(H)(H)–N(H)(H)

Noradrenaline

Diagram

These catecholamines are formed from amino acids, tyrosine and phenylalanine by hydroxylation and decarboxylation. Steps and enzymatic processes involved in the synthesis of catecholamines from phenylalanine and tyrosine have been presented in Fig. 13.19.

Phenylalanine —(Pheny lalanine hydroxylase)→ Tyrosine —(tyrosin e hydroxylase)→ DOPA

DOPA —(Aromatic L– aminoacid decarboxylase)→ Dopamine

Dopamine —(dopa min e B– oxidase)→ Norepinephrine —(Phenylethano– –lamin e–N– metyl transferase)→ Epinephrine

Fig. 13.19 : Schematic representation of biosynthesis of catecholamines.

Epinephrine (Adrenaline) : It is one of the active principles of adrenal medulla. Epinephrine content of the resting gland is about 0.1% mg of its moist weight. Total store in both glands is about 10 mg in man.

Actions of epinephrine : Its action on different tissues and systems are briefly summarised below:

(1) On Circulation

(A) Heart

1. Rate, force and output increase.
2. Myocardium-excitability increased.
3. Bundle of His-conductivity raised.

(B) Blood vessels

All constricted except coronary vessels and those of skeletal muscles. Although splanchnic vessels constrict, yet the intestinal vessels are believed to dialate.

1. *Constriction of :* (a) skin and splanchnic vessels mainly (volume of limb, kidneys, intestine, etc., diminishes) and of (b) cerebral and pulmonary vessels. But these are less affected due to poor sympathetic supply. They passively may dilate due to raised blood pressure.
2. Dilation of (a) coronary vessels, (b) vessels of skeletal muscles.

(C) Blood pressure

Rises sharply and comes down slowly and even below the basal level. Systolic blood pressure rises. Diastolic blood pressure may fall. But mean arterial blood pressure is raised. Total peripheral resistance is increased due to vasoconstriction in the skin and splanchnic area causing decrease of total vascular capacity of the body.

(2) On Respiration

(A) Bronchial muscles relax causing dilatation of bronchioles and cause shrinkage of the mucosa and diminution of secretion of mucus (hence, its therapeutic use in Asthma). The rate and depth of respiration are increased. The metabolic rate is accelerated, hence RQ is increased.

(B) *Epinephrine apnoea :* This is not seen in man. In animals, respiration becomes shallow and even may cease at the height of raised blood pressure following epinephrine injection.

(3) On Anterior Pituitary

Epinephrine stimulates anterior pituitary to liberate ACTH, which again helps in the release of glucocorticoids mainly.Glucocorticoids increase blood sugar through a process of gluconeogenesis.

On skeletal muscles :

A. Excitability and contractility raised.

B. Onset of fatigue delayed.

C. Muscles glycogen converted into lactic acid and discharged into the blood stream.

D. Exert anti-curare action (curare paralyses myoneural junction).

(4) On liver

Glycogen is mobilised due to increased breakdown of liver, glycogen.

(5) On Blood

A. Blood sugar raised due to : (1) Glucogenolysis from liver, (2) Formation of glucose from lactic acid of muscles (3) Increased gluconeogenesis due to increased liberation of glucocorticoids.

B. Blood lactate increases due to breakdown of muscle glycogen.

C. Coagulability raised (coagulation time reduced).

D. A rise in serum potassium.

E. Red cell, white cell, platelet count, percentage of haemoglobin, as also blood volume raised, due to contraction of spleen. It causes a fall in the number of circulating eosinophils.

F. Plasma proteins concentrated.

(6) On Kidneys

A. Urine volume reduced.

B. Renal circulation diminished (caused by constriction of renal vessels, specially the efferent glomerular vessels).

C. May cause glycosuria (due to hyperglycaemia).

(7) On Metabolism

A. Basal metabolic rate is increased by moderate doses of epinephrine, large doses cause a fall.

B. Respiratory quotient. O_2 consumption rises by 20-40 % and CO_2 production by 30-50 %. Hence, respiratory quotient rises.

C. Carbohydrate metabolism. Blood sugar is raised due to breakdown of glycogen (glycogenolysis) in the liver and muscles. Epinephrine activates phosphorylase in the liver and skeletal muscles, and hence blood sugar rises.

(8) On Smooth Muscle

A. Intestine-Movements inhibited, spincters closed.

B. Gall bladder-Contraction of gall-bladder.

C. Urinary bladder-Relaxation of bladder and constriction of sphincter.

D. Uterus-Effects not uniform. In labour and puerperium inhibited.

E. Spleen-Contraction.

F. Eye-Dilation of pupils, due to contraction of dilator pupillae muscle and retraction of lids due to contraction of the smooth muscle of the lids.

(9) On Skin

A. Contraction of arrectores pili causing standing of the hairs. Other smooth muscles of the skin also contract.

B. Sweat gland-In human beings sweating can be induced by intradermal administration of epinephrine in small amount. But in some animals, though the glands are innervated by sympathetic nerves, yet sweating cannot be induced.

(10) On Nervous System

Epinephrine but not norepinephrine produces a sense of restlessness, anxiety and fatigue.

(11) On Spinal Cord

Large doses of epinephrine diminishes muscle tone and somatic reflexes (knee jerk, etc.). This is due to a direct depressant action of the cord, independent of any circulatory or other changes.

(12) On Salivary Gland

Salivary glands have got both sympathetic and parasympathetic innervations. The two nerves act synergistically and for the same reason their respective neuro-humours, norepinephrine, likewise epinephrine and acetylcholine have got synergistic effects on the secretion of salivary glands. Epinephrine or norepinephrine stimulates thick mucinous secretion and aceylcholine stimulates profuse watery secretion. Thus total volume of salivary secretion is increased when epinephrine and acetylcholine are administered at a time.

(13) On Lacrimal Gland

Lacrimal glands receive secretory fibres from the parasympatheic but not from the sympathetic. Stimulations of the parasympathetic always cause secretion,. but sympathetic stimulation has got no such effect. Epinephrine likely has got no effect on lacrimal secretion.

(14) On Melanophores

The effects of MSH on the dispersion of melanin granules within melanophores are antagonised by catecholamines through adrenergic α-receptors.

Control of Epinephrine Secretion

Nervous control : Hypothalamus is the higher centre which controls the sympathetic and epinephrine secretion. This centre may be affected in two ways : (a) directly, and (b) reflexfy.

(I) The following factors affect the centre directly :

(a) Higher centre. Excitement generally stimulates secretion.

(b) O_2 lack, CO_2 excess, increased H-ion concentration, etc. stimulate. They also exert reflex effects through sino-aortic mechanism.

(c) Blood sugar level. Hypoglycaemia stimulates, hyerglycaemia depresses the centre.

(II) The following factors affect the centre reflexly :

1. *Sino-aortic reflexes* : (i) Raised blood pressure depresses, lowered blood pressure (haemorrhage, etc.) increases epinephrine secretion, (ii) O_2 lack, CO_2 excess, increased H-ion concentration stimulate. The sino-aortic nerves exert a tonic inhibitory control over adrenal medulla, section of these nerves stimulates secretion.
2. Exposure to cold stimulates epinephrine secretion reflexly. This helps in two ways : (a) Vasoconstriction of the skin-reducing heat loss. (b) Increased metabolic rate - raising heat production. Thus in cold climates, epinephrine plays a great part in heat regulation.
3. Any acute sensation, viz, pain, heat, etc., stimulates reflexly.

Nor-epinephrine (nor-adrenaline) or levarterenol or levophed : Nor-epinephrine is another hormone, discovered from adrenal medulla. It is the immediate precursor of epinephrine. It is supposed to be the actual sympathetic transmitter produced at the endings of the adrenergic fibres.

Commercial epinephrine, as usually extracted from the adrenal medulla, contains about 18% nor-epinephrine. Hence, the effects of the commercial epinephrine is due to the presence of both. Normally, when adrenal medulla secretes, it liberates both the hormones. Consequently, the effects of stimulation of adrenal medulla (or sympathetic) in the body is due to both the hormones.

Action : Except for a few instances, the actions of epinephrine and nor-epinephrine are very similar. The chief differences are as follows Table 13.2.

Table 13.2

Human Systems	Epinephrine	Norepinephrine
1. Heart		
a. Rate	Increased	Slightly increased
b. Output Raised	Raised	No change
c. Blood pressure systolic pressure	Raised	Raised
Diastolic pressure	No change	Raised
Mean arterial pressure	Increased	Raised
2. Vessels	Dilator for some (muscle) constric--tor for others.	Entirely constrictor
3. Respiration	Stimulated	Stimulated
4. Kidney	Constrictor of renal vessels.	Constrictor of renal vessels.
5. Uterus		
Non-pregnant in rat or cat	Inhibited	Inhibited
6. Central nervous system	Increased mental anxiety	No effect
7. Metabolism		
a. O_2 consumption	Increased	Increased
b. Blood sugar	Increased	Increased
c. Free fatty acid release	Increased	Increased
8. Eosinophil count	Increased	No effect
9. Intestine	Increased	Inhibited.

Control of nor-epinephrine secretion : Adrenergic endings continuously secretes nor-epinephrine which is essential for the normal control of vascular tone and so, blood pressure. It is believed that changes in the blood pressure level regulate the liberation of nor-epinphrine from both the adrenergic endings and the adrenal medulla. The increased liberation of this hormone in emergent condition is not of primary importance.

From these observations the following facts about epinephrine secretion are known :

(1) *Continuous tonic secretion at rest* : Nerve impulses from different parts of the body are constantly stimulating adrenal medulla and so it is believed that small amounts of epinephrine are continuously being secreted.

(2) *Emergency secretion* : *Cannon* and his associates have shown that adrenal medulla liberates its secretion in emergent condition which disturbs the mental or physical state of the subJect, *e.g.*, in times of stress, emotion threatened dangers, etc. Any other emergent condition which disturbs the normal mental or physical state of the subject stimulates epinephrine secretion, for instance, physical exercise, exposure to cold, fall of blood pressure, asphyxia, anoxia, cerebral anaemia, hyoglycaemia, anaesthesia, stimulation of afferent nerves, acute sensations like pain, heat, cold, etc., and so on.

Epinephrine secreted under such conditions, reinforces the already mobilised sympathetic action and prepares the whole body in such a way that the subject can cope with the situation successfully. For this reason, it is called the gland for *fright, fight and flight*. During muscular exercise the secreted epinephrine causes the following changes : (i) Redistribution of blood from one part to another. (ii) Increases coronary flow rate and force of heart beat, raises blood pressure and cardiac output-thus assuring adequate blood supply to the muscles .and enabling the heart to deal effectively with the increased venous return.

(3) Increases pulmonary circulation for carrying more oxygen.

(4) Increases cerebral circulation to maintain an adequate cerebral control.

(5) Raises the red cell count and thereby the O_2 carrying capacity of blood, thus; ensuring more oxygen supply to the muscles.

(6) Increases coagulability of blood assuring quicker coagulation in case of bleeding.

(7) Delays the onset of fatigue.

(8) Dilatation of bronchioles-helping pulmonary ventilation.

(9) Mobilises liver glycogen and raises blood sugar, so that tissue cells may get enough fuel.

(10) Stimulates tissue oxidation and raises basal metabolic rate.

In this way epinephrine prepares the subject in such a way that, muscular activity can be carried on with advantage for a longer time.

The secretion of nor-epinephrine from adrenal medulla during emergency has secondary importance only.

Summary of the functions of adrenal medulla : From the above observations, functions of adrenal medulla can be summarised as follows:

1. Reinforce sympathetic action (sympathomimetic).
2. Helps to keep the normal resting blood pressure at a steady level by adjusting the rate of epinephrine secretion. Fall of blood pressure stimulates, rise of blood pressure depresses secretion via sinoaortic nerves.
3. Secretes more epinephrine during emergency and enables the subject to fight out the situation successfully.
4. Takes part in heat regulation.
5. Takes an important part in metabolism-specially in carbohydrate metabolism.

Adrenaleotomy : Total adrenalectomy usually follows the death of an animal within 10 to 15 days. Like cortex, removal of medulla is not so fatal and animal can survive without it under laboratory care. Adrenal cortex, on the other hand, is extremely essential for the life. Insufficiency of the adrenal cortex can also arise because of (i) destructten of the cortex by disease, (ii) Failure of adenohypophysis to secrete ACTH, or (iii) congential failure of steroid secretion (*virllism*). Chronic adrenal malfunctioning is called *Addison's disease* in which secretions of both cortisol (glucocorticoid) and aldosterone (mineralocorticoid) is insufficierit. Generalized features in the adrenal deficiency can be summarised as :

1. Loss of appetite, vomiting, fall of blood pressure and muscular weakness.
2. Subnormal body temperature and lowered BMR.
3. Excessive renal loss of sodium chloride and bicarbonate. At the same time there is a diminished clearance of potassium. The excretion of sodium is accompained by a diuresis. Excessive loss of bicarbonates decreases pH of the blood with subsequent acidosis. Thus, there is an increase in the blood potassium calcium, phosphate and non-protein nitrogen.
4. Hypoglycemia, *i.e.,* decreased level of the blood sugar.
5. Signs of the renal failure.

Injections of the adrenal extract or *overactivity* of the adrenal cortex bring about a series of metabolic complications. Clinical manifestation of *adrenal overactivity* is called, as *Cushing's syndrome*. The main features of Cushing's syndrome are :

1. Wasting and weakness of the skeletal muscles, especially of the limbs. This in turn is due to the breakdown of muscle proteins and lowered level of plasma calcium.
2. Centripetal redistribution of fat with wasting of the extremities. The face appears moon shaped, *i.e.,* rounded with narrow eyes and fish-like mouth. The abdomen becomes pendulous.
3. State of hyperglycemia usually depends on the efficiency of patient's pancrease, if sufficient insulin is secreted hyperglycemia may not be evident.
4. There are sexual changes such as impotence and hypogonadism in the male and amenorrhea in the female.
5. There is a little change in the ionic concentration of plasma. however, tendency of sodium chloride as well as chloride retention is enhanced.

Endocrine Pancrease

Pancrease is found between stomach and duodenum and in addition to its digestive functions, secretes two important hormones, insulin and glucagon.

Histology : the pancrease is composed of two major types of tissues, as shown in Fig. 13.20. (i) The acini, which secrete digestive juices into the duodenum, and (ii) The Islets of Langerhans, which do not have any means for emptying their secretions externally but instead secrete insulin and glucagon directly into the blood.

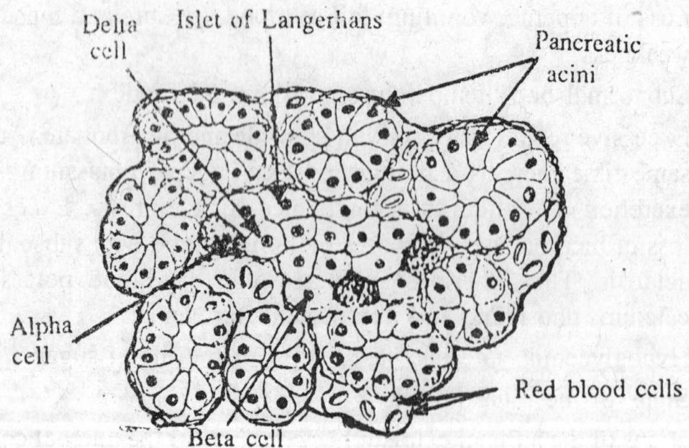

Fig. 13.20 : Physiologic anatomy of the pancrease.

The pancrease of the human being has almost a million islets of Langerhans, each only a hundred or so microns in diameter and organised around small capillaries into which its cells secrete their hormones. The islets contain three major types of cells, the *alpha* (α), *beta* (β), and *delta* (γ) cells, which are distinguished from one another by their morphology and staining characteristics. The beta cells, constituting about 60% of all the cells, secrete Insulin. The alpha cells, about 25% of the total, secrete *glucagon*. And the delta cells, about 10% of the total, secrete a more recently discovered hormone, *somatostatin*. In addition, atleast one other type of cell called PP cells, is present in small numbers in the islets and secrete a hormone of doubtful function called *pancreatic polypeptide*.

The close interrelationships among these different cell types in the islets of Langerhans allow direct-control of secretion of some of the hormones by the other hormones. For example, insulin inhibits glucagon secretion, and somatostatin inhibits the secretion of both insulin and glucagon.

Insulin : Insulin was first isolated from the pancrease in 1922 by *Banking* and *Best*. It is a small protein with a molecular weight of 5808 for human insulin. It is composed of two amino acid chains, connected to each other by bisulfide linkages. There are 51 amino acid residues arranged in two chains, the A-chain containing 21 and the B-chain 30 residues.

Function of insulin : In condition of insufficient insulin, there are increased gluconeogenesis, glycogenolysis, hyperglycaemia, ketogenesis, polyuria and etc. The functions of insulin can be summarised as follows:

(1) Effect of Insulin on Carbohydrate Metabolism

(a) *Oxidation of sugar* : Insulin increases combustion of sugar in the tissues and also helps in the transport of glucose into the cells.

(b) *Glycogen formation and storage* : Insulin increases synthesis of glycogen from sugar and lactate both in the liver and muscles. This is called the directive effect of insulin.

(2) Effect on Protein Metabolism

(a) *Prevents gluconeogenesis* : Glucose is normally formed from proteins and lipids in the liver. In diabetes, this process is enhanced.

(b) Insulin stimulates protein synthesis (proteogenesis) and growth, *e.g.*, nitrogen retention bone formation, etc.

(c) Insulin increases the synthesis of messenger RNA. It is possible that insulin is concerned with the activity of intracellular structures, *e.g.*, ribosomes involved in protein biosynthesis.

(d) During insulin lack, amino acids are catabolised (proteolysis) providing source of energy.

(3) Effect on Fat Metabolism

(a) Prevents formation of ketone bodies : In advanced diabetes, excess ketone bodies are formed in the liver, due to incomplete combustion of fatty acids. After administration of insulin, more sugar burns and liver glycogen increases displacing the lipids. Hence, lipid combustion is discouraged and ketosis disappears.

Glucagon : Glucagon is also known as *hyperglycaemic glycogenolytic factor*, (HGF) and is secreted by the α-cells of the islets of Langerhans. It is a polypeptide hormone with 29 amino acids having molecular weight of 3,485. It has following *Functions* : (i) This hormone stimulates *glycogenolysis, gluconeogenesis* and glucose release by the liver as other defenses against glucose starvation of tissues. (ii) It is also an important regulator of amino acid metabolism. It activates gluconeogenesis and promotes adaptive synthesis of enzymes within the liver cells. These actions enable the hormone to provide long term protection against hypoglycema. (iii) It is responsible for lower blood levels of calcium, higher excretory levels calcium, an increase in heart rate, and an increase in the force of cardiac contractions. (iv) It reduces the intestinal motility and gastric secretion.

Control of Secretion of Islets Cells

(1) *Nervous control* : There is some evidence that stimulation of vagus increases insulin secretion. Normally blood sugar adjusts the vagal tone and modifies insulin secretion. High blood sugar stimulates and low blood sugar depresses the vagus. But this mechanism is least effective and is only a means for fine adjustment.

(2) *Control by blood sugar level* : The blood sugar concentration of arterial blood entering the pancrease is the best controller for the secretion of insulin by islets cells. High blood sugar stimulates while low blood sugar depresses. This action is perhaps direct on the islets tissues independent of nerves.

The hypoactivity of the gland or removal of pancrease results in the following:

Hypoglycaemia is a condition in which blood sugar level is present below the normal level *i.e.,* below 80 mg per 100 ml. Since the nerve cells have very little stored food and since they use sugar mostly as the sole source of energy. Hypoglycaemia will, therefore, affect the nerve cells first. Hence, the earliest symptoms will be nervous in origin. For instance: (1) A feeling of fatigue, weakness and hunger. (2) Extreme anxiety and irritability. (3) Abnormal behaviour as in alcohol poisoning. (4) Tremores develop and fine movements are not possible. (5) Vasomotor disturbances such as flushing, perspiration chillness. (6) There may be diabetic coma and convulsions and loss of deep relfexes.

Hyperglycaemia is a condition in which blood sugar increases above the normal level *i.e.,* above 120 mg per 100 ml and sugar appears in the urine. Lack or diminished secretion of insulin is the main factor which produces hyperglycaemia and *glycosuria* as in *diabetes mellitus.*

Glycosuria is a condition when the blood glucose level exceeds 180 mg glucose per 100 ml blood above the normal blood glucose level (60-100 mg) glucose per 100 ml blood. At this time the renal tubule cells are not able to reabsorb all the glucose. Some glucose reaches the urinary bladder and glycosuria results.

Diabetes mellitus : The term *diabetes* means that a large volume of urine is passed. The term *mellitus* (= sweet) dates from the time when the urine was tested by tasting and the urine in this condition is sweet to the taste.

Hyperglycaemia, glucosuria, ketosis, acidosis, diabetic coma (unconsciousness). Polyuria, weight loss in spite of polyphagia (condition of increased appetite) and polydipsia (condition of increased thirst) are the abnormal characteristics of diabetes. Diabetes mellitus is a disorder of metabolism characterised by high blood sugar level and excretion of sugar in urine.

The Pineal Body

The pineal body (epiphysis cerebri or conarium) of human brain is a somewhat flattened, cone-shaped, grey body measuring about 5-8 mm in length and 3-5 mm in breadth. It is attached by a short hollow stalk to the roof of third ventricle. It is covered by a capsule formed from piamater.

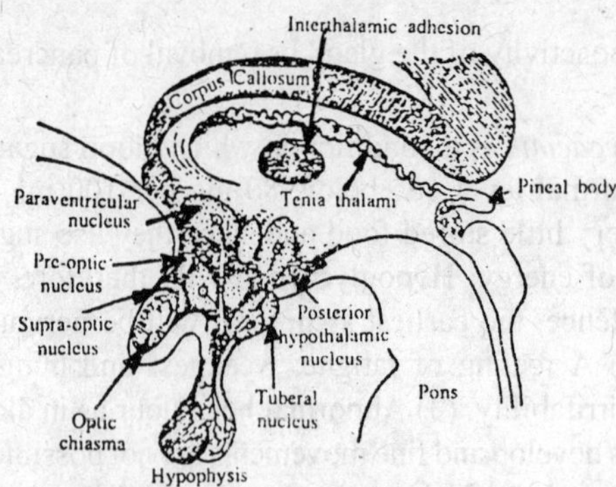

Fig. 13.21 : Segittal section of human brain stem showing the anatomical position of pineal body.

In some lower vertebrates like *sphenodon*, the gland consists of two bodies, para pineal organ which is exposed through the roof of the skull as a "third eye" and a deep lying epiphysis.

Histology : The cells of the pineal are neural in origin, but bear little resemblance to nerve cells when fully differentiated. There are atleast two types of a major cells : (i) *parenchymal* or chief cells (pinealocytes) have large irregular nuclei and a moderately basophilic cytoplasm, (ii) *Interstitial* or *supportive cells* or *glial cells*. These are stellate in appearance and lie between the clusters of pinealocytes and in perivascular spaces. The cytoplasm is somewhat more basophilic.

Connective tissue cells, mast cells, Sehwann cells, and axons of autonomic nerves are also present in the pineal.

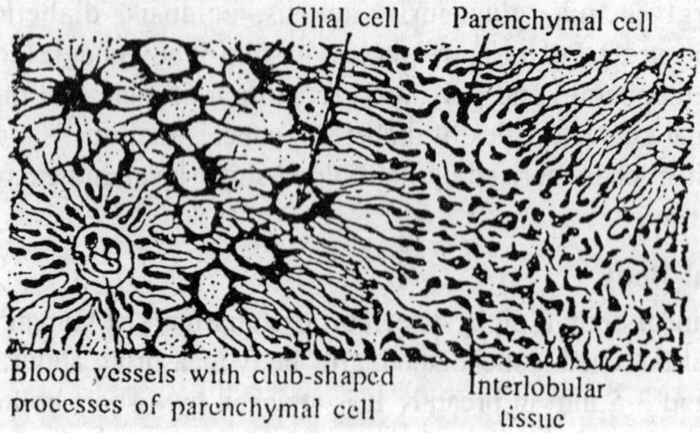

Fig. 13.22 : Semidiagrammatic representation of an adult human pineal body showing two lobules.

Functions : It has been reported that pineal gland contains high concentration of melatonin. It is *N-acetyl-5-methoxytryptamine.* It has been named melatonin because it lightens the skin of the tadpoles by an action on the melanophores. Melatonin is synthesized from *5-hydroxytryptamine-the serotonin.* Serotonin is converted into melatonin by the enzyme *hydroxyindole-o-methyl transferase* (HIOMT).

It is source of growth inhibited factor.

The pineal body seems to have a neuroendocrine function. The pineal seems to participate in the regulation of the rythmic activity of the endocrine system, by the elaboration of specific hormone or compounds such as methoxyindoles. The main stimulus for this secretion may well be mediated by visual reflexes.

It has been discovered that melatonin inhibits the activities of the ovaries. During daylight hours, light entering the eye stimulates neurons to transmit impulses to the pineal that inhibits melatonin secretion. Witthout melatonin interference, the ovaries are free to step up their hormone production. But at night, the pineal gland is able to release melatonin which slows down the estrous cycle and slows down ovarian development. The removal of pineal body or its non-functional state in children is associated with premature (precocious) puberty. An excellent case of precocious puberty has been reported in human-being. The youngest mother on record gave birth to a full term healthy infant by cesarean section at 5 years, 8 months,

Another function of the pineal gland might very well by regulating the activities of the sexual endocrine glands, particularly the *menstrual cycle.*

The pineal may also secrete a hormone called *adreno-glomerulotropin.* This hormone may stimulate the zona glomerulosa of the adrenal cortex to secret aldosterone.

Feedback Mechanism of Hormone Secretion

The principal function of endocrine system is to maintain the internal environment of body constant in fluctuating external environment. For the maintenance of such constancy many homeostatic mechanisms come into play.

None of the endocrine glands is completely independent. They are closely interrelated and interdependent. The interrelationship may be synergistic or complementary, permissive and inhibitory. They live like a hormonious family, guiding and controlling one another, being complementary to some and antagonistic to others. Consequently, hypoactivity or hyperactivity of a gland will lead to corresponding changes in the other related endocrines. For instance, hyperpituitarism (anterior) may lead to hyperthyroidism. A reciprocal relation is often observed, *e.g.*, if a gland A stimulates another gland B, then B depresses A, directly or indirectly through other glands. For instance, anterior pituitary stimulates thyroid, gonads and adrenal cortex; while the secretion of any one of three glands depresses the particular trophic hormone of anterior pituitary. Means, a hormone often regulates its own secretion indirectly through other glands. This is known as the *feedback* or *push-pull* mechanism. This may be a fundamental rule of endocrine regulation. Feedback may be defined as *the influence of the output of a system upon its input*. Two types of feedback mechanisms are known: (1) *negative* and (2) *positive*.

Most of the vertebrate endocrine glands are the examples of negative feedback and a few are of positive feedback type.

(1) *Negative feedback* : Negative, feedback mechanism works as follows : (i) The endocrine gland has a natural tendency to oversecrete its hormone. (ii) Because of this tendency, the hormone, exerts more and more of its control effect on the target organ. (iii) The target organ in turn performs its function. (iv) But when too much function occurs, usually some factor about the function then *feeds back* to the endocrine gland and causes a *negative effect* on the gland to decrease its secretory rate. Thus, the function of the hormone is monitored, and this information in turn provides negative feedback control of the secretory rate by the gland.

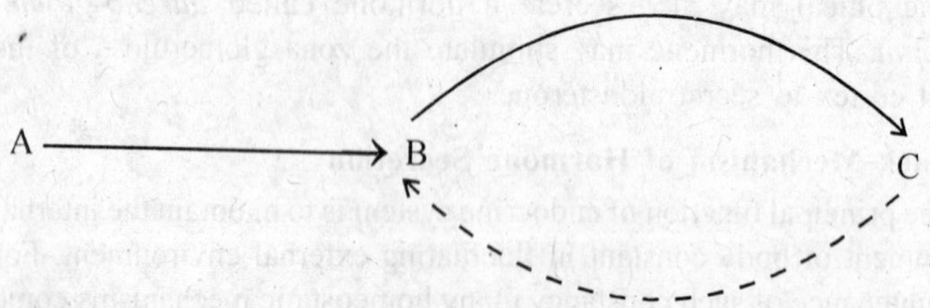

Fig. 13.23 : Negative feedback showing when variable A increases, variable B increases lading to an increase in variable C. But an increase in variable C leads to a decrease in variable B.

Fig. 13.23 demonstrates that A stimulates B, and B stimulates the formation of C. But increased formation of C inhibits B.

Negative feedback mechanism can be explained by taking the example of pituitary-thyroid interrelationship. The pituitary secretes the tropic hormone thyrotropin (TSH) which stimulates the thyroid gland to increase the rate of production of its hormone, thyroxine. As the amount of thyroxine rises in the blood, a concentration level is reached that begins to feedback directly on the pituitary to suppress the production of TSH. This leads to stoppage of stimulation of the thyroid gland and the level of thyroxine does not rise further. As the thyroid hormone is utilised, catabolised and excreted, its concentration falls. This soon leads to release of the pituitary from feedback inhibition by the thyroxine and it once again starts producing thyrotropin. In this way a delicate balance is established between the pituitary and the thyroid gland, and which more or less automatically controls the rate of secretion of thyroid hormone.

Similar type of negative feedback mechanisms operates between the pituitary and other target organs, viz, adrenal cortex, ovary and testis.

Some times, this typical negative feed back system is known as "closed-loop control system". The signal from the controlled variable is feed-back into system, forming a closed loop and is used to maintain a steady state.

(2) *Positive feedback* : Positive feedback mechanisms are rare. Fig. 13.24 demonstrates the positive feedback. Here A stimulates B, and B stimulates the formation of C and again C stimulates B.

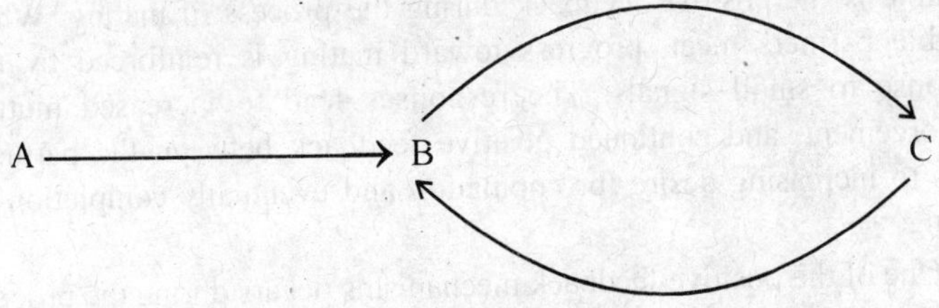

Fig. 13.24

A positive feedback makes a system change more and more rapidly toward some extreme state.

A well known example of positive feedback is the digestive enzyme *trypsin*, which is secreted from the pancrease as inactive *trypsinogen*. Trypsinogen is transformed into active trypsin by the intestinal enzyme *enterokinase*. However, trypsinogen is also activated by trypsin, and as more trypsin is formed, the activation of trypsinogen proceeds more and more rapidly. This is known as autocatalytic activation of the enzyme and is a typical case of positive feedback. A similar autocatalytic reaction applies to the activation of *pepsin* in the stomach, again a case of positive feedback.

There is an interesting example of positive feedback in the generation of the *menstrual cycle*. Low levels of estrogens stimulate the secretion of *follicle-stimulating hormone* (FSH), which, in turn, stimulates the secretion of *follicle-stimulating hormone* (FSH), which in turn, stimulates the secretion of estrogen—a positive feedback relationship that increases the levels of both estrogen and FSH in the blood. As the hormone levels rise sufficiently, positive feedback is terminated as negative feedback. This happens because high concentrations of the estrogen inhibit FSH production, causing a change in feedback sign. Secretion of both FSH and estrogen is thereby largely curtailed until another cycle of positive feedback begins to build up the concentrations of these hormones.

Apart from endocrine system, the positive feedback occurs in other system also, as in the generation of a nerve impulse. We know that a slight decrease in the membrane potential of a nerve increases its permeability to sodium ions, and the consequent increased influx of sodium inturn further decreases the membrane potential, giving a positive feedback situation that results in a full action potential in the nerve. Positive feedback thus can serve to amplify a small signal and bring about a full response.

Positive feedback often is useful in synchronizing events. A familiar example is the positive feedback during the process of mating. When suitable partners meet, progress toward mating is reinforced by the response to small signals. The responses lead to increased mutual reinforcement, and continued positive feedback between the partners leads to increasing desire for copulation and eventually completion of mating.

One of the positive feedback mechanisms occurs during the process of coagulation . There are three important stages of blood coagulation, (i) formation of prothrombin activator, (ii) conversion of prothrombin into thrombin, and (iii) conversion of fibrinogen into fibrin by thrombin. In addition to converting fibrinogen into fibrin, thrombin increases the formation of prothrombin activator. This causes formation of more and more amount of prothrombin activator so that the process of coagulation is accelerated and blood loss is prevented quickly. Positive feedback mechanism occurs during milk ejection reflex and parturition also, by the secretion of oxytocin.

14

CHRONOBIOLOGY

Life of organisms including man, evolved on a planet that rotates on its polar axis every 23 hours 56 minutes and 4 seconds to provide a diurnal cycle of day and night, while it revolves around the sun once in 365, 26 days to create a progression of seasons from summer through winter and back again to summer. At the same time, the more complicated movements of the moon in relation to the earth and sun produce our lunar month and the tidal cycles. These diurnal and annual periodicities, the lunar and the tidal cycles have been exploited by animals and plants during their phylogeny to measure time and to use this temporal information advantageously. *Chronobiology*, is the recent branch of biology which deals with the study of internal rhythmic mechanisms for linking physiological and behavioral events to predictable environmental conditions (such as summer or winter day or night).

Many moths and butterflies emerge from their cocoons at dawn when the still, somewhat moist air provides the best conditions for slowly drying their unfolding wings. Bats emerge from their caves or roosts at dusk each evening to forage for insects or fruits and return before dawn to sleep during the daylight hours. These activities and a host of other animal behaviour patterns occur on a regular daily basis. Many songbirds of north temperate deciduous forest fly southward during the autumn, over winter in tropical or subtropical zones and begin their return flight northward as spring approaches. Woodchucks emerge from their winter dens in spring, remain active for four to six months, and return to hibernation by late autumn. During their months above ground they mate, produce offspring, rear the young, and prepare for another winter. These and other activities occur on an animal cycle. These rhythmic and cyclic activities of organisms depends on environmental factors like day and night, tides, lunar phases etc. which acts as clocks for controlling the behavioural activities, so called *biological clocks*. Biological clocks are internal timing mechanisms that involve both a self sustaining physiological pacemaker and an environmental cyclic synchronizer. *Biological rhythms* are those animal activities and behaviours which can be directly related to distinct environmental frequencies. Biological rhythms are the external manifestations and are regulated by biological clocks.

History

About 300 years before Aristotle, men wrote about plants that raise their leaves to the sky during the day and fold them at night. But it was not noticed for another 2,400 years that the leaves would rise and fall even when the plants were indoors under artificial light and apparently deprived of environmental information regarding the time of day. Then it was found that even in plants that were kept in total darkness and at a constant, temperature, the leaves would continue to rise and fall with a startling regularity. This mean, of course, that the organisms were somewhat able to keep time, and so the search for the "biological clock" was on.

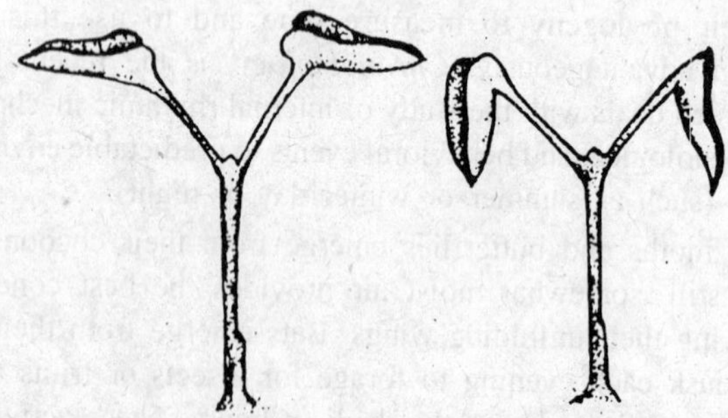

Fig. 14.1 : The normal sleep movements of plants. The leaves rise mórning and fall at night. Such movements persist even the plant is placed under constant artificial light or in total darkness and even temperature.

The first reports of biological clocks from America come from *John Welsh*, at Harvard (working with crustaceans) and *Orlando Park* at Northwestern (working with insects) in 1934. The response to their work was unfortunate. The scientific community greeted their reports with distinct coolness, and their evidence was almost ignored. For the most part, biologists simply found it very difficult to accept either of the two proposed hypotheses : independent internal timers, or the ability to read exceedingly subtle environmental clues. It was generally though that the fault may with experimental techniques. Then, in 1948, *Dr. Frank A. Brown*, stated that organisms time themselves by environmental clues. The major work in India is in much progress at Madurai Kamraj University.

Biological Rhythms

Any regularly oscillating process is called *rhythmic* or *periodic*; it may follow a sine wave pattern or it may be asymmetric. The physical characteristics of a rhythm are described using following terms:

Cycle : The shortest part of a rhythm which repeats itself indefinitely: it may be taken from trough to trough or peak to peak.

Period : The time occupied by a cycle;

Amplitude : The distance between the extremes, *i.e.,* the trough and crest

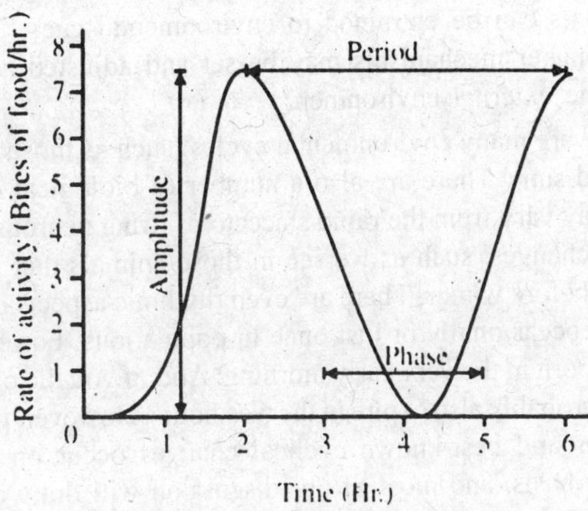

Fig. 14.2 : Biological rhythm including period, phase and amplitude.

In addition, the following terms are applied to rhythmic physiologic processes:

Diurnal : A rhythm whose period is a day.

Circadian : A more recently introduced term describing a rhythm whose period is around 24 hr.

Nycthermal : The alternation of day and night. Biological rhythms may be characterised by several specific properties. First, whereas temperature changes after the rate of most chemical reactions and cellular processes, biological rhythms are *temperature-compensated.* Generally the rate of a chemical reaction doubles for each 10°C increase in temperature. However, biological rhythms are relatively insensitive to change in temperature. This is significant, for if biological rhythms were speeded up or slowed down by ambient temperature changes, they would not keep accurate time.

Second, biological clocks are generally unaffected by metabolic poisons or inhibitors that block biochemical pathways within cells. We might expect that, application of a metabolic poison, such as sodium cyanide, would alter the period of biological rhythm, yet this does not happen.

A third properly is that the periods of biological rhythms occur with approximately the same frequency of one or more environmental features. Fourth biological rhythms are self-sustaining, maintaining approximately their normal cyclicity even in the absence of environmental clues. Lastly, biological rhythms can be entrained to environmental cues. The self-sustaining pacemaker mechanisms may be set and adjusted according to input from the external environment

Just as there are many environmental cycles (such as those imposed by the moon and sun). There are also a number of biological rhythms. Such rhythms may vary from the rapid staccato of firing neurons to slow yearly seasonal changes, such as we see in those animals that build up fat or store food before winter. There are even rhythmic aspects of events that occur. Only occasionally or just once in populations. For example, most people are born in the very early morning. And, if you die of natural causes, you will probably also expire in the wee hours. However, probably the most obvious and best-known cyclical changes occur on about a twenty-four-hour basis, and most of our discussion will draw on these daily changes.

It should be pointed out that rhythms may not be solely related to abiotic (nonliving) influences such as temperature and light. They may also be coordinated with the activities of other organisms, which may be, in turn, locked in step with the environment. Bees time their visits to flowers so that they arrive at the time when they are beginning their daily period of nectar secretion. This means the bees can gather the maximum amount of food with a minimum effort, and it means the flowers, which open with the sun, need not waste energy by continuously secreting their enticing nectar. There are numerous examples of rhythms of one species coordinating its activities with another groups. Owls hunt mostly at night when the mice are out, and mice come out at night when they can't be seen.

Differences in the rhythms of two species occupying the same range may be important in reducing competition. Fly-catching birds and bats are not in direct competition because of the time differences in their feeding behaviour.

Some animals show an interesting age-dependent rhythmicity. They may operate on one time schedule early in their lives and on another one later. For example, badgers play in the sun near their den when they are young. As they grow older, they gradually shift their period of greatest activity toward evening and night. Such shifts are accompanied by other changes in behaviour. The younger badges are quite calm during the day, but as they grow older, they become more uneasy during the day and increasingly bolder at night. In some cases, night time activity may be a function, not so much of photo period, but of the amount of moonlight that is illuminating the environment. Prey animals can be seen far more easily in moonlight than starlight and therefore some of them tend to restrict their activities to periods when the moon is down.

It is not entirely correct to speak of the rhythm of an organism. Since several cyclic events may be taking place simultaneously within a single organism. Furthermore, such rhythms may be entirely out of phase with each other. Proper co-ordination in timing called *phase-relationships* among the various internal physiological processes are sometimes critical. Substrates, enzymes, energy resources, and information-carrying molecules must appear in a properly spaced sequence if the body is to function on a coordinated whole. For example, in chick embryos the importance of the phase relationship of cellular constituents is indicated by the rather sudden appearance of a great many enzymes, on about the eleventh day of incubation. After their rapid formation in the watery embryonic tissues, they begin functioning in proper phase relationship to each other.

As an indication of the complex nature of the biological clocks, it has been found that all the cycles occurring within a single individual may not be in step with the same aspects of the environment. For example, intertidal crabs change colour in time with local day-night cycles, and they also vary cyclically in their "running periods", the time of greatest activity. Interestingly, the light dark period takes place over about a 24 hour interval and corresponds with the appearance of the sun; but there are two running periods, one usually at night. The other during the day. The running periods arrive fifty minutes later each day and correspond with the rise and fall of the tide, so we see that crabs are able both on solar day and lunar day.

Biological rhythms are not always coordinated with the onset of some ecological event. In some cases, the adaptiveness of a particular rhythmic pattern is not apparent when the pattern begins. There are instances when a certain behaviour must begin at such a time that it will end at a critical period. Here, the environmental event is "predicted", for example a wide-ranging nocturnal animal must stop hunting and begin its trek home so that it will reach the protection of its burrow before day break. It may not be immediately apparent to an observer why an animal abandons a promising hunt to turn homeward.

So, from above discussions we can conform that biological clocks are self-sustaining pacemaker mechanisms which may set and adjusted according to input from the external environment.

Types of Rhythms

Depending on the period, duration of day and night, tidal activities, lunar cycles, etc., biological rhythms can be divided into following types.

(1) *Epicycles :* Different organisms exhibit a variety of biological activities with varying frequencies and periods. Some of these patterns are of relatively *short duration* and are generally called as epicycles for example, *Lug worms (Arenicola marina)*, living in burrows on sand flats in the intertidal zones, feed every 6 to 8 minutes. Some small mammals like *meadow voles (microtuspennsylvanicus)*, which are active primarily during the day light hours, show bursts of activity followed by periods of rest in short cycles that vary from 12 to 20 minutes up to about 2 hours.

Tidal Rhythms : Tides are the result of gravitational forces associated with the moon. Tidal rhythms affect activity periods in many organism that inhabit these zones. The tidal rhythms are of two types (a) Those associated with twice a day ebbing and flowing movement of sea. (b) Those associated with 14/28 day (spring and neap tides) cycle of moon.

Animals that live in the tidal zone show an activity rhythms that corresponds to the daily rhythms of the tides, *e.g.*, the isopod *Exicirolana chiltoni* when exposed to constant conditions without a tidal rhythm displays a periodicity in daily swimming activity which corresponds to tidal rhythm. The free running period lasted 24 hrs 55 minutes and was roughly 5 minutes longer than normal tidal rhythm.

The sand beach happer *syncheledium* exhibits an activity rhythm of swimming and digging in, at the sandy coasts of California, that corresponds exactly to local tidal rhythm. Numerous marine animals show rhythms of behaviour that coincide with the tidal cycle, and continue under constant laboratory conditions; the shanny (*Blennius pholis*) a littoral fish, shows a rhythm of swimming activity with an approximately 12 hr period; fiddler crab (*Uca*) emerge from their burrows at low tide and become very active foraging, courting etc., creeping back to their burrows with each flood tide. The crab's rhythm of activity can persist for up to 5 weeks under constant laboratory conditions. There is considerable amount of evidence that the endogenous clock controlling the tidal rhythms of many marine animals is of a chemical nature. In same cases it is clear that the behaviour of the animal is controlled by both a tidal clock and a 24 hr. clock. The shore crab (*calcium maenas*) for example, often shows a daily rhythm of activity which is superimposed upon a tidal rhythm. It appears that the super-imposition of two rhythms can allow the animal to adapt to the irregular changes of high and low tide that occur in some parts of the world. On the California coast, for example, a time interval of 13.80 hr. between high tides is followed by one of 10.43 hr. and these two periods alternate with each other. Another spectacular example is the beach spawning of the pacific grunion, *Leuresthes tennis*, which swims up on the beaches, spawns, and then flips back into the water just after the turn of the tide on the second, third, and fourth nights after the full moon in the months of March, April, May and June. Precision of this sort greatly increases the chances of successful reproduction and may also synchronize the hatching of larvae with suitable plankton blooms.

Lunar Rhythms : As the travels around the earth on a cycle of about 29½ days. It reflects the maximum amount of solar illumination to the earth at the time of the "full moon" its "size" progressively increases before the "full moon" while it gradually decreases from night to night until it "disappears" thereafter. This lunar cycle is also of potential significance in the evolution of cyclical natural phenomena. Many lunar or full lunar cycles have been recorded, as well as physiological events which occur only once or a few times during the year but always in association with some particular phase of moon. One of the classical examples is the *Palolo worms (Leodice)* which is a tube dweller in coral reefs. The West Indian species, *L. fucaia*, spawns only during the third quarter of the June-July moon. The anterior part of the animal remains in its burrow beneath the sea, but the posterior ends, distended with ripe gametes, break off and wriggle to the surface in such vast numbers that the waters are milky for an hour or two with the eggs and sperms. This swarming occurs at dawn and thus is precisely timed both to sun and moon. In the sea hare *Aplysia* a marine mollusc nerve cells have been found which have a rhythm of activity with a period exactly half that of the lunar cycle. Although most laboratory studies have been carried out with marine animals, other cases are known. The fresh water guppy *(Poecilia reticuluta)* has a rhythm of change of spectral sensitivity which corresponds to the lunar cycle and the terrestrial beetle *Calendra granaria* has cycles of phototaxic responsiveness which correspond to the lunar cycle.

Circannual Rhythms

In many animals, seasonal physiological rhythms have apparently become independent of the environmental controls and are endogenously regulated *i.e.,* self-sustaining internal pacemakers; they persist under constant conditions or may depend on the environment only for the "correction" of the endogenous clock and that occur with a period of about one year.

Circannual rhythms are evidently widespread in the animal kingdom, and it is generally assumed that they enable animals to anticıpate seasonal changes in environmental conditions. Such a mechanism clearly facilitates the accurate liming of months, especially under conditions where climatic factors may vary from year to year. Such precision is particularly important in the timing of migration, and various aspects of reproductive activity. Some mammals enter a condition of deep sleep and reduced metabolic activity, or *hibernation*, during the winter months. By doing so they avoid the harsh conditions of winter. Many bird species escape the rigorous of winter in northern and temperate climates by migrating to southern latitudes. The annual life cycle of many insects that live where there are seasonal climatic shifts incorporate a *diapause phase* a period of *dormancy*-during the more rigorous portions of the climatic cycle. For example, silkworm moths (*Bombyx spp*) and mosquitoes (*Aedes spp.*) lay eggs that are dormanant during the winter, nymphs of the dragonfly (*Tetragneura cynosura*) over winter as larvae forms a complete development in the following spring; both the parasitic wasp (*Nasonia vitripennis*) and its host the flesh fly (*Sacrophage argyrostoma*) enter, diapause as larvae; still other insects go through diapause in the pupal stage or as adults.

In birds, endogenous circannual rhythms have been established in European Warblers. Some of the Warblers, such as the garden Warbler (*Sylvia borin*), the subalpine warbler (*Sylvia cantillans*), and the willow warbler (*Phylloscopus trochilus*) are long distance migrants which show marked seasonal changes in body weight, moult, testis size, nocturnal restlessness and food preferences. It appears that there is an *innate* endogenous Circannual clock, which is responsible for the timing of the physiological and behavioural changes associated with migration. Warbler species that migrate only short distances, such as the blackcap (*Sylvia atricapilla*) and the chiff chaff on the Sardinian Warbler (*S. melanoce phaia*) also show circannual changes when reared in the laboratory but these are not as marked as those of the long distance migrants.

There have been many studies of the seasonal rhythms of reproductive activity in birds, and some of these suggest that an endogenous process is involved. In most of these studies, concern species that breed exclusively in the temperate zone, and at these latitudes an annual breeding cycle is likely to have high *survival value* because of the alternation between seasons, favourable and unfavourable for the survival of the offspring. At equatorial latitudes, however, where there are seasonally stable food supplies, and less marked seasonal changes in climate, it might be of advantage to maintain reproductive condition continuously. Nevertheless, some equatorial species do show a marked breeding rhythm that appears to be unconnected with seasonal changes, several sea birds, including the sooty tern (*Sterna fuscata*), the brown body (*Sulfa teucogaster*), and the lesser noddy tern (*Anous tenuirostris*), breed at intervals of 8-10 months under equatorial conditions. The progressive shift between such breeding cycles and the seasonal cycle suggests that no one season is preferable, but that there is some benefit inherent in the breeding rhythm itself. Perhaps the energy required for continuous reproductive activity is prohibitive, and a periodic rest during which moult can occur is beneficial.

In mammals, there is evidence of endogenous circannual rhythms in a few species. In the Western European hedgehog (*Erinaceous europaeus*) and in man too, there are marked physiological changes, which are correlated with the seasons and may well be endogenous. In the golden mantled ground squirrel (*Citellus lateralis*) there is marked circannal rhythm, which is evident even when the animals are maintained under constant laboratory conditions. This small rodent is found in Western North America at altitudes of 1500-3600 m, ranging from northern British Columbia to Southern California. Under natural conditions they hibernate for a 3 or 4 month period, during which their body weight falls considerably. Food consumption increases rapidly after hibernation, reaching a peak in midsummer, and body weight increased up to the onset of hibernation in October. In laboratory experiments on these animals all external factors are maintained as constant as possible, and all disturbances kept to a minimum. The rhythm of hibernation has been observed to continue for over 2 years under these conditions, clearly showing that a circannual clock is involved. The period of the rhythm under laboratory conditions is actually a little shorter than the natural period. Normally the clock is reset to the rhythm of external events by some particular time setter, such as the duration of the daylight period. This has been clearly demonstrated in the woodchuck (*Mormota monax*). Which is also known to exhibit a circannual rhythm of hibernation. Woodchucks from eastern USA have an annual rhythm of deposition of fat which is maintained under laboratory conditions when transported to Australia and exposed to the natural light and temperature conditions there, but with food and water freely available, woodchucks were found to reverse their normal rhythm within 2 years, bringing them into line with local conditions.

Circadian Rhythms

It is an endogenous oscillation with a natural period (t) close to, but not necessarily equal to that of the solar day (24 hours). Within the daily cycle, some animals exhibit peak activity during the day light (diurnal) : some are active primarily at night (*nocturnal*); still other exhibit peak activity around dusk and or dawn (*crepuscular*). Activity periods may shift periodically. Many bird species that are year-round residents of northern temperate zones are primarily crepuscular throughout late spring and summer, but they shift to a more diurnul pattern during the colder winter months, thus avoiding the very cold temperatures of early winter mornings. Circadian activity periods may also show age-dependent shifts. Young *woodchucks* restrict most of their activity to early evening hours, whereas adult *woodchucks* are most diurnal in their pattern. Similarly, young dragonflies fly during the few hours just after dawn, but adult of the species fly mostly in the middle of the day.

Endogeneity of circadian rhythms is confirmed by *translocation* experiments conducted by *Brown* and his co-workers. Transportation of the animal longitudinally around the earth to a new location should then result in immediate resynchomization of the rhythm to the new local time. For example, the circadian cycle of colour change in the integument of fiddler crabs, which persists in continuous darkness; when crabs were, flown in darkened boxes from the Atlantic coast of the United States to the pacific coast, the rhythm of colour change maintained the original timing, despite of the 51 degrees of longitudinal translocation, equivalent to a time change of 3.3 hours. A similar result was obtained with a tidal rhythm of water propulsion in mussels.

The most elaborate translocation experiments are those conducted by *Renner* with bees instead of working with bouts of activity throughout the day, *Renner* exploited the tendency of individual honey bees to visit flowers or a feeder regularly at a particular time of day. *Renner* (1957) constructed a small portable room with constant light and temperature. A colony of bees placed inside could forage in the completely enclosed room at artificial feeders. In such a room in *Paris* a group of bees was trained to come to a feeder at a particular time of day. Then the hive was sealed and flown overnight to *New York.* A replicate room was set up in advance in New York, and after an overnight flight the bees were released in it. For three days the bees continued to visit the empty feeder at intervals of approximately 24 hours and at the hour they were accustomed to feeding in *Paris*. Local conditions imposed no immediate change in timing, thus demonstrating the independence of the circadian rhythm from local time. Translocation in the opposite direction gave the same result. Such translocation experiment demonstrate both the existence of an endogenous element.

Inheritance of Circadian Rhythms

Several kinds of animals raised under constant conditions, in same instances for several generations, show a circadian rhythm at some stage in their life cycle. Domestic chicks, hatched in an incubator with constant light and temperature; showed a circadian activity cycle when they hatched. Similarly, lizards hatched from eggs incubated under constant conditions showed a clear circadian activity rhythm. The impression of endogenety is reinforced by *Hoffmann's* (1959) studies of lizards. Lizard eggs were kept on 18-hour (9 light 9 dark) and 36-hour (18 light, 18 dark), days with corresponding temperature cycles. When the lizards were transferred to constant light and temperature the various treatments were found to have had no effect on subsequent activity cycles. These studies suggest heritable variability on circadian rhythms, but the genetic mechanism involved remains to be worked out. No studies have been made of the activity of animals born to parents with different circadian rhythms. Only breeding experiments of this type can lead to definite statements about the contributions of inheritance to behaviour.

Pacemakers for Controlling Biological Rhythms

Great progress has been made during the past several decades on locating the pacemakers for biological rhythms and studying their physiology. Much of us work has been done by Brady (1982); Menaker, Takahashi and Eskin (1978), Aschoff (1981) and De Coursey (1983) on cockroaches, sea hares, birds and rodents. Brady (1969), while working on transection studies in cockroaches demonstrated that optic lobes and the lateral brain neurosecretary cells play a key role in circadian rhythms. Experiments on the sea hare (*Aplysia*) have provided additional evidence about the relationships between neural structures, the optic system, and biological rhythms. Sea hare's isolated eyes, kept in total darkness in sea water, exhibits a circadian rhythms of optic nerve impulse. Eyes taken from sea hares maintained in conditions of twelve hours of light and twelve hours of dark prior to the eye excision show a peak firing frequency at "dawn" on the day after removal. Eyes from sea hares kept in constant light prior to surgery exhibit regular rhythms of optic nerve impulses. Thus, some type of oscillator, possibly related to neurosecretory processes, must be present in the eye.

Investigations of biological rhythm mechanisms in vertebrates comes from birds and mammals. Research on Rats (*Rattus norbegicus*) have led to the finding that a direct neural connection exists between the retina and the hypothalamus, a pathway that terminates in the *suprachiasmatic nuclei* (SCN), a specific region of the hypothalamus. When investigators made lesions to cut off connections to these nuclei, the rats lost circadian rhythms for drinking behaviour and wheel-running activity. These studies on the SCN lead some investigators to hypothesize that the SCN are the pacemakers. There is now ample evidence to indicate this is not the case, there must be at least one other pacemaker located somewhere else in the animal. Several bits of evidence suggest that another pacemaker may be located in the ventromedial nucleus of the hypothalamus (VMH). Evidence suggests some form of mutual coupling between the various pacemakers; there are neural pathways connecting the SCN and VMH.

Investigations of rhythms in birds and mammals have implicated the pineal gland as a probable receptor of light stimuli that *entrain* and affect circadian patterns. Recent reviews have supported the hypothesis that both neural processes and hormonal-neuroendocrine products are involved in the mechanisms underlying biological rhythms in vertebrates.

The pineal gland in mammals lies within the brain, near the midline, but in some earlier forms of terrestrial vertebrates this structure was positioned at the top of surface of the brain and served as a third or median eye. In today's reptiles, birds and amphibians the pineal gland is located just under the skull-indeed, it is still sensitive to light in many of these organisms. It is not surprising then that the pineal plays a key role in regulating certain rhythms based on photo period (the light cycle).

Ultradian Rhythms

Ultradian rhythms are those with time sequences shorter than circadian rhythms or also called as short-term rhythms with frequencies in the range of 10^{-3} to 5.10^{-5} Hz, that is, with periods in the range of 20 min to 6 hr. Short-term rhythms in activity are known in laboratory rats and mice but occur more conspicuously in other small mammals, such as shrews and valves. They characterize the alternation of grazing and rumination in cattle and other ruminants, such as roedeer. Ultradian rhythms in locomotion have also been described in free-ranging howler monkey's and in caged rhesus monkeys.

In most instances, short-term activity patterns, are related to foraging and food intake. Bouts of activity, commonly are times of concentrated feeding, alternating with other behaviours, for example, incubation, sleep, or rest. Both casual and functional analysis of short term rhythms have scarcely begun. It is known only in some instances that the rhythm reflects the natural behaviour of the species in the field and is not a pattern induced by a constant laboratory environment.

Typical examples of ultradian rhythms in man are provided by the repetition of phase of rapid eye movements (REM) during sleep in about 90 min intervals, and by cycles of similar duration that can be observed during wakefulness, for example, in oral activity, in performance, in renal excretory activity, or in the perception of apparent motions. However, the great variability in frequency, and a progressive elongation of intervals observed in some of these rhythms, render their interpretation difficult. In the rhesus monkey, behavioural ultradian rhythms have been reported with periods of about 45 min and of 90 min duration.

Rhythms in Man

Sleep : In the late 1960s sleep research began to consider sleep and sleep subcharacterstics within the context of biological rhythms. Clearly, there is growth of interest in sleep as a biological rhythm. Since 1968, the Brain Information service of the UCLA centre for Health Sciences has published as annual bibliography of worldwide sleep literature (1972). Recent studies confirmed that sleep is a part of ultradian rhythm. There are two major objective components of sleep the patterns of sleep and the structure of sleep. The term *patterns of sleep refers* to the interrelation between sleep and waking. The basic unit of sleep pattern is defined by sleep onset and termination. These units are typically measured in a 24 hr or circadian context, and a number interacting components result: total sleep time, number of sleep episodes, episode lengths, and placement descriptors (*e.g.,* diurnal ratios or onset and termination time averages).

Sleep structure refers to within-sleep characteristics, and these are conventionally indexed by the electroencephalogram (EEG). The EEG patterns are the result of varying extracellular current flows in the patch of cerebral cortex which underlies the recording electrode, the current flows reflecting varying degrees of activity of the individual cortical neurons. The EEG is largely due to summed postsynaptic potentials, particularly in the large neurons whose processes are perpendicular to the cortical surface. The wave patterns of the EEG are about 100 times smaller than the amplitude of an action potential, and the frequency of the waves may vary from 1 to 30 Hz, the patterns being distinguished from one another by both their frequencies and amplitudes. Changes in EEG patterns are correlated with changes in behaviour spanning the entire normal range from alertness to sleep.

The Waking State

Behaviourally, the waking state is far from homogeneous, comprising the infinite variety of things one can be doing. The prominent EEG wave pattern of an awake, relaxed adult whose eyes are closed is a slow oscillation of 8 to 13 Hz, known as the *alpha rhythm*, recorded best over the parietal and occipital lobes. The alpha rhythm is associated with decreased levels of attention, and when alpha rhythms are being generated, subjects commonly report that they feel relaxed and happy. A high degree, of alpha rhythm is also associated with meditational states.

When people are attentive to an external stimulus, the alpha rhythm is replaced by lower, faster oscillations (*the beta rhythm*). This transformation is known as EEG arousal and is associated with the act of attending to stimuli rather than with the perception itself; for example, if people open their eyes in a completely dark room and try to see.

Sleep

The EEG pattern changes profoundly in sleep. As a person becomes increasingly drowsy, the alpha rhythm is gradually replaced by slow-wave patterns and sleep begins. This phase of sleep, called *slow-wave* sleep, is itself, divided into stages, each having an EEG pattern characterized by progressively slower frequency and higher voltage. The depth of sleep also varies with the different stages, stage 1 corresponding to *light sleep* and stage 4 to *deep-sleep*. Sleep always begins with an initial progression from stage 1 into a period of deep sleep (stage 4).

The passage from stage I to stage 4 takes 30 to 45 min, and then the process reverses itself, taking the same length of time to return to stage 1.

Throughout the night there occurs a sequence of light-and deep-sleep episodes. Except for the initial period of light sleep, the light-sleep (stage 1) periods are invariably associated with rapid movements of the eyes behind closed lids and an EEG pattern similar to that of an awake, alert person. Because the person is asleep but has an EEG pattern similar to that of an awake, alert person this type of sleep is called *paradoxical sleep*.

At the onset of paradoxical sleep, there is an abrupt and complete inhibition of tone in the postural muscles, although periodic episodes of twitching of the facial muscles and limbs and movements of the eyes occur. Paradoxical sleep is therefore also called *rapid-eye-movement* or REM sleep. Respiration, and heart rate are irregular, and blood pressure may go up or down. When awakened during paradoxical sleep, 80 to 90% of the lime subjects report that they have been dreaming.

Continuous recordings show that the two states of sleep follow a regular 30 to 90 min cycle, each episode of paradoxical sleep lasting 10 to 15 min. Thus, slow-wave sleep constitutes about 80% of the total sleeping time in adults, and paradoxical sleep about 20%. The time spent in paradoxical sleep increases toward the end of an undisturbed night.

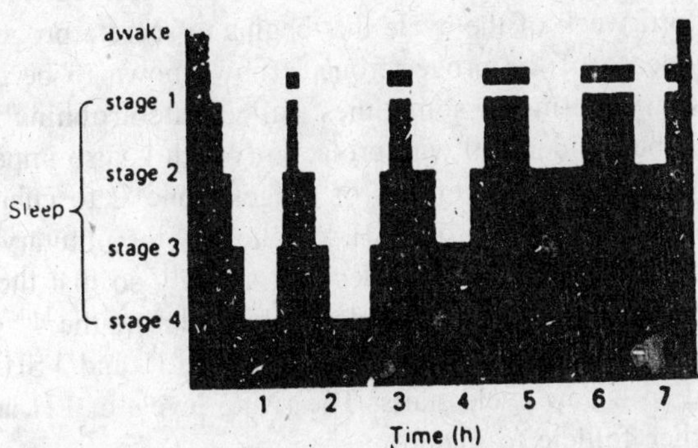

Fig. 14.3 : A typical night of sleep in a young adult. The heavy lines indicate periods of paradoxical sleep, which are characterized by low-voltage EEG patterns and rapid eye movements.

Menstrual Cycle

As discussed earlier that based on the approximately 28 day cycle of the moon, lunar rhythms are clearly related to the tidal rhythms and one of the best example of these rhythms is the menstrual cycle of women having a periodicity of 28 days.

In the human the menstrual cycle starts at puberty and normally occurs regularly every 28 days until the menopause somewhere in late middle age. The cycle starts with the secretion of FSH from the anterior pituitary, which stimulates the development of (usually) a single primary follicle in one or other ovary.

LH (luteinising hormone) is also secreted in small amounts at this time and works together with the FSH in causing the follicle to ripen. Meanwhile the ripening follicle starts to secrete the female sex hormone oestradiol, which is one of a class of hormone collectively called oestrogens. Oestradiol stimulates the development of the mammary glands and causes the development of the muscle and endothelial layers of the uterus; the latter becoming glandular and well vascularised with extensive crypts. The living of the vagina becomes cornified and the mammary glands enlarge.

Rising oestradiol concentrations in the bloodstream cause further release of LH from the hypothalamus-pituitary complex; it is this hormone that is necessary for actual maturation of the Graffian follicle and ovulation. Ovulation usually occurs on day 15 of the 28-day cycle.

LH then brings about the luteinisation of the ruptured follicle and during the third week of the cycle this begins to secrete progesterone. The actual release of the progesterone is now known to be due to a further pituitary hormone sometimes called luteotrophin but now recognised as being identical with prolactin (which is also important in milk secretion). One of the effects of progesterone is to enhance the negative effects of oertradiol on FSH secretion by the pituitary. As the oestradiol level falls the LH level declines as well, so that the corpus luteum is no longer maintained and degenerates during the 4th week of the cycle. The inhibition on the gonadotrophic LH and FSH is thus removed and so a new cycle starts. The rising levels of LH and FSH causing another follicle to mature.

It should be noted that besides its negative effects on the pituitary, progesterone has positive effect on the uterus and mammary glands in a way which prepares them for pregnancy. When the level declines, as it does when conception does not occur, the living of the uterus is lost (hence the menstrual blood loss) and the mammary glands recede.

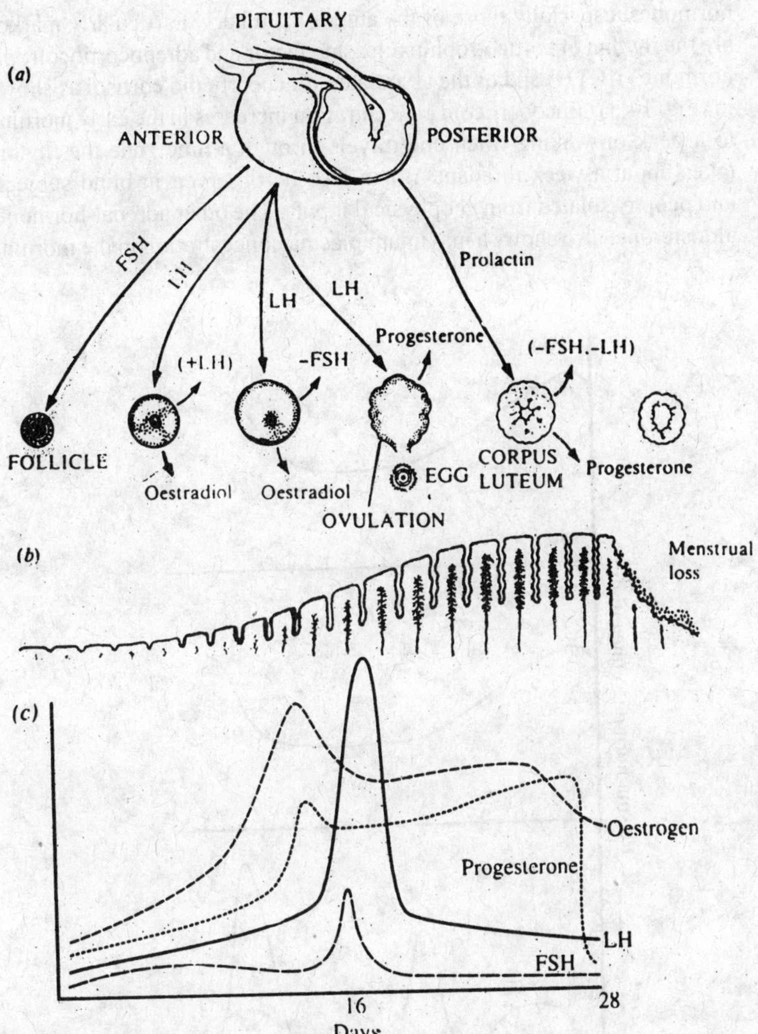

Fig. 14.4 : The human oestrous cycle : (a) the hormones involved; (b) the changes in the lining of the uterus; (c) hormone levels in the blood.

Plasma

Another series of parameters which have long been known to exhibit circadian rhythms are fluctuations in plasma levels of different endocrine hormones: especially those of the anterior pituitary. Particularly marked are the rhythm of corticotrophin releasing factor and adrenocortiocotropic hormone (ACTH) and of the associated glucocorticoid cortisol as shown in (Fig. 14.5) Glucocorticoid concentration increases in the early morning to a peak on waking when one travels through a time zone the rhythm takes about a week to adapt. It can also be observed in blind subjects and people isolated from geophysical inputs. The other adrenal-hormone, aldosterone, also shows a maximum plasma concentration in the morning

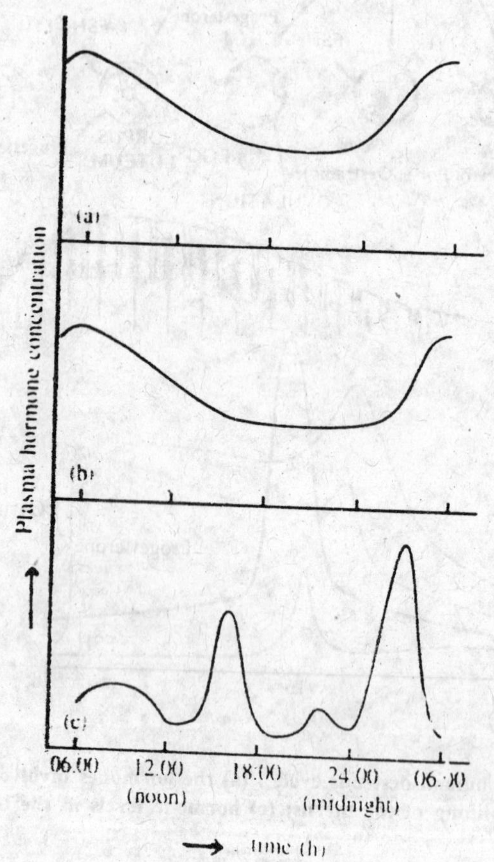

Fig. 14.5 : Fluctuations in plasma levels of three hormones. (a) ACTH (b) Cortisol. (c) Growth hormones.

and a minimum-on retiring. In contrast to the glucocorticoid rhythm, it is abolished by enforced recumbency and reversed within one day of reversing the light-dark pattern. The rhythm of potassium coincides with that of aldosterone but persists when the aldosterone pattern is shifted. Many other hormones show enhanced secretion during the evening as, for example, prolactin and growth hormone, which are elevated during the early onset of sleep, particularly in children. The hormone pulses are not seen if sleep is delayed. Circadian changes in gonadotropins are complex and show species differences, depending on a number of factors. For example, the onset of puberty in the human is marked by increased LH pulses, especially during the night. Even the delivery of human infant is most likely to occur in the early morning.

Melatonin

A striking characteristic of many bodily functions is the rhythmical changes they manifest. Body temperature, for example, fluctuates considerably during a normal 24-h period. Some rhythms have periods that are much longer than 24 h. The menstrual cycle is the best-known longer cycle, but there may be others with even greater time spans.

The rhythmicity of reproduction is one of its most characteristic biological features. With the refinement of radio immunoassay techniques, it has been possible to monitor circadian as well as seasonal cycles of pituitary and gonadal hormones. In search for the pacemaker or clock responsible for this rhythmic activity, many workers have focussed on the pineal gland. It has been reported that pineal gland contains high concentration of melatonin. It seems to have a neuroendocrine function. The pineal seems to participate in the regulation of the rhythmic activity of the endocrine system, by the elaboration of specific hormone or compounds such as methoxyindoles. The main stimulus for this secretion may well be mediated by visual reflexes. It has been discovered that melatonin inhibits the activities of the ovaries. During daylight hours, light entering the eye stimulates neurons to, transmit impulses to the pineal that inhibits melatonin secretion. Without melatonin interference, the ovaries are free to step up their hormone production. But at night, the pineal gland is able to release melatonin which slows down the oestrous cycle and slows down ovarian development. The removal of pineal gland or its non-functional state in children is associated with premature (precocious) puberty. Another function of the pineal gland might very well by regulating the activities of the sexual endocrine glands, particularly the menstrual cycle.

Body Temperature

The effect of temperature upon circadian cycles under constant conditions has been studied intensively for a good reason. Since the rate of many physiological processes increases appreciably with rising temperature, the limited temperature dependence of circadian rhythms is of special interest. Since man's habits are largely governed by social and environmental rhythms, it is not surprising to find that many physiological measurements show a more or less regular periodicity. Rhythmic variations in blood pressure, pulse rate, and body temperature could result simply from a regular alternation of rest and exercise. Body temperature is a parameter which shows a circadian rhythm, a fact

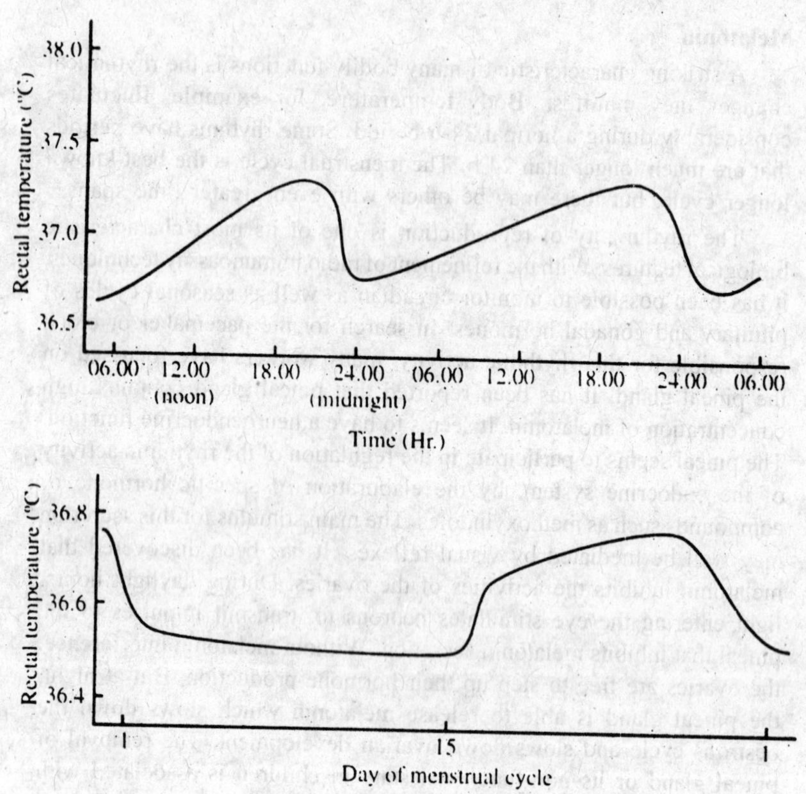

Fig. 14.6 : (a) Variation in body temperature 24-h day human. (b) Variation in temperature over 28-day menstrual cycles (human).

reported by *Davy* in 1845. One could argue that it is due to the heat production associated with activity, but it is still seen in people confined to bed and therefore other factors such as heat loss through cutaneous blood flow must be considered. In fact the temperature rhythm is indeed endogenous and is maintained even after a phase shift, though it will finally adapt to the new time.

In the human the temperature on waking is generally lower than on retiring and in women, temperature rises slightly on ovulation and remains elevated until the next menstruation. The centre for temperature regulation lies in the preoptic region of the hypothalamus, where the central thermoreceptors are located. Information is also provided by the thermoreceptors in the skin. For the sake of simplicity one can imagine a hypothalamic thermostat. In the development of a fever the thermostat is reset to a higher level through the action of progens. These pyrogenic stimuli result in the release of interleukins, which act on the hypothalamus. The effect of aspirin, which in reducing body temperature inhibits prostaglandin synthesis, suggests that prostaglandin's may also be involved. A feeling of cold is experienced and heat is produced until the new set point is reached. When the fever breaks, the set point is returned to the normal level and heat is lost from the body. The appropriate responses to bring about these changes are initiated in the hypothalamus.

Significance of Rhythmicity

Polar biology : Two enormous accumulations of glacial ice on earth are the Greenland and Antarctic ice sheets on north and south poles respectively.

Many Millions of years ago, Antarctica was an ice free continent. Scientists have found fossils of trees and of dinosaurs and small mammals that once lived there. Glaciers began to form in the polar regions about 30 million years ago. They slowly advanced over parts of the earth during a period known as the ice age. Although ice-age ended about 10,000 years ago ice sheet still cover Antarctic and Greenland.

Antarctica is nearly barren land forms the coldest and iciest region in the world. It is slightly colder than north pole. Antarctica covers-about 5,400,000 square miles. Icy cap, which -averages approximately 7,100 feet thick, the average elevation of Antarctica is 7500 feet above sea level. Temperatures in Antarctica rarely reaches above 0°C and may go below-80°C, it receives no rain and hardly any new snow each year. Antarctica's climate varies from extremely cold, dry conditions on the inland plateau to middle moisture conditions along the costs, many people call the plateau as *'polar desert'*. There are no any seasons like winter, summer and monsoon, as well as there is no twenty four hour day night cycle as there is six months day and six months night. So in short monotonous climatic conditions are seen which affect on the plant and animal life. Few plants like mosses, algae, lichens could grow in this ice-covered and harsh climate. Animal life includes few insects, most common are krill, a small shrimp like animal feeding on tiny floating organisms; all other animals like whales, seals, penguins and different birds depends on krill for their food; and they do not show any rhythmicity in their behaviour *i.e., arhythmicity* is seen in animal life.

More man 75 years passed before explorers proved that the south pole is located on land. During that time scientific interest in Antarctica region was increased. First man to reach the south pole was *Roald Amundsen*, a Norwegian explorer. His expedition set off from Antarctica's Bay of Whales on Oct., 19, 1911, and reached the pole on December 14,1911. Scientific knowledge of Antarctica increased worldwide during *International Geophysical* Year (IGY), a programme in which scientists carried out research and shared their findings. The IGY began on July 1,1957, and ended on December, 31, 1958 from then onwards near about 26 nations have established Research stations on continent and nearby islands. India has also established his research stations at *Dakshin Gangotri* in 1984 under the leadership of Dr. S. Z. Kasim, Dr. Sachdera and many other geologists, physiologists, chronobiologists for further research. Recently in 1996, India has settled a second research station namely *dakshin Maitri*, particularly for research in mineral exploration, chronobiology and ozone depletion. Some Antarctic studies concern all the continents. Significant research deals with ozone, a form of oxygen, ozone is most concentrated in a layer that varies in altitude from about 14 to 19 miles. This layer protects an living things from certain harmful ultraviolet rays of the sun. In mid-1980's scientists discovered that ozone layer above Antarctica is becoming less concentrated. Evidence pointed to manufactured compounds called chloroflurocarbons as a major cause of this "ozone hole."

Space Exploration

One of the most obvious expression of rhythmicity in animal behaviour is the periodic change in amount of locomotor activity. Locomotion, however, consists not only of amount (*i.e.,* frequency of movements and velocity) but also direction, and inevitably, it changes the relationship between the animal and its spatial environment. Thus, in some cases in which the amount of movement, and in all cases in which the direction of movement, is influenced by the periodically changing inner state of an organism, the underling rhythm directly effects the animal's orientation in space. Most research on this subject has been done in the 20 years following the discovery of the sun compass in 1950 by *K. Von Frisch* in bees and G. *Kamer* in birds.

Biological Clocks in Astro-Orientation

There are several reasons that the use of extraterrestrial cues for orientation in a terrestrial environment may be profitable.

1. The sun and the moon are very prominent "landmarks" that can easily be distinguished from all other environmental features and that can be localized without highly developed mechanisms of visual discrimination.
2. The uniqueness of celestial (about space or sky) cues and the wide-range, constancy of their appearance allow generalizations that would never be possible with respect to the manifold structures of the immediate environment.
3. The large distance of a celetial cue guarantees that maintaining a constant angle to it will result in a straight course and not in a spiral, as it would in most cases if the animal were to rely on an object in its close vicinity.
4. Theoretically, celestial bodies can be used not only for determining and maintaining directions but also for determining the observer's position on the earth.

There are certain disadvantages in extraterrestrial cues, that their location in the sky varies, dependent on the daily rotation of the earth, on season, and on geographic latitude.

The Sun as Orientational Cue

The time-compensated sun compass : Light-compass reaction or photomenotaxis in a classical sense, means that an animal maintains, over a period of time, a constant course angle with respect to a light source. This light source may be the sun, and it not only involves the use of the sun as an orientational cue but also takes into account its daily movement. In order to maintain a constant compass course, the animal has to change its menotactic light angle periodically in an appropriate manner. Sun-compass orientation, in this sense, has been found in many species of arthropodes and vertebrates (fishes).

The well-established ability of animals to determine a direction based on the sun and to maintain this direction by compensating for the cycle of solar directional change has been termed *sun compass orientation.* Where experimental evidence has been obtained the compensation has been found to be intimately related to the biological clock.

Von frisch discovered that worker bees, having found a rich source of nector, return with a full load of pollen or nector to the hive to communicate accurately the location of their find. This they did by dancing in the dark side of the hive on the vertical combs. The distance, and directions of honey-water feeders were correlated with the dances of marked bees when they returned to the hives.

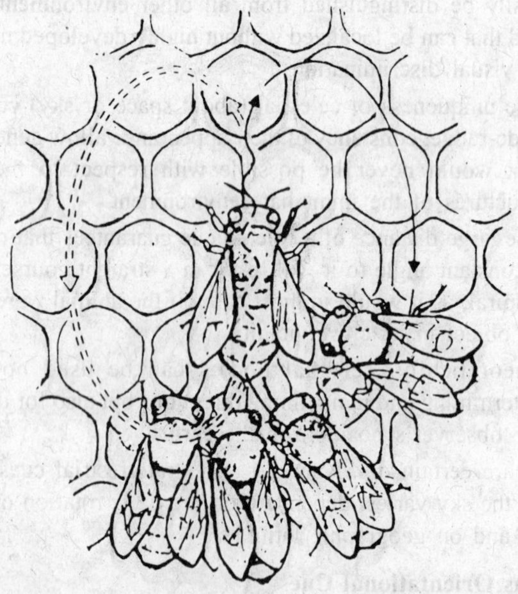

Fig. 14.7 : The Waggle dance of the honey bee.

The angle between the waggle run and the vertical is determined by the position of the sun relative to the food. This angle changes during the day as the sun travels across the sky. *Von Frisch* and his co-workers demonstrated by observation and experimentation that bees can compensate for sun movement (1953). *Lindaur* (1961) studied the selection of new hive sites by swarming bees. He discovered that scout bees (workers) communicate the location of possible sites by the same dances that are used to announce food, except that they last much longer, sometimes several days. During the course of these persistent dances the relative direction of the sun changes and the orientation of the dance does so as well.

Ants also use this type of orientation in moving to and from their nests, but they cannot compensate for movements of the sun. If an ant is held for 2½ hrs in a dark box while it is on its way home, the sun will have travelled approximately 37°. When the ant is released, it shifts its direction approximately 37°, maintaining its original angle to the sun. This direction will not take it to its nest, but it may discover other clues along the way and adjust its path appropriately.

Lunar Orientation

The possibility of lunar orientation has received comparatively little attention. The first demonstration of moon compass orientation was the report by *Papi and Pardi* (1953) on the beach happer, *Talitrus saltator* when these amphipods are placed in a cylindrical chamber they immediately respond with a phototactic orientation toward the *moon.* But when they are tested on a dry substrate they shift to a backward orientation. Tests at night revealed a persistence of the geographically appropriate orientation as long as the moon was visible. When the moon was not visible eventhough the sky was clear, directional orientation failed.

The lunar orientation emerges even after exposure to 24 hrs of constant darkness before testing. Thus the orientation is apparently based on an ability to compensate for the movement of the moon across the sky similar to the sun compensation mechanism.

Enright (1961) studied another amphipod, *Orchestoidea corniculata*, on the pacific coast of North America. He found that animals held in constant darkness before testing tend to maintain a fixed angle relative to the moon. Since a moon-compensated orientation appeared when these amphipods were pretreated by exposure to a natural day-night cycle. *Enright* suggested that orientation might be based on nightly rephasing of the compensation mechanism.

Star Orientation in Birds

More birds migrate at night than during the day. Following the initial discovery that a caged bird will orient by reference to the sun, *Kramer* attempted to apply this method to night orientation. But nocturnal migrants such as the blackcap warbler, *sylvia atricapilla* performed inconsistently. Often they fluttered in the direction of city lights. *Sauer* (1957) subsequently investigated this problem with hand and wild-raised garden warblers, *sylvia borion.* A vertical screen restricted the view to less than 90° the sky. With the distracting city lights and city glow from the horizon effectively cut off, they oriented in the migration directions, southwest in the fall, north-esterly in the spring. When the sky was overcast the fluttering Waned and they oriented randomly.

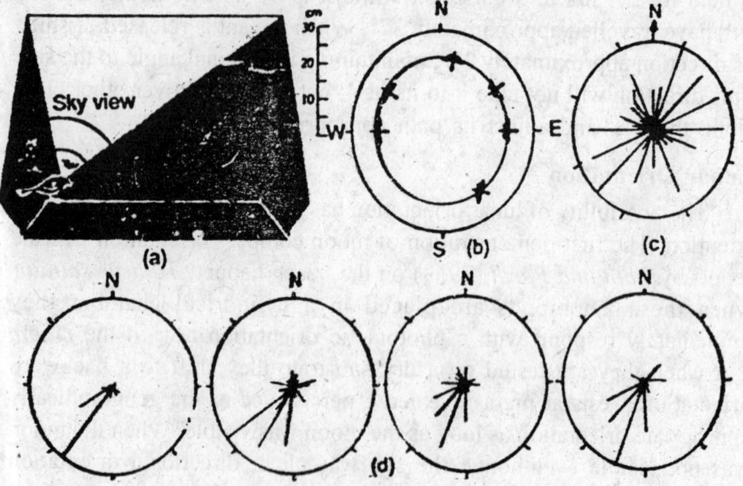

Fig. 14.8 : The Orientation of birds provided with a view of the natural night sky.

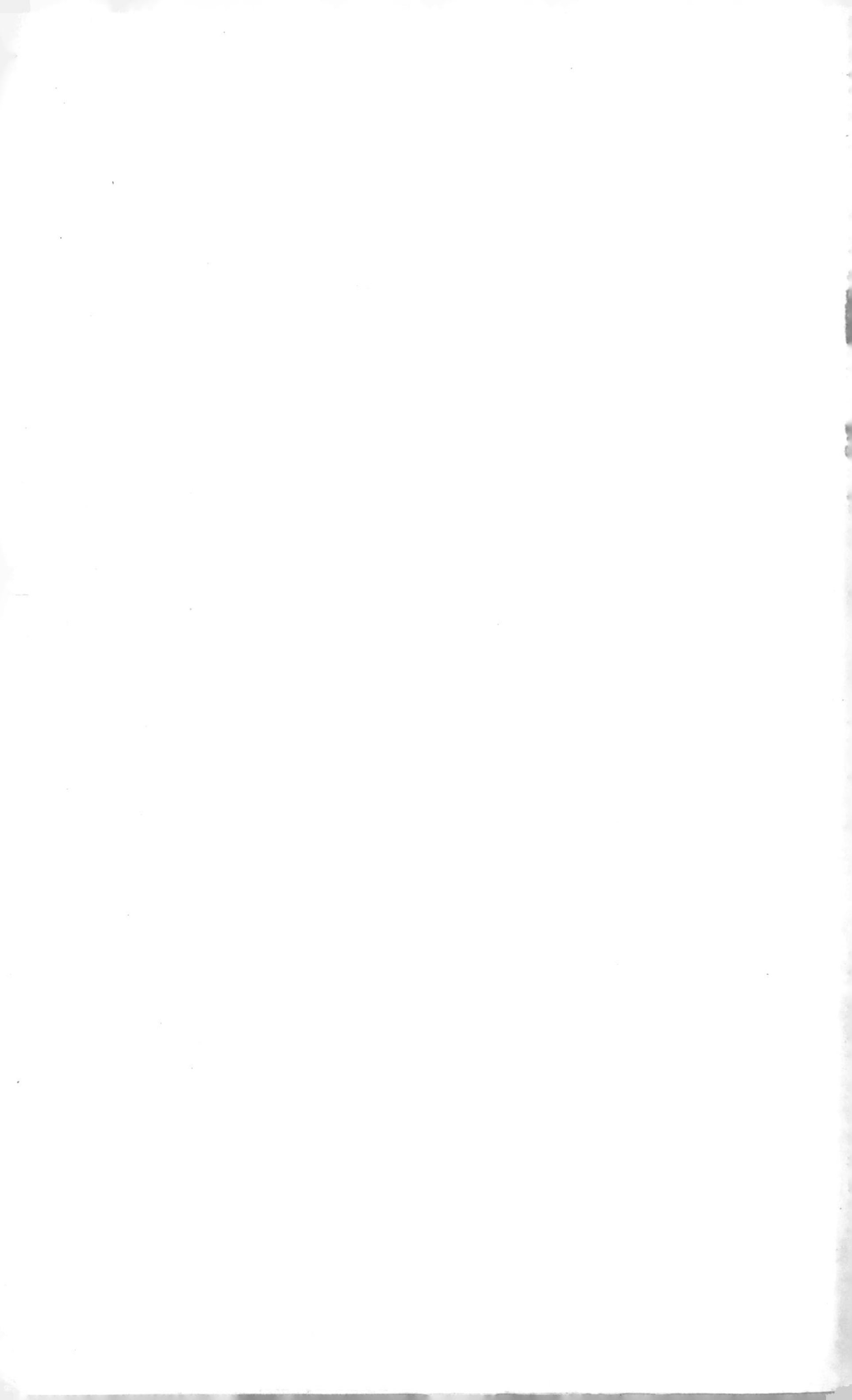